Checklist Workbook to Accompany

CLINICAL SKILLS AND ASSESSMENT TECHNIQUES IN NURSING PRACTICE

Checklist Workbook to Accompany

CLINICAL SKILLS AND ASSESSMENT TECHNIQUES IN NURSING PRACTICE

Vicki Vine Earnest
COMMUNITY COLLEGE OF DENVER

Scott, Foresman / Little, Brown College Division
Scott, Foresman and Company
Glenview, Illinois   Boston   London

ISBN 0-673-39871-4

2 3 4 5 6 7 8 9 10—MKN—94 93 92 91 90 89

Printed in the United States of America

PREFACE

This workbook is a learning tool to supplement *Clinical Skills and Assessment Techniques in Nursing Practice.* To aid in identifying and managing client problems, this workbook allows the student to self-evaluate both his or her understanding of the theory supporting clinical actions by doing the quizzes, and his or her problem-solving abilities by answering the questions in the case studies. Answers to the quizzes and case studies at the back of the book provide immediate feedback for the student. Performance checklists of the clinical skills and assessment techniques comprise the main portion of the workbook.

Learning takes place in several ways and on several levels. Reading information, writing notes, and participating in classroom discussion are common forms of cognitive learning. Evaluation methods such pencil-and-paper tests are universally applied as methods of determining the extent of learning, but if they are used by the student for self-evaluation, they can reinforce learning that has already occurred. Most psychomotor learning takes place with demonstration and practice; it is often evaluated by a return demonstration. Some learners benefit most from the checklists: written instructions suggesting step-by-step actions for performing an activity. This workbook also offers the student several methods of self-evaluation and guidance through the quizzes, case studies, and performance checklists.

Each workbook quiz corresponds to a chapter in the textbook. To maintain variety and hold the student's interest, different types of questions are used: short-answers, fill-in-the-blanks, matching, and data analysis with diagnostic formulation. Several levels of knowledge are evaluated: simple definitions at the lowest level, and analysis of complex problems at the highest.

The case studies correspond to units of study. Each case study describes a client and his condition and is followed by a series of questions designed to guide the student toward more complex data analysis, diagnostic formulation, or insight into client behavior. Integrated into the case study are the theory and skills presented in that particular unit.

The performance checklists correspond to the suggested steps in the textbook. These checklists may be used by the student to guide his or her actions in a laboratory or clinical setting, they may be used by the instructor to evaluate the student's performance.

Ultimately, learning can be enjoyable if the proper tools are used. Activities such as group discussion or projects, guest speakers, audiovisual aids or computer-assisted instruction can add variety and interest for the learner. Each of these activities reinforces the others. Combined with a variety of other teaching strategies, the pencil-and-paper exercises in this workbook offer a method of reinforcement and self-evaluation, creating a complete learning program and offering the best possible outcome for the learner.

CONTENTS

PERFORMANCE CHECKLISTS 125

Checklist Workbook to Accompany

CLINICAL SKILLS AND ASSESSMENT TECHNIQUES IN NURSING PRACTICE

SELF-TESTS AND CASE STUDIES

Unit I SELF-TESTS

CHAPTER 1 UNDERSTANDING NURSING

1. Fill in the blanks in the following statements:

   Some nurses work in ______________________ agencies, which manage the health care needs of clients who cannot care for themselves because of serious or life-threatening illnesses and who require continuous nursing care.

   Other nurses work in ______________________ agencies, which offer supportive or therapeutic care for clients at home.

   Nurses also work in ______________________ agencies, which conduct health research, education, and specialized types of health care in the community.

2. Match the description in Column II with the type of nursing care delivery system in Column I.

   I. System

   _____ functional nursing

   _____ team nursing

   _____ total client care

   _____ primary nursing

   II. Description

   A. Several nurses work together under the guidance and supervision of a responsible leader to provide nursing care for all clients.

   B. Each nurse performs a particular task or skill for each of the clients.

   C. The nurse identifies the client's problems, plans his care, and implements all subsequent nursing actions while working with him. The nurse assures the continuity of the client's care by becoming the client's advocate for the duration of his association with the agency.

   D. The nurse performs all tasks and accepts responsibility for the nursing needs of one client during the time she is assigned to him.

3. Identify three functions of the state nurse practice act.

   1)

   2)

   3)

4. Explain the difference between negligence and malpractice.

5. What is meant by the Patient's Bill of Rights?

6. Explain the nursing implications of these terms:

   professional liability

   confidential communication

   informed consent

7. Match the phase of the nursing process in Column I with its description in Column II.

I. Phase	II. Description
_____ Assessment	A. Data analysis and identification of the client's actual or potential health problem
_____ Nursing Diagnosis	B. Examination of the client to determine if the desired outcomes have been achieved
_____ Planning	C. Data collection
_____ Implementation	D. Development of desired outcomes and determination of strategies to achieve them
_____ Evaluation	E. Coordination and execution of the physician's and nurse's orders

8. In the following situations, the nurse is demonstrating some phase of the nursing process. Identify the correct phase.

   a. The nurse is helping the client walk so that the client can regain his strength after surgery. This is ______________________.

   b. The nurse is meeting with the client and his family to discuss how they will help him return to work after discharge from the hospital. This is ______________________.

   c. The nurse is measuring the client's height and weight upon admission to the hospital. This is ______________________.

   d. One hour after giving the client medication to relieve pain, the nurse asks him if he is feeling relief. This is ______________________.

   e. After interviewing the client and examining him, the nurse prepares a list of health problems that have been identified. This is ______________________.

CHAPTER 2 CARING FOR THE CLIENT IN THE HOME

1. Fill in the blanks in the following statements:

   In home health care, a ______________________________ is the time when the nurse sees the client in his home for management of his health care needs.

   The person who accepts responsibility for providing direct nursing care to the home-bound client is the identified ______________________________.

2. Identify three socioeconomic trends that have contributed to home health care and explain their impact on health care.

   1)

   2)

   3)

3. Explain the differences between home care health maintenance, intermediate services, and intensive services.

4. Name at least three of the roles of the home care nurse:

   1)

   2)

   3)

CHAPTER 3 COMMUNICATING

1. Explain the difference between a social conversation and a therapeutic interaction.

2. Identify the three components that must be present for communication to occur:

   1)

   2)

   3)

3. List at least five characteristics that suggest a nursing diagnosis of impaired verbal communication:

   1)

   2)

   3)

   4)

   5)

4. Explain the purpose of these therapeutic communication skills:

   broad opening

   general lead

   silence

   focusing

   seeking clarification

   sharing observations

   offering self

   suggesting collaboration

   giving information

5. Why do these techniques block communication?

   reassurance

   giving approval

   introducing an unrelated topic

   interpreting

agreeing

rejecting

disapproving

disagreeing

advising

defending

6. What is the difference between a therapeutic communication and an interview?

7. Explain the difference between a nursing history and a medical history.

8. Match the example question in Column II with the type of question indicated in Column I.

I. Type of Question	II. Example Question
A. indirect	_____ "Tell me about your illness."
B. direct	_____ "Do you have pain or are you comfortable right now?
C. double-barreled	_____ "Are you married?"
	_____ "Why don't you talk to your doctor about this?"
	_____ "You mentioned that your husband is ill . . . "
	_____ "Have you walked yet or are you too tired to-day?"

CHAPTER 4 TEACHING THE CLIENT

1. Explain what is meant by

   affective domain.

   cognitive domain.

   psychomotor domain.

2. What client characteristics suggest the nursing diagnosis of knowledge deficit?

3. Fill in the blanks:

   Before teaching a client, the nurse must determine that the client has sufficient

   ____.

   If the client is unable to speak, hear, or see, the nurse must develop ________

   ______________________________ approaches to teaching.

   A client's ______________________ for learning may be confirmed when he expresses an interest in the topic for discussion.

4. What are some techniques conducive to learning?

CHAPTER 5 REPORTING AND RECORDING

1. Explain what is meant by the term *health record* or *medical record*.

2. Identify five uses of the health record.
   1)
   2)
   3)
   4)
   5)

3. Explain the difference between ownership of the information in a health record and ownership of the physical document of the health record.

4. Explain the difference between a source-oriented health record and a problem-oriented health record.

5. Match the components of the health record in Column I with their function in Column II.

I. Record Part	II. Function
A. admission sheet	_____ Grants legal permission for therapy.
B. health history	_____ Documents nursing goals and strategies for client management.
C. physician's orders	_____ Records continuing assessment data on a single form for several hours or days.
D. graphic record	
E. medication administration record	
F. progress notes	

G. consent form

H. nursing care plan

_____ Documents the client's demographic data.

_____ Records names, doses, times, and method of drug administrations.

_____ Records information about the client's previous health status.

_____ Records all current subjective and objective data on the client.

_____ Records the physician's instructions regarding treatment of the client.

6. What is the purpose of the nursing Kardex?

7. Circle S if the client information is subjective and O if the information is objective:

S O Pain and numbness in the feet.

S O Elevated body temperature.

S O Nausea.

S O Burning when passing urine.

S O Pale skin that is cool to the touch.

S O Smiling and laughing.

S O Bruise located on the arm.

CHAPTER 6 WRITING A NURSING CARE PLAN

1. List four purposes of a nursing care plan.

   1)

   2)

   3)

   4)

2. What is the difference between a standardized care plan and an individualized care plan?

3. In each of the following situations, several client problems are identified. Underline the problem that is *most urgent.*

   a. Susie Garcia, 17 months old, is brought to the emergency room by her parents. Upon examination, you find that Susie

   - wears a wet, soiled diaper.
   - is blue around the mouth and seems unable to breathe.
   - has a bloated abdomen.

   b. Mr. Holden, age 86, is hospitalized for pneumonia. During the nursing history and examination, you learn that he

   - lives by himself and doesn't like to cook.
   - has lost 23 pounds in the past year.
   - has a frequent productive cough accompanied by chest pain that leaves him exhausted.

   c. Mrs. March, age 65, has severe arthritis in her hands. While you are teaching her how to use a special fork for eating, she tells you

   - the pain is not new and she doesn't think anything will help.
   - she hasn't had a bowel movement in four days.
   - she can't concentrate now because she is worried about her husband who hasn't visited in two days.
   - she would like to lose weight.

   d. James Arthur, age 16, broke his leg two days ago, which is now in a hip-to-toe cast. While you are helping him with his bath, he tells you

   - he's unhappy to be missing so much school.
   - his parents are getting a divorce and he's very upset.
   - the skin on his casted leg itches so much he can't rest.

4. Circle YES if the client outcome is measurable; circle NO if it is not.

YES	NO	The client has normal respiratory function.
YES	NO	The client is free of infection as evidenced by normal body temperature, normal white blood cell count, and absence of pain, redness, swelling, and dysfunction of a body part.
YES	NO	The client's pain is at a tolerable level as confirmed by his verbal and nonverbal behavior.
YES	NO	The client has normal bowel movements.

5. Underline the word or phrase that represents a condition in these outcome statements:

   The client walks with assistance from his room to the elevators three times each day.

   The client demonstrates how to change his dressing two times before he leaves the hospital.

   The client eats all of the food on his breakfast tray each morning.

Unit I CASE STUDY

COMMUNICATION SKILLS

This case study is an analysis of a conversation between a home care client and a nurse. The conversation reads like a play. The actual words of the client and nurse are in quotation marks; their behaviors are described in parentheses. At the conclusion of the interaction, your task is to answer questions referring to parts of the interaction. As you read, look for communication skills or blocks and analyze the effectiveness of the nurse's communication.

Setting: This conversation takes place in the living room of the Juarez home, a two-bedroom apartment. The room has a sofa, two chairs, several tables, a television, and several components of a stereo system. The room is clean although cluttered with toys, children's clothing, and magazines and newspapers. The home care nurse, Betty, is making her second home visit since mother and baby came home. She has just entered the home when the action begins.

Description of the Client: Mrs. Juanita Juarez, age 26, gave birth to her third child, a boy named Carlos, Junior, seven days ago. Her other two children are girls, ages 4 and 2 years. Her husband of six years, Carlos, is a construction worker. Mrs. Juarez has not worked since the birth of her first daughter. She has long dark hair, a clear complexion, and dark brown eyes that appear tired. Only the baby is at home with her today; the other children are visiting her mother-in-law. Mrs. Juarez is sitting on the sofa holding the baby; the nurse is sitting in a nearby chair.

Nurse: "Tell me about your baby." (Looking at the baby in Mrs. Juarez's arms) [1]

Client: (Smiling) "He's just wonderful! Little Carlos weighed 6 pounds and 2 ounces. His dad adores him and the little girls love him, too."

Nurse: "He must be a welcome member of this family." (Smiling at the client) [2]

Client: "Oh yes." (Sighing)

Nurse: "Since I last saw you, have you any questions or concerns regarding his care?" (Looking at the client) [3]

Client: "No, I don't think so. (Laughing) After all, he's my third baby! (Pauses for a few seconds) Everything is okay, I guess . . . " (Voice trailing off; staring at the floor)

Nurse: (Gently) "Do you mean you have some doubts that everything is okay?" [4]

Client: "Well, I am a little tired. . . . " (Sighing, face looks solemn)

Nurse: "Tell me about your fatigue." (Looking concerned) [5]

Client: "Oh, I'm okay; I was tired when the girls were babies too. (Pauses) But there's so much more to do now with three . . . and my husband is working two jobs. He doesn't have much time left over for me. Little Carlos is hungry all the time."

Nurse: "It sounds like you have a heavy load." (Looking thoughtful.) [6] "You mention that the baby is hungry all the time. Tell me about his feeding schedule." [7]

Client: "He takes a few ounces almost every other hour and falls asleep right away. I wish he'd sleep longer! I can't get any sleep myself. Maybe if I could breastfeed him. . . . " (Hesitant, questioning sound in voice)

Nurse: "Breast-feed?" (Slight frown, looking at client) [8]

Client: (Long pause, looking down at the floor) "Carlos, my husband, doesn't want me to breast-feed . . . (Pausing again). He thinks it isn't the modern way to be a mother." (Looking at nurse with tears in her eyes)

Nurse: "I see. (Pause) What do you feel?" [9]

Client: (Sobbing) "I breast-fed my little girls and all went well . . . But now Carlos doesn't want his little boy on the breast. (Looking at the nurse, sounding angry) He says it isn't right for a boy. . . . " (Wiping eyes with tissue)

Nurse: (Sitting quietly, watching the client cry. After a long pause) "Perhaps you could change his formula. He may drink more and prolong the time between feedings so you could get some rest." [10]

Client: (Wiping eyes, taking a deep breath, looking away from the nurse) "Well, I suppose I could talk with my doctor about it."

Nurse: (Very quickly) "That's a good idea. I'm sure the baby will start sleeping longer soon and you'll feel better." [11]

Client: (Sadly) "Perhaps you're right. . . . I guess the nurse knows best."

End of interaction

Answer these questions:

1. What type of question is [1]? Is it effective for getting information?

2. What type of communication is [2]?

3. What type of question is [3]? Is it effective for getting information?

4. What type of communication is [4]? Is it effective in furthering conversation?

5. What type of communication is [5]? Is it effective in furthering conversation?

6. What type of communication is [6]?

7. What type of question is [7]? Is it effective for getting information?

8. What type of communication is [8]? Is it effective in furthering conversation?

9. What type of skill or question is [9]? Is it effective?

10. What type of communication is [10]? Is it effective in furthering conversation?

11. What type of communication is [11]? Is it effective in furthering conversation?

Unit II SELF-TESTS

CHAPTER 7 PROVIDING PHYSICAL AND BIOLOGIC SAFETY

1. Suggest one nursing action to protect the client from

   fire

   falls

   accidental poisoning

2. Indicate with a checkmark whether the siderails should be in use or not in the following situations:

   a. Mr. Parr, 75 years old, has normal vision and hearing but is very weak from a long illness and leaves his hospital bed only to use the bathroom.

      Siderails in use _____ or not in use _____.

   b. Jane Moore, 21 years old, has never been hospitalized until giving birth to her baby boy just 30 minutes ago. She is to remain in bed until the effects of her anesthesia wear off in about two hours.

      Siderails in use _____ or not in use _____.

   c. Mrs. Clancy, 52 years old, had surgery two days ago to remove her gall bladder. She wears corrective glasses and has normal hearing. She may be out of bed whenever she wishes, but she continues to experience pain and is receiving pain medications regularly that make her sleepy.

      Siderails in use _____ or not in use _____.

3. Before applying restraints, the nurse assesses the client to identify potential for injury. In the following list, draw a line through those factors that are *not* important when assessing a potential for injury.

   wakefulness of the client

   awareness of the environment

   amount of urine passed

   judgment

   ability to eat by himself

   medications

   history of falls or accidents

   body temperature

4. What type of restraint would be applied to each of these clients for their protection?

   a. Ms. Bergen, 72 years old, is very weak and confused and cannot move by herself in bed, but she can move her arms and has removed several tubes from her body. What type of restraint would you apply? ________________

____

b. George Kearney, 81, is also weak and confused and can't use the call signal to ask for help. He has tried to climb over his siderails on several occasions but you found him before he fell. What type of restraint would you apply?

____

c. Baby Jenny, 9 months old, is receiving fluids through a tube attached to her scalp because she is dehydrated from severe diarrhea. Jenny has tried to remove the needle because it irritates her. What type of restraint would you apply? ____

5. Use these words to fill in the blanks in the statements about the chain of infection: host, reservoir, infectious agent, portal of entry, portal of exit, method of transmission.

A bacterial microorganism, which is the ________________________, is growing and multiplying in a wound drainage fluid, the ________________ ________________. The drainage fluid seeps through a small skin opening, ________________________, and dampens a dressing. The nurse removes the contaminated dressing with her bare hands and discards it in a trash container. She does not wash her hands before the client in same room asks for a drink of water. She pours the water in a cup and hands it to the other client. This is the ________________________. The client holds the cup with a hand that has a wound, which is the ________________________. Some time later the client reports swelling, pain, redness, and drainage from his wound. The client is the ________________________.

6. Indicate if the following situations demonstrate **A**, clean technique (medical asepsis), or **B**, sterile technique (surgical asepsis):

_____ The nurse washes her hands before serving breakfast trays.

_____ The nurse uses packaged sterile supplies and sterile gloves to change a wound dressing.

_____ The nurse pours a liquid medication into a sterile cup before giving it to the client.

_____ The nurse swabs the skin with a disinfectant before giving an injection with a sterile needle.

_____ The nurse introduces a sterile tube (catheter) into the bladder of the client using sterile gloves.

7. Circle the T if the statement is true; circle the F if it is false.

T F Only sterile objects are used in or on a sterile field.

T F Sterile objects are considered no longer sterile if they come in contact with other sterile objects.

T F A sterile object is no longer considered sterile if it is wet.

T F Sterile objects are not contaminated by airborne particles.

T F Sterile objects are still considered sterile even when beyond the range of vision.

T F The worker may reach across a sterile field without contamination.

8. Match the purpose of category specific isolation in Column II with the name of the isolation in Column I.

I. Type of Isolation	II. Purpose
A. strict	_____ Prevents infections transmitted by airborne particles.
B. contact	_____ Prevents transmission of highly contagious or virulent infections spread by air or direct contact.
C. enteric	_____ Prevents infections transmitted through direct or indirect contact with infected body fluids.
D. bloody/body fluids	_____ Prevents infections transmitted through contact with feces.
E. respiratory	_____ Prevents transmission of highly contagious infections not requiring strict isolation.

CHAPTER 8 ASSISTING THE CLIENT TO DRESS

1. What client characteristics are assessed to determine if the nursing diagnosis of self-care deficit: dressing and grooming is present?

2. Mr. Jones has weakness and paralysis on the right side of his body. When helping him to put on a client gown, which arm does the nurse place through the sleeve first: right or left?

   When removing the hospital gown from Mr. Jones, from which arm does the nurse remove the sleeve first: right or left?

3. These are steps to follow as you remove and replace a gown from a client with an intravenous tubing attached to her left wrist. Indicate the correct order of the steps (1, 2, 3, etc.).

   a. _____ Help the client remove her right arm from the right gown sleeve.

   b. _____ Draw the IV bottle or bag through the bundled left sleeve of the gown.

   c. _____ Help the client place her right arm through the right sleeve of the fresh gown.

   d. _____ Remove the gown sleeve from the left shoulder and arm and bundle it into your hand around the IV tubing.

   e. _____ Draw the sleeve up the client's IV arm and over the shoulder.

   f. _____ Gather fresh gown in your hands and draw the IV bottle/bag and tubing through the sleeve from the inside of the gown.

   g. _____ Discard the soiled gown and pick up a fresh one.

4. What is the purpose of elastic stockings for the client who is in bed?

CHAPTER 9 ASSESSING AND BATHING THE SKIN

1. List four functions of the skin:

   1)

   2)

   3)

   4)

2. Match the term in Column I with the definition in Column II.

I. Term	II. Definition
_____ melanin	A. Substance that gives elasticity to skin
_____ elastin	B. Plumpness or tension of skin
_____ turgor	C. Pigment that colors the skin
_____ collagen	D. Substance that gives support or structure to skin tissues
_____ albinism	E. Absence of skin pigmentation

3. What are some normal skin changes that occur with aging?

4. Mrs. Turpin, 67 years old, is in bed most of the time because she is unable to walk due to paralysis. She is very thin for her body size and her skin is quite dry. During her bath, you notice that she has a reddened area over the coccyx. Mrs. Turpin reports that this skin area is painful. Her nursing diagnostic category is

5. What is the primary purpose of AM and PM care?

6. You will assess for what characteristics to determine if the client has self-care deficit: bathing?

7. Describe nursing activities that may be accomplished during the bed bath in addition to actually bathing the client.

8. When bathing the female perineum, why is the cleansing motion from the pubis to the anus?

9. Name at least three nursing diagnostic categories that may be treated with back massage.

   1)

   2)

   3)

10. Fill in the blanks:

    ______________________ is the massage stroke that is smooth and evenly applied over large body surfaces. ______________________ is the kneading motion performed by picking up the tissue between the fingers and thumbs.

    ______________________ is rubbing superficial tissues over the underlying tissues.

    ______________________ is the use of percussion to beat or pound on the body tissues.

CHAPTER 10 PROVIDING HYGIENE FOR THE MOUTH, EYES, HAIR, AND NAILS

1. Define these terms:

   mucosa

   mucus

   saliva

   papillae

   dentin

   plaque

   caries

   gingiva

2. What are the characteristics that suggest a potential alteration in oral mucous membranes?

3. Explain how to position the unconscious client for mouth care.

4. How do you remove dentures from a client who is unable to do so himself?

5. Indicate the *function* of these parts of the eye:

   sclera

   iris

   pupil

   lacrimal apparatus

6. Fill in the blanks:

   The client's eyes may be at risk for injury during periods of unconsciousness if his ______________________________ is absent.

The eye is cleansed by moving from the ______________________

canthus toward the ______________________ canthus.

To remove hard contact lenses from the eyes of a client unable to do so himself,

maneuver each lens so that the ______________________ that holds it in place is broken.

Contact lenses are stored in ______________________ solution.

7. Explain the difference between terminal and vellus hair.

8. What is the function of a shampoo board?

9. Mrs. Carter, a 50-year-old Black woman, has been very weak during her hospitalization and asks you to comb and braid her hair. Her hair is very tightly curled. How will you comb and braid it?

10. Circle the T or F to indicate if these statements are true or false:

T F If the client is receiving anticoagulant therapy, the nurse may check agency policy before shaving a client.

T F General body nutrition may be partially assessed through the condition of the nails.

T F Fingernails grow at a rate of approximately 1 mm daily.

T F Toenails grow faster than fingernails.

T F Hard nails may be softened by soaking in water for a period of time before cutting.

T F Generally the nurse never cuts the nails of a client with peripheral vascular disease.

Unit II CASE STUDY

MANAGEMENT OF SAFETY AND HYGIENE

Three weeks ago, George Powers, age 76, became very weak on the right side of his body and within an hour, could not move his right arm or leg. Gradually he lost consciousness. His wife called for an ambulance, which brought him to the hospital. After examinations and tests, his physician determined that Mr. Powers had suffered a cerebral vascular accident, commonly known as a stroke. He was admitted for treatment and rehabilitation.

Today, Mr. Powers continues to have weakness and paralysis of (inability to move) his right arm and leg. Even though he tries, he is unable to move from side to side in bed; you help him turn every two hours. He is unable to get out of bed by himself or to walk. He likes to sit in the chair but cannot keep himself properly positioned and falls to his right side.

Before his stroke, Mr. Powers was right-handed. He has been trying to eat with his left hand but finds it very awkward. He is unable to take off or put on his pajamas without help. He would like to brush his teeth, comb his hair, and shave by himself but cannot. His left hand just does not work as well as his right hand before his stroke. He is able to wash his hands, face, and neck but cannot bathe the rest of his body.

Mr. Powers is 5 feet 11 inches tall and weighs 145 pounds, which is underweight for that height. His skin is very dry and appears almost paper thin in some areas. He bruises easily. When he sits in the chair for an hour, he reports that his "backside" hurts. After he is returned to bed, you notice that he has a reddened area on the skin over his coccyx.

Answer these questions:

1. Because of Mr. Powers's weakness, paralysis, and inability to move purposefully, which affects his safety, he has a nursing diagnosis of: (State a two-part nursing diagnosis.)

2. Write a desired client outcome related to the nursing diagnosis in question 1.

3. What nursing measure(s) will you implement to achieve the outcome in question 2?

4. Because of Mr. Powers's inability to dress without assistance, he has a nursing diagnosis of: (State a two-part nursing diagnosis.)

5. Write a desired client outcome related to the nursing diagnosis in question 4.

6. Because of Mr. Powers's immobility and reddened skin area, he has a nursing diagnosis of: (State a two-part nursing diagnosis.)

7. Write a desired client outcome related to the nursing diagnosis in question 6.

8. What nursing measure(s) will you implement to achieve the outcome in question 7?

Unit III SELF-TESTS

CHAPTER 11 USING TECHNIQUES OF PHYSICAL EXAMINATION

1. List at least four characteristics that are required of the examiner when using examination techniques:

   1)

   2)

   3)

   4)

2. Identify the type of information that will be obtained by each of the techniques of examination:

   inspection

   palpation

   percussion

   auscultation

3. Indicate which technique(s) of examination you will use to obtain more information about these conditions:

   a. skin rash

   b. lung sounds

   c. painful joint

   d. abdominal pain

   e. heart sounds

   f. location of the liver

   g. lump in the breast

   h. skin wound

CHAPTER 12 ASSESSING THE VITAL SIGNS

1. Match the heat transfer mechanism in Column I with its examples in Column II.

I. Heat Transfer Method	II. Mechanism
A. radiation	_____ Body surface chilling in a cold wind
B. conduction	_____ Perspiration
C. convection	_____ Application of heat to a wound
D. vaporization	_____ Body surface warming in the sunlight

2. Explain the effect of a circadian rhythm on body temperature.

3. What is the medical term for an elevated body temperature? What is the most common cause of this condition?

4. On each of the thermometers drawn below, draw a line at the level that is normal body temperature.

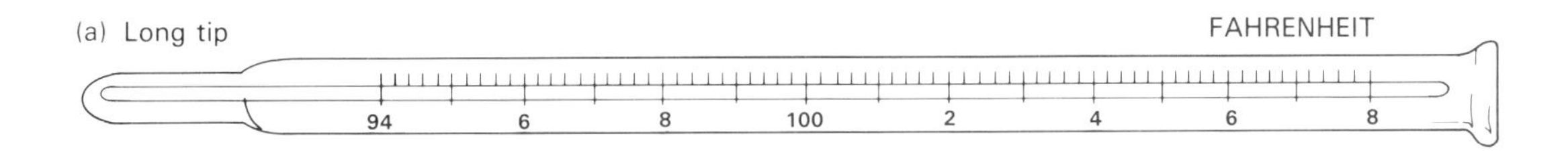

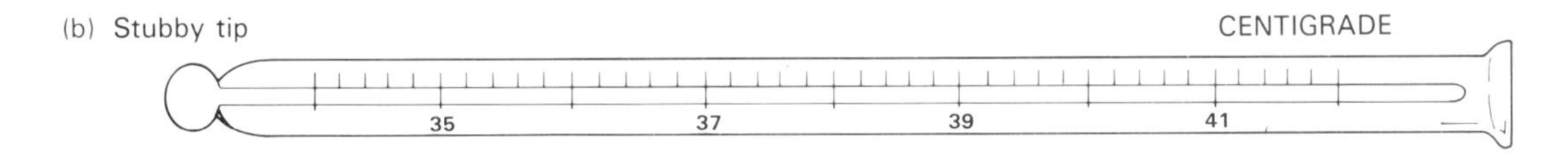

5. Designate the correct length of insertion time necessary to record body temperature for each of these temperature sites:

oral glass ________________

rectal glass ________________

axillary glass ________________

6. Explain how each of these variables affects the pulse *rate:*

   exercise

   emotions

   body temperature

   pathology

7. Define these terms that describe respiration:

   tachypnea

   bradypnea

   hyperpnea

   apnea

   dyspnea

   orthopnea

8. Fill in the blanks:

   Arterial blood pressure peaks during ______________________ when the left ventricle ______________________. The lower level of arterial pressure occurs during ______________________ when the ventricle ______________________.

9. Explain how each of these hemodynamic factors affects arterial blood pressure:

   circulating blood volume

   peripheral vascular resistance

   blood viscosity

   vascular tone

10. What is the auscultatory gap when monitoring arterial blood pressure? What significance does it have clinically?

CHAPTER 13 ASSESSING WEIGHT AND HEIGHT

1. Briefly describe the effects of these variables on the proportion of tissue weight to total body weight:

   age

   sex

   morphology

   nutrition

2. Briefly describe the effect these factors have on individual body height:

   age

   sex

   race

   heredity

   nutrition

CHAPTER 14 ADMISSION, TRANSFER, AND DISCHARGE

1. Explain the purposes of these parts of the admission process:

   introduction of nurse to the client

   orientation of the client to his room and facilities

   orientation of the client to the agency

   information regarding Patient's Bill of Rights

   admission interview

   assessment of vital signs

2. Each of these clients has just been admitted to a hospital. Through analysis of their statements or situations, identify a nursing diagnosis each is demonstrating:

   a. Mrs. Allen, age 23, in the final stages of pregnancy, is admitted to the labor and delivery unit to give birth to her first child. She states to the admitting nurse, "Do you know how long my labor will take? Can my husband stay with me in the labor room and be with me when I deliver? Will my doctor be here soon?"

Her nursing diagnosis is

b. Thomas Gandy, age 87, who lives by himself, has been admitted to the hospital after his daughter, Mrs. Carter, learned he hadn't eaten for three days and seemed confused. Through interviewing both Mr. Gandy and his daughter, the nurse learns that he had not been taking his medications for a week because his prescriptions ran out and he didn't have money to renew them. Mrs. Carter worries that he can no longer live independently.

His nursing diagnosis is

c. Mrs. Walton, 38, has just been admitted to the hospital to have surgery to remove her gall bladder later in the day. She has never had surgery or other hospitalization except for the deliveries of three children during her twenties. She states, "I am worried about surgery. My doctor has told me everything that will happen but I have never had surgery before and am scared. I don't want to remain in the hospital, away from my children, longer than necessary."

Her nursing diagnosis is

3. What is the purpose of a referral when a client is transferred to another agency? What pieces of information might it contain?

4. Mr. Nichols, age 73, is recovering from a stroke that left him weak and partially paralyzed in his right arm, which is his dominant arm. He is hypertensive and on several medications. He is going home where he lives with his wife. Both Mr. and Mrs. Nichols are worried about how they will manage. What are some specific nursing measures that may be implemented prior to his discharge?

Unit III CASE STUDY

FUNDAMENTAL ASSESSMENT SKILLS

John Lowe, age 79, is a pleasant gentleman who lives by himself in a two-room apartment with a small kitchen; he does his own cooking and has a pet dog. Until recently, he took his dog for a daily walk, often walking nearly two miles at a time. He enjoys reading but has failing vision.

You are a home care nurse assigned to visit Mr. Lowe because of his physician's concern about him. During your initial nursing history, you learn that Mr. Lowe has become short of breath in the past year and noticed his ankles swell in the afternoon and evening. In the past three weeks, he has had difficulty breathing when lying down; if he uses two or three pillows, his breathing eases somewhat and he is able to sleep. He also reports a sensation that he calls "palpitations" in his chest occasionally. Several months ago, his physician told him he has high blood pressure and a rapid heart beat. He reports feeling "dizzy" when he has the palpitations. Since yesterday, he has been feeling "hot" and "sweaty" and in general, states that he "just plain feels sick."

You take Mr. Lowe's vital signs. His pulse is 100 and irregular; his respirations are 24 and even; his temperature is 38.2°C; his blood pressure is 142/70. You notice that his skin temperature feels warmer than your own. His ankles are so swollen that an impression remains after you press your thumb against the skin. You weigh Mr. Lowe on his bathroom scale. He tells you that he weighed 156 pounds at his physician's office a week ago; today he weighs 168 pounds.

Answer these questions:

1. List all of the objective and subjective data identified above.

   Objective **Subjective**

2. What technique of physical examination will you use to assess Mr. Lowe's:

   breathing rate?

   breath sounds?

   skin color?

   skin temperature?

   heart rate?

   blood pressure?

3. What is the medical term for each of these problems?

   difficulty breathing

discomfort in breathing except in an upright position

slow breathing

high blood pressure

low blood pressure

slow heart beat

swelling of the soft tissues

4. Is Mr. Lowe's pulse normal? Give the correct terms to describe its rate and rhythm.

5. Is Mr. Lowe's respiration normal? Give the correct term to describe its rate.

6. Is Mr. Lowe's temperature normal? What is the term for this temperature?

   Is he febrile or afebrile? What is his temperature in Fahrenheit?

7. Concerning Mr. Lowe's blood pressure, which value is the systolic? Which is diastolic?

Unit IV SELF-TESTS

CHAPTER 15 ASSESSING MUSCULOSKELETAL FUNCTION

1. Match the musculoskeletal processes identified in Column I with their descriptions in Column II.

I. Process	II. Description
_____ hemapoiesis	A. Muscle shortening
_____ erythropoiesis	B. Bone development
_____ ossification	C. Production of blood cells
_____ articulation	D. Production of red blood cells
_____ contraction	E. Bone contact

2. Fill in the blanks:

   ______________________ is the dense connective tissue that creates a framework in the body, which is the ______________________. The ______________________ is a protective fibrous membrane that covers the bones. Inside the bones is a fatty material called the ______________________ that is involved with white blood cell production. Bones are held together with ______________________ and ______________________. Muscles attach to bones with fibrous bands called ______________________.

3. General examination of the client's musculoskeletal function will include what characteristics?

4. Explain what is meant by "activities of daily living" and identify at least four examples.

5. Explain the difference between activity orders for bedrest and "up ad lib."

6. Identify the nursing diagnosis for these clients:

   a. Robbie Albert, age 21, is in a coma following a motorcycle accident. He has no voluntary movement and is completely dependent.

      His nursing diagnosis is

   b. Mr. Jenkins, age 78, is very short of breath and unable to walk because of his respiratory disease. He is able to eat by himself but needs help with bathing and dressing.

      His nursing diagnosis is

   c. Sally Marsh, 35 years old, has an inner ear disorder that has affected her balance so that she cannot walk. She is dizzy all the time.

      Her nursing diagnosis is

CHAPTER 16 POSITIONING, MOVING, AND TRANSFERRING

1. Fill in the blanks:

   ____________________ is the force of attraction of two objects, such as the earth and an object on the earth. The ____________________ ________ of an object is the area of the object on which its weight rests. The ____________________ is the point on an object on which its whole weight rests. The ____________________ is an imaginary vertical line drawn from the center of gravity to the base of support.

2. Match the term in Column I with its definition in Column II.

I. Term	II. Definition
_____ motion	A. Condition in which all opposing forces are equal
_____ force	B. Force acting through a distance
_____ momentum	C. Increasing force through use of a machine
_____ work	D. Object that produces work by changing the application of energy
_____ machine	E. Fixed point around which work occurs
_____ lever	F. Resistance to motion
_____ fulcrum	G. Process of making change
_____ leverage	H. Force of motion acquired by a moving object
_____ friction	I. Strength or energy to cause motion or change
_____ equilibrium	J. Simple machine that increases work

3. Give at least four indicators of proper body alignment for each position:

   standing

   sitting

   lying

4. Suggest one application of each of these principles of body mechanics:
   a. More force or work is required to lift an object than to push or pull it.

   b. A lower center of gravity and wider base of support increases the stability of the body.

   c. Friction between two moving objects increases the amount of effort required to move one or both of them.

   d. Working with gravity requires less effort than working against it.

5. In your own words, describe the body posture in these positions:

   supine

   dorsal recumbent

   prone

   lateral

Fowler's

Sims'

dangling

6. Explain when the following body positions may be used:

   Trendelenberg

   reverse Trendelenberg

   lithotomy

   knee-chest

7. Indicate at least three basic but critical factors that must be kept in mind when transferring the client in any circumstance:

   1)

   2)

   3)

8. Mr. James, 71, is hospitalized because he had a stroke seven days ago. You are the nurse managing his care. Indicate at least five factors that you will assess to determine his activity and mobility status.

   1)

   2)

   3)

   4)

   5)

9. Mr. James has right hemiplegia, which means complete paralysis and weakness on his right side. Because he normally is right-handed, Mr. James is unable to eat or dress without assistance and cannot walk at the present time. His nursing diagnosis is:

CHAPTER 17 BEDMAKING

1. Explain these terms:

   unoccupied bed

   occupied bed

   open bed

   closed bed

   anesthesia bed

2. Indicate at least three factors you will assess prior to making the client's bed:

   1)

   2)

   3)

3. What is the purpose of the drawsheet?

4. List three actions taken by the nurse to limit transfer of microorganisms while changing bed linens:

   1)

   2)

   3)

5. List three actions taken by the nurse to reduce back strain or muscular strain on herself:

   1)

   2)

   3)

CHAPTER 18 EXERCISING AND AMBULATING

1. Fill in the blanks:

   The resting position of a joint is called its ______________________ position. The opening and closing of the joint is called its ______________________. The ______________________ muscles contract and shorten while the ______________________ muscles relax to close the angle of the joint. To open the joint angle, the ______________________ muscles contract and shorten and the ______________________ muscles relax. This entire process is called ______________________. The joint stiffening process is ______________________. The permanent shortening of the muscles is called ______________________. Muscle wasting is called ______________________.

2. Match the joint action in Column I with its description in Column II.

Action	Description
_____ flexion	A. Moving the toes toward the knee
_____ extension	B. Turning palm upward
_____ abduction	C. Moving the bone around its longitudinal axis
_____ adduction	D. Turning palm downward
_____ hyperextension	E. Bending the joint
_____ supination	F. Moving the bone away from the body midline
_____ pronation	G. Straightening the joint
_____ circumduction	H. Moving the bone toward the body midline
_____ plantar flexion	I. Moving the toes away from the knee
_____ dorsiflexion	J. Straightening the joint beyond its functional position

3. Explain what is meant by passive range of motion.

4. Compare the positive and negative effects of active and passive range of motion exercises.

5. Indicate at least three factors assessed prior to performing passive range of motion exercises:

   1)

   2)

   3)

6. Explain the advantage gained from isometric exercise.

7. What is the difference between gait and pace?

8. Explain these terms:

   progressive ambulation

   assisted ambulation

   independent ambulation

9. List at least two nursing diagnoses that suggest the client needs help with walking.

10. Suggest at least three factors necessary to determine the appropriate assistive device when the client has impaired physical mobility related to inability to ambulate safely.

    1)

    2)

    3)

CHAPTER 19 PROTECTING THE IMMOBILE CLIENT

1. List at least two effects of immobility on these body systems:

   cardiovascular

   1)

   2)

   respiratory

   1)

   2)

   musculoskeletal

   1)

   2)

   urinary

   1)

   2)

   integumentary

   1)

   2)

2. What variables determine the effect of immobility on the person?

3. Suggest at least two actions to limit the effect of immobility on these body systems:

   cardiovascular

   1)

   2)

   respiratory

   1)

   2)

musculoskeletal

1)

2)

urinary

1)

2)

integumentary

1)

2)

4. What are pressure points on the body? Where are they located?

5. Identify the factors that suggest a nursing diagnosis of potential impairment of skin integrity:

6. Explain the purposes of these therapeutic beds:

turning frame

CircOlectric bed

Clinitron bed

CHAPTER 20 MAINTAINING THERAPEUTIC IMMOBILITY

1. Describe these bone or muscle injuries:

   strain

   sprain

   laceration

   dislocation

   fracture

2. Match the terms in Column I with the definitions in Column II.

I. Term	II. Definition
_____ callus formation	A. Artificial body part
_____ open reduction	B. Surgical realignment and stabilization of bony fragments
_____ closed reduction	C. Bone scar tissue formation
_____ prosthesis	D. Realignment of bony fragments through immobilization devices
_____ arthroplasty	E. Surgical joint replacement

3. Explain how these devices immobilize a body part:

   splint

   brace

   cast

4. Explain the three aspects of the neurovascular status of a distal extremity and how they are assessed.

   1)

   2)

   3)

5. Explain the differences between a plaster of paris and a synthetic cast.

6. Johnny, 10 years old, has just had a synthetic cast placed on his left forearm because of a radial fracture. The cast encases the palm of his hand, with fingers and thumb protruding, and immobilizes his elbow in a 90° angle. You are the

nurse teaching Johnny and his mother how to care for the cast. List at least five suggestions that you will make.

1)

2)

3)

4)

5)

7. Explain the difference between skin and skeletal traction.

8. List at least five assessments that must be routinely made when the client is in traction.

1)

2)

3)

4)

5)

Unit IV CASE STUDY

MANAGEMENT OF ACTIVITY AND MOBILITY

Three days ago, Jessica Thorne, age 87, slipped on ice as she was walking with a nurse's aide outside of the nursing home where she resides. She reported excruciating pain when she fell, and was unable to move her right leg. An ambulance brought her to the emergency room where x-rays showed she had fractured the head of the right femur. Upon admission, the fracture was reduced with Buck's extension traction with 15 pounds weight. Presently Mrs. Thorne remains in traction, waiting for surgery to fix the fracture or replace the hip joint.

Mrs. Thorne is slender with white hair; she wears bifocals and a hearing aid. She is friendly and talkative. She reports she likes this "hotel" because the "maids" look so clean and fresh in their "white uniforms." She states she wants to "get out of this contraption" because "there's a war on and I've got work to do." Two years ago, her family arranged for her admission to the nursing home because they felt it was unsafe for her to live alone due to increasing confusion and disorientation. Except for occasional respiratory infections, Mrs. Thorne's only health problem has been osteoarthritis, a degenerative joint disease common among older people. She reports pain and stiffness in most of her joints, and as a result, sometimes has difficulty grasping small objects, such as silverware or a hairbrush.

Currently, the physician's activity orders for Mrs. Thorne are

Bedrest with right leg in Buck's extension traction with 15 pounds.
Passive joint range of motion exercises to all joints except right hip and knee four times a day

Because of the traction device that immobilizes her right hip and knee joint, Mrs. Thorne remains supine in bed. She has a trapeze attached to the traction frame on the bed, and is able to lift her upper body off the mattress slightly. Her head may be elevated to a mid-Fowler's position (45° angle) for brief periods, such as mealtime. The traction limits her from turning side to side.

Answer these questions:

1. List the subjective and objective data identified in the case study.

   Subjective Data | **Objective Data**

2. Mrs. Thorne's confinement to bed, placement in traction, and joint movement limitations due to arthritis suggest a nursing diagnosis concerning her mobility needs. Write this two-part nursing diagnosis.

3. Suggest a client outcome for the nursing diagnosis in question 2.

4. List as many nursing actions or measures as you can think of to achieve the client outcome in question 3.

5. Mrs. Thorne's confusion, disorientation, and immobilization suggest another nursing diagnosis about her safety. Write this two-part nursing diagnosis.

6. Suggest a client outcome for the nursing diagnosis in question 5.

7. List as many nursing actions or measures as you can think of to achieve the client outcome in question 6.

8. Mrs. Thorne's immobilization, slender body frame, age, and joint injury suggest a nursing diagnosis about her skin. Write this two-part nursing diagnosis.

9. Suggest a client outcome for the nursing diagnosis in question 8.

10. Explain how you will assess the neurovascular condition of Mrs. Thorne's right leg.

Unit V SELF-TESTS

CHAPTER 21 MANAGING ANXIETY

1. List characteristics of fear and anxiety in columns under these terms:

   Physiologic Manifestations **Behavioral Manifestations**

2. Identify the defense mechanism demonstrated by each of the following clients:

   a. Mr. Carter is in the intensive care unit because he had a heart attack. Even though his physician has told him that he must rest in bed, Mr. Carter insists on walking up and down the hallway. You notice that he grimaces and clutches his chest after a brisk walk. You ask, "Mr. Carter, are you having chest pain?" His response is, "No, not at all. I'm just a little short of breath. I'm really fine. These doctors don't known anything."

      His defense mechanism is

   b. Ms. Helen Gray has been having menstrual-like bleeding even though she experienced menopause several years ago. Her mother had similar symptoms before she died of uterine cancer. Ms. Gray has made several appointments to see her physician but never remembers to keep the appointment.

      Her defense mechanism is

   c. Although John Jeffries manages a large office with 20 workers, his father, who owns the business, criticizes virtually every decision John makes. John never responds to his father's criticism, thinking he may lose his job if he does. After a critical discussion with his father over a minor decision John made, John angrily fires his secretary because she forgot to mail a letter he requested.

      His defense mechanism is

   d. Peter Downing, 15 years old, has acne, which embarrasses him. He refuses to attend school functions, telling his parents, "None of the kids like me. They think I'm ugly to look at."

      His defense mechanism is

3. List at least five identifying characteristics of the nursing diagnosis, anxiety:

   1)

   2)

   3)

   4)

   5)

4. The first task when managing the anxious client is to create a therapeutic environment. How will you do that?

5. Indicate at least three ways in which you, the nurse, can facilitate the client's expression of feelings.

   1)

   2)

   3)

CHAPTER 22 MANAGING PAIN

1. List four types of physical stimuli that cause sensations of pain and give an example of each:

   1)

   2)

   3)

   4)

2. Fill in the blanks:

   The free nerve endings found throughout the body are called ____________ ____________. When stimulated by ______________________, these nerve endings cause a sensation of pain when the impulse is transmitted to the spinal cord via an ______________________ sensory fiber. The type of sensation perceived depends on which type of ____________ ____________ conducts the impulse. The ______________________ theory of pain suggests that some fibers may ______________________ other impulses from getting through. The pain ____________ is the point of pain intensity at which the individual perceives the sensation as pain. Sometimes this is also called pain ______________________.

3. Define these terms that are used to characterize pain:

   pain intensity

   intermittent pain

   intractable pain

   diffuse pain

   localized pain

   radiating pain

   referred pain

   phantom pain

4. List some objective (may be observed by the examiner) physical indicators of pain.

5. List some behaviors that are suggestive of pain.

6. Match the pain therapy in Column I with its description in Column II.

I. Pain Therapy	II. Description
_____ therapeutic touch	A. Using suggestion to relieve pain while person is in an altered state of consciousness
_____ guided imagery	B. Controlling breathing and relaxing muscle groups
_____ relaxation	C. Focusing thoughts on pleasing images
_____ distraction	D. Stimulating tissue through manipulation of needles placed in the body at specific points
_____ thermotherapy	E. Touching or rubbing a painful area
_____ biofeedback	F. Consciously controlling body functions that are not normally consciously controlled
_____ acupuncture	G. Applying heat or cold
_____ hypnosis	H. Providing an alternative to the pain stimuli

Unit V CASE STUDY

PROVISION OF COMFORT

Joan Maynard, age 43, learned she has cancer of the ovaries nine months ago; when surgery was performed to remove the tumor, the surgeons found that she had other tumor growth throughout the abdomen. In the six months following surgery, Joan underwent extensive chemotherapy, which alleviated her symptoms of abdomen pressure and pain somewhat. She decided to stop further chemotherapy three months ago when it became apparent that the tumors continued to grow. Now tumors have spread to her pelvis and lumbar spine. For six weeks she has been unable to walk because of the pressure of the tumor against her spinal cord; she can no longer control her urination and defecation.

Joan returned to her home after her surgery and has remained at home ever since. She lives with her husband, Jack, and their four children. The oldest child, Susan, age 19, commutes to a junior college nearby. Jeff, age 17, is a high school senior. Jared, age 13, and Eric, age 12, attend a neighborhood junior high school.

You, a home care nurse, have just visited the Maynard family for the first time. From your initial interview, you have determined that each family member knows that Joan has cancer and can see that her condition is worsening but you also see that each family member is coping differently. Jack states, with a broad smile, that he is optimistic for a recovery. "Joan is going to make it. She has a lot of spirit and I know she can beat this thing." Jeff hardly talks at all during the interview and never looks directly at you. His answers to your questions are brief. When his father leaves the room, he says, "Dad just wants to control everything, especially me. I'm furious with him for not helping Mom more." His voice quivers as he talks. Susan almost dominates the conversation with her eagerness to express her thoughts. Matter-of-factly she tells you in rapid-fire words, "I know we may not have Mom much longer, but we're nearly grown up now and can take care of ourselves. She's a great Mom and has taught us a lot. I'm not worried about losing her; I know we'll be okay." Eric remains quiet and never expresses himself in any way; he looks at the floor throughout the time you are with the family. Jared won't talk about his mother either, but he does tell you about his soccer team with great enthusiasm. "We're the best in the league and I know we'll win the state championship. I'm a great player; I usually make four or five goals every game." At this point, Jack interrupts. "Stop exaggerating, Jared," he says rather harshly; he shrugs his shoulders as he turns to you.

Later, you interview Joan privately. She reports that her pain is considerable and she really never gets any relief. To understand her pain, you take a pain history. Joan reports that the pain is primarily located in her pelvis but when the pain is intense, she feels her entire body trunk and lower legs are "on fire." Most of the time, she ranks her pain level as "5 on a scale of 0, no pain, to 10, the worst possible pain." The pain is at its worst when she is alone. To date, Joan has taken very little analgesic medication because, "I want to wait until I really need it." She asks, "Please help me deal with this pain. I don't want to be drugged; I want to be awake when I'm with my family, but I also want some measure of comfort so that I can enjoy them."

Answer these questions:

1. Each of the Maynards is experiencing anxiety regarding Joan's illness. Which defense mechanism is Jack using? ____

   A. rationalization
   B. denial
   C. projection
   D. introjection

2. Susan's defense mechanism is ____.

   A. repression
   B. suppression
   C. rationalization
   D. fantasy

3. Jeff is using the defense of ____.

   A. displacement
   B. denial
   C. sublimation
   D. undoing

4. Jared's defense mechanism is ____.

   A. denial
   B. sublimation
   C. undoing
   D. fantasy

5. Eric's behavior doesn't give enough information to identify a defense. What does his behavior suggest to you?

6. Each member of the Maynard family is experiencing anxiety that is preventing him or her from developing some coping skills for dealing with Joan's illness. Prepare a client outcome that is suitable for the entire family, in response to their anxiety.

7. Suggest some nursing measures to achieve the client outcome.

8. Joan's immediate problem is alteration in comfort: pain related to her malignancy. Prepare a client outcome for this nursing diagnosis.

9. Suggest some nursing measures to achieve the desirable outcome for Joan.

Unit VI SELF-TESTS

CHAPTER 23 ASSESSING FLUID BALANCE AND NUTRITION

1. Fill in the blanks:

   Between ____________________ and ____________________ ________ percent of body weight is water, which varies according to ________ ____________________ and ____________________. The water found inside the body cells is called ____________________; water found outside the cells is ____________________.

2. Name at least three sources of body fluid loss:

   1)

   2)

   3)

3. Identify the nursing diagnostic category for these clients:

   a. Mr. Garcia, 79 years old, has been confused and sleepy in the past 24 hours. His fluid intake has been 860 cc for the past 24 hours (1,450 cc the previous 24 hours) with an output of 930 cc of concentrated urine (1,500 cc the previous 24 hours). His lips are dry and chapped; his skin turgor is diminished. His pulse is 92 (yesterday 80) and his temperature is 99.3°F (yesterday 98.6°F).

      His nursing diagnostic category is

   b. Mr. Marsh, 72 years old, has swollen feet, ankles, and lower legs. The skin over the swelling is taut. Today his blood pressure is 150/88; upon admission three days ago, his blood pressure was 138/80. His weight today is 168; upon admission it was 156.

      His nursing diagnostic category is

4. You are keeping a food and fluid intake record for Mrs. O'Casey to monitor her calorie count. Calculate her total fluid intake for your 700 to 1500 shift from this food and fluid intake record:

Time	Food or Drink	Amount
800	coffee	1 cup (150 cc)
	orange juice	4 oz. (120 cc)
	cooked oatmeal	3/4 cup
	milk	1/2 pint (240 cc)
	toast	1 slice
	jelly	1 tablespoon
900	water	2 oz. (60 cc)

Time	Food or Drink	Amount
1000	ginger ale	4 oz. (120 cc)
1200	creamed soup	6 oz. (180 cc)
	gelatin	1/2 cup (about 4 oz. or 120 cc)
	bread roll	1
	tea	1 cup (150 cc)
1400	ice cream	1/2 cup (about 4 oz. or 120 cc)
		TOTAL: ____________ (in cc)

5. Define these terms:

   nutritionist

   diet history

   food intake study

   anthropometrics

6. Identify the anthropometrics that are used to evaluate nutritional status:

7. For each of these body parts, indicate at least two changes suggesting altered nutritional status:

   hair

   eyes

   mouth

   skin

   nails

   heart

8. Identify the nursing diagnostic category for these clients:

   a. Mr. Jeffries, 35 years old, weighs 230 pounds, is 5 feet 8 inches tall, works as an accountant and does little physical activity other than walking to and from his automobile to home or office. He states he really enjoys eating and consumes at least four meals each day. Upon examination, you find that his triceps skinfold is approximately 25 cm.

      His nursing diagnostic category is

   b. Jane Hudson, 19 years old, weighs 98 pounds and is 5 feet 9 inches tall. She states she has a "good appetite" but you notice that she barely eats lunch and dinner and refuses breakfast entirely.

      Her nursing diagnostic category is

CHAPTER 24 HELPING THE CLIENT EAT

The nursing diagnostic category, actual or potential self-care deficit: feeding, may be easily overlooked unless the nurse is alert to the identifying characteristics. For each of these clients, indicate:

A. for a potential self-care deficit: feeding
B. for an actual self-care deficit: feeding
C. no deficit is present

1. ____ Wendy Burton, 4 months old, is hospitalized with croup, a respiratory infection.

2. ____ Matthew Jackson, 5 years old, has chronic kidney failure. He is anorexic.

3. ____ Mary Wilson, 15 years old, broke her right arm and left leg while skiing. Her arm has a cast from the fingertips to the shoulder and her leg is in traction. She is right-handed.

4. ____ Jason Heath, 25 years old, has a spinal cord injury from a motorcycle accident and is completely paralyzed from the neck down.

5. ____ Jennifer Morrison, 36 years old, has multiple sclerosis. She has intact arm and hand movement but is unable to walk and is blind.

6. ____ Mel Chase, 55 years old, has diabetes. He is hospitalized with a skin infection on his left foot.

7. ____ Maria Lopez, 60 years old, is in the hospital because of hypertension.

8. ____ Leonard Franklin, 88 years old, is hospitalized because of dehydration, confusion, and a failing heart. He has been living by himself. His family reports that he doesn't eat or drink unless reminded, and sometimes he refuses to eat and drink.

CHAPTER 25 MANAGING THE CLIENT WITH A GASTROINTESTINAL TUBE

1. Match the anatomic placement in Column II with the name of the gastrointestinal tube in Column I.

I. Tube	II. Placement
_____ orogastric	A. From the abdominal wall to the stomach
_____ nasogastric	B. Through the nose to the jejunum
_____ nasojejunal	C. From the abdominal wall to the jejunum
_____ gastrostomy	D. Through the mouth to the stomach
_____ jejunostomy	E. Through the nose to the stomach

2. Gastrointestinal intubation is done for several reasons. Explain what these terms mean:

   decompression

   gavage

   lavage

   compression

3. Explain the effect of these factors on the flow rate of fluids in and out of tubes:

   suction

   force of gravity

   tube diameter

   viscosity

   tube length

4. How do you determine the length of the tubing to insert before placing a nasogastric tube?

5. Describe three methods for determining accurate placement of a nasogastric tube:

   1)

   2)

   3)

6. Explain the reasons for irrigating a nasogastric tube used for decompression and removal of gastric contents.

7. Fill in the blanks:

   ______________________ nutrition is the term used to describe the instillation of liquid food into the stomach through a tube. Formulas used contain ______________________, ______________________, and ______________________ as well as vitamins and minerals. The exact nutrients used depend on ______________________. A common side effect of this type of feeding is ______________________, which happens because of the high osmolarity of the formulas used.

8. Explain why the nurse checks for gastric residual feedings at intervals.

CHAPTER 26 MANAGING INTRAVENOUS FLUID THERAPY

1. Describe the clinical characteristics of these problems:

   fluid volume depletion (dehydration)

   fluid volume overload (overhydration)

   fluid concentration disturbances

   fluid composition disturbances

2. Explain these terms:

   replacement therapy

   open line

   keep open rate

3. Fill in the blanks:

   Nutrient intravenous solutions are given to ________________. Solutions that maintain or alter body pH are called ________________ ________________ solutions. Normal saline is a ________________ solution. Blood volume expanders are given to ________________ ________ when severe blood loss occurs. Examples of blood volume expanders are ________________, ________________, and ________________.

4. Match the part of intravenous administration equipment in Column I with its function in Column II.

I. Device	II. Function
____ bottle or bag	A. Controls flow rate by manually regulating size of tubing.
____ drip chamber	B. Contains solution.
____ drip tube	C. Determines volume of drips.
____ tubing	D. Pierces skin, tissues, and vein to deliver solution.
____ catheter	E. Uses pressure to deliver solution into vein.
____ clamp	F. Permits observation of the drops from the container to the tubing.
____ controller	G. Controls flow rate by automatically changing tubing diameter by electronic sensor.
____ pump	H. Delivers solution from bag or bottle to catheter or needle.

5. List at least four factors considered when selecting a venipuncture site.

   1)

   2)

   3)

   4)

6. List at least three factors, besides a preset drip rate, that affect the actual rate of infusion?

   1)

   2)

   3)

7. Mr. Carson is receiving intravenous fluid replacement therapy because of severe dehydration following a gastrointestinal illness. The physician has ordered 1,000 cc of D_5W to be infused in five hours. You use an administration set with a drip factor of 10. What is the drip rate? ______________

____

8. Joshua Beggs is receiving intravenous fluids to replace electrolytes. His order is 500 cc of D_5S with KCl 20 mEq in four hours. You use an administration set with a drip factor of 15. What is the drip rate? ______________

____

9. Mrs. Elkhart is receiving intravenous fluids at a slow rate to keep open a line for intermittent administration of medications. She is receiving 500 cc of D_5W over eight hours. The administration set has a drip factor of 60. When monitoring her infusion, you note that the infusion drips about 80 drops each minute. Is the infusion too fast, too slow, or right on time? ______________

____

10. Mr. Joyce is receiving continuous intravenous fluids with heparin for anticoagulation. He is to receive 8,000 units of heparin in eight hours. It is added to a 500 cc bag of D_5W. To ensure administration of 1,000 units per hour when the administration set delivers 12 drops per minute, what is the desired drip rate? ______________________________

CHAPTER 27 MANAGING TOTAL PARENTERAL NUTRITION

1. Define these terms:

   total parenteral nutrition

   hyperalimentation

   nitrogen balance

   catabolism

2. Explain what causes negative nitrogen balance.

3. Name three conditions that may cause negative nitrogen balance.

   1)

   2)

   3)

4. Why is a central vein a more desirable site for the infusion of parenteral nutrition than a peripheral vein?

5. Infection is a major complication of TPN therapy. What clinical manifestations will you observe for?

6. While assisting the physician to insert a central line, you observe the client having sudden, sharp chest pain, difficulty breathing, and coughing. What complication do these signs suggest?

7. If bright red, pulsating blood returns in the catheter during insertion, what complication is suggested?

What is the treatment for this problem?

8. You have been managing the TPN therapy for Mrs. Grey, who receives TPN because of Crohn's disease. While changing her dressing, you notice the insertion site is red and slightly swollen. It didn't appear red at the last dressing change two days ago. Her vital signs are within normal range and she has not reported any unusual symptoms. What is her nursing diagnosis, on the basis of what you know?

Unit VI CASE STUDY

MANAGEMENT OF NUTRITION AND FLUIDS

Sylvia Livingstone, age 52, was admitted to the hospital yesterday because she had been vomiting every few hours for three days without relief. In the health history, Mrs. Livingstone stated that she had been having nausea and severe epigastric cramps before she started vomiting. She had been unable to eat or drink anything for four days. Her weight dropped from 138 pounds to 124 pounds during the three days of vomiting. Upon examination, her mucous membranes were dry and sticky and her skin had diminished turgor. Radiologic examination confirmed the physician's suspicions that Mrs. Livingstone has an obstruction in the proximal jejunum that prevents the products of digestion from passing. The backed-up partially digested foods and fluids accumulated in her stomach until vomiting began to relieve the distention.

Shortly after Mrs. Livingstone entered the hospital at 1000 yesterday morning, you placed a 14 French double lumen nasogastric tube which you attached to continuous suction, following the physician's instructions. The tube began to drain dark greenish-brown fluid with flakes immediately. As of 0600 this morning, the gastric drainage totaled 2,575 cc. Other fluid output during that same time period was 225 cc of urine.

At 1030 yesterday, you started an intravenous infusion, selecting a vein on the back of her left hand as the venipuncture site. Mrs. Livingstone is to receive 3500 cc dextrose 5 percent in water over 24 hours. As of 0600 this morning, she had received two 1,000 cc bottles of intravenous infusion plus the infusion of 275 cc of a third 1,000 cc bottle. Mrs. Livingstone has been NPO since her admission.

At 0800 this morning, you assess Mrs. Livingstone's condition. She tells you that she continues to feel nauseated and have pain. She points to the epigastric region to show you where the pain is located. She also tells you that the tube irritates her nose. The nares appear red and dry. The NG tube has drained only 50 cc of dark green fluid in two hours. It presently doesn't seem to be moving anything. Her intravenous infusion is on a controlled pump. The venipuncture site is red, tender, and swollen.

Answer these questions:

1. List all the objective and subjective data identified in the first paragraph.

   Objective | **Subjective**

2. What nursing diagnosis is suggested by the above data? Make it a two-part statement.

3. Suggest a client outcome to treat the problem identified in question 2.

4. What is Mrs. Livingstone's total intake and output until 0600 this morning?

______

5. Explain the purpose of the second lumen on the nasogastric tube.

6. If Mrs. Livingstone is going to receive only a nutrient solution such as dextrose in water, what size needle or catheter is used for the venipuncture? ______

______

7. At what hourly rate will you set the infusion controller pump? ______

______

8. Suppose the physician changes the infusion order to 3,000 cc of dextrose 5 percent in water per 24 hours. At what hourly rate will you reset the infusion controller pump? ______

9. What comfort measure may you institute to relieve Mrs. Livingstone's irritated nostril?

10. At 0800, what has been the hourly average of nasogastric drainage since the insertion of the nasogastric tube? ______

______

11. If the drainage in two hours was 50 cc and the tube doesn't appear to be draining, what is the patency of the tube? What nursing action does this suggest?

12. What do the signs of redness, swelling and pain at the venipuncture site suggest? How can you further check?

Unit VII SELF-TESTS

CHAPTER 28 ASSESSING GENITOURINARY FUNCTION

1. Fill in the blanks.

   The urinary system has the capacity to control the composition of ________ ________ and regulate water, electrolyte, and ________ ________ balance of the body. The urinary system has two ________ ________ and two ________, plus a bladder and urethra. The kidneys also are part of the regulatory system for ________ by the production of ________ ________.

2. Describe the mechanism for eliminating urine from the bladder.

3. Match the process in Column I with its description in Column II.

I. Process	II. Description
____ perfusion	A. Physical process of moving urine from the kidney to the bladder
____ filtration	B. Process by which water and solutes that are filtrated by the kidney tubules are returned to the blood
____ reabsorption	C. Passage of blood through an organ
____ tubular secretion	D. Removal of particles from the blood
____ transportation	E. Expulsion of urine from the body
____ micturition	F. Process in which distal tubular cells regulate pH of blood through secretion of hydrogen ions in exchange for sodium ions

4. Define these terms:

   urgency

   dysuria

   hesitancy

   nocturia

   enuresis

   incontinence

5. Identify the nursing diagnostic category for these clients:

   a. Mrs. Joyce Sorenson, 58 years old, reports that she "leaks" urine whenever she coughs or does heavy lifting.

      Her nursing diagnostic category is

   b. Mr. Cohen, 72 years old, reports that he has difficulty passing his urine even though he feels the urge. When he does void, the stream is weak and he feels like his bladder never completely empties. He feels like he has to urinate all the time; he does urinate every hour and a half, day and night.

      His nursing diagnostic category is

CHAPTER 29 TOILETING

For each of these clients, indicate if the nursing diagnosis is

A. Actual self-care deficit: toileting.
B. Potential self-care deficit: toileting.
C. Neither nursing diagnosis is present.

1. ____ Mrs. Chin, 78 years old, is unable to walk to the bathroom without assistance because she is weak and short of breath. She is able to use a bedside commode but only with assistance.

2. ____ Jess Kearney, 14 years old, broke both his wrists while skateboarding. He has casts from his fingers to his mid-upper arm and cannot flex his fingers.

3. ____ Mr. Leopold, 59 years old, had his larynx removed because of a malignancy. He is unable to speak. He is on bedrest with bathroom privileges.

4. ____ Mrs. O'Malley, 74 years old, broke her right hip and is in skeletal traction. She uses a trapeze to raise herself from the bed surface.

5. ____ Ms. Martin, 31 years old, has a degenerative muscle disease that has limited her ability to walk because of weakness and paralysis in all extremities.

CHAPTER 30 INSERTING AND MANAGING URINARY CATHETERS

1. What size urinary catheters are used for

   adult women?

   adult men?

   children?

2. Why is the urinary catheterization done with sterile technique?

3. Maria Garcia, 48 years old, had a hysterectomy (her uterus removed) in surgery earlier today. She has not voided since her return from the recovery room two hours ago. Her postoperative orders state, "Straight catheterization for urinary retention p.r.n." What assessments will you make to determine whether she should be catheterized? List at least three factors.

   1)

   2)

   3)

4. The nurse, Bill, is catheterizing Mr. Thompson, who is unable to void because of an enlarged prostate gland. Indicate if Bill's technique maintains sterility (check Yes) or contaminates the field (check No) in the following: After the catheterization set is opened, Bill puts on sterile gloves and arranges the catheterization tray on Mr. Thompson's thighs.

   Does this maintain sterility? Yes _____ No _____

   Bill unfolds the perineal drape and centers it over Mr. Thompson's penis, taking care to handle only the upper side of the drape with his sterile gloved hands.

   Does this maintain sterility? Yes _____ No _____

   With his sterile gloved hands, Bill checks through the equipment in the catheterization tray. He opens the antiseptic package and pours antiseptic solution over the cotton balls; he drops the solution packing into a waste receptacle at the bedside.

   Does this maintain sterility? Yes _____ No _____

   Bill picks up the penis in his left hand and uses his right hand to cleanse the glans and meatus with the cotton balls.

   Does this maintain sterility? Yes _____ No _____

When the glans and meatus are cleansed, Bill transfers the penis to his right hand. He uses his left hand to guide the catheter into the meatus.

Does this maintain sterility? Yes _____ No _____

5. As Bill, in the above situation, guides the catheter into the urethra, resistance is met. What two techniques can Bill use to overcome this resistance?

6. What is the difference between the use of a straight catheter and an indwelling retention catheter? Explain their physical differences.

7. Identify two nursing diagnostic categories that suggest the use of an external urinary catheter.

8. Explain the difference between a catheter irrigation and a catheter instillation.

9. List two purposes of three-way bladder irrigation (also called continuous bladder irrigation):

   1)

   2)

10. Mr. Jackson has a continuous bladder irrigation following prostate surgery. At the beginning of your shift, the irrigation bottle contained 1,900 cc of bladder irrigant and his urine collecting container was empty. During your shift, you empty his urine collecting container of 1,500 cc. Later, the irrigation bottle emptied and you added an additional 2,000 cc bottle. Just before the end of your shift, you must determine his urinary output. His irrigation bottle now contains 750 cc of irrigant and his collecting bag has 1,275 cc. What is his urinary output? _______________

CHAPTER 31 ASSESSING BOWEL ELIMINATION FUNCTION

1. Fill in the blanks.

   ______________________ is the mixture of partially digested food and digestive secretions that moves through the intestine by a process called ______________________. It becomes a solid mass called ______________________ in the distal ______________________. Evacuation of waste materials occurs when the bulk distends the intestinal walls and increases ______________________. This opens the internal anal sphincter and signals a ______________________ urge to defecate. Peristalsis is stimulated by the introduction of food, a mechanism called the ______________________.

2. List at least five factors that influence bowel elimination patterns.

   1)

   2)

   3)

   4)

   5)

3. Define:

   melena

   steatorrhea

   impaction

   flatus

   eructation

4. Identify the nursing diagnostic categories for these clients:

   a. Mr. Roberts, age 78, has noticed that he has infrequent bowel movements. He passes hard, dry stools only with abdominal cramping and difficult effort.

   His nursing diagnostic category is

   b. Ms. Henry, age 32, reports she has abdominal cramping and a sense of urgency for defecation. She has 10–12 stools a day, all watery. Upon examination, you find that she has hyperactive bowel sounds.

   Her nursing diagnostic category is

5. What is rebound tenderness? How do you assess for it?

CHAPTER 32 REMOVING FECES AND FLATUS

1. Suggest three ways the nurse assists the client to maintain or achieve natural bowel elimination.

   1)

   2)

   3)

2. What is the difference between a laxative and a cathartic?

3. Explain the purpose of these enemas:

   cleansing

   retention

   return-flow

4. Suggest three ways the nurse assists the client to pass flatus.

   1)

   2)

   3)

5. Describe the clinical signs and symptoms that would suggest the client has a fecal impaction.

CHAPTER 33 MANAGING THE OSTOMY

1. Match the definition in Column II with the term in Column I.

I. Term	II. Definition
____ stoma	A. Opening made from the ileum to the abdominal surface
____ effluent	B. Health care provider who specializes in teaching and supporting ostomates
____ colostomy	C. Artificial opening from a body cavity to the surface of the body
____ ileostomy	D. Person who has an ostomy
____ enterostomy therapist	E. Material discharged from an ostomy
____ ostomate	F. Opening made from the colon to the abdominal surface

2. Describe characteristics of the effluent of these ostomy types:

   sigmoid colostomy

   colostomy in the cecum

   ileostomy

   urostomy

3. Explain the purpose of this ostomy equipment:

   appliance

   faceplate

   skin barrier

   skin sealant

4. Identify four factors that will affect how the client responds to an ostomy.

   1)

   2)

   3)

   4)

5. Each of these clients recently had an ostomy. Name the probable nursing diagnostic category suggested by the given data:

   a. Mr. Griego, age 67, has had a sigmoid colostomy because of a rectal malignancy. After surgery, he expresses relief that his tumor was found early enough so that it could be removed but says he had never heard of a colostomy procedure before. He asks many questions about the management of his stoma.

His probable nursing diagnosis is

b. Sally Larson, age 24, had an ileostomy because of chronic inflammatory bowel disease. She is relieved that her long-term problems of abdominal pain and frequent diarrhea are past, but she reports being "worried" about her continuing relationship with the young man that she expects to marry. "I'm afraid he won't want to live with me, now that I am mutilated." She cannot bear to look at her stoma or surgical incision.

Her probable nursing diagnostic category is

c. Rick Altman, age 30, had an ileostomy three months ago because of chronic inflammatory bowel disease. Although he has learned how to apply the pouch, he has had difficulty maintaining a seal and subsequently his appliance has leaked effluent on the skin. His stoma is bright, glistening, moist, and red but the peristomal area is red and excoriated in some areas.

His nursing diagnostic category is

6. Which types of colostomies are irrigated?

7. Match the description in Column II with the type of urostomy in Column I.

I. Urostomy Type	II. Description
_____ cutaneous ureterostomy	A. A "bladder" is constructed from portion of the bowel which collects urine before it drains from the body.
_____ ileal conduit	B. An opening is made from ureters to abdominal surface.
_____ continent urostomy	C. Ureters are implanted in the sigmoid colon, which acts as a bladder.
_____ uretosigmoidostomy	D. A "bladder" is constructed from a portion of the bowel; it has a nipple valve that prevents urine leakage.

Unit VII CASE STUDY

MANAGEMENT OF ELIMINATION

Edna Jeffries, age 77, lives in an extended care facility for elderly people because she has failing vision. Until recently, her only other health problem was arthritis that gave her early morning stiffness and soreness. Mrs. Jeffries is a widow; she has five children who live in the nearby community and visit frequently. She is bright, alert, and frequently the center of lively conversation among the residents.

As the nurse who manages the wing where Mrs. Jeffries lives, you have noticed lately a smell of urine in her room. She occasionally appears with moist spots on her clothing and you suspect she has been dribbling urine but may not be aware of it. You decide to assess the situation. During your interview with Mrs. Jeffries, she reports that she has a full feeling in the area of her bladder; she feels like she has to urinate often but often can't pass her urine when she does reach the bathroom. She feels burning when she passes her urine. She has noticed that her underwear often feels wet. She has stopped drinking as much liquid as she normally does to try to control this problem of "dribbling."

Although her urinary problem annoys her, Mrs. Jeffries confides that she is more worried about her bowels. She doesn't have a bowel movement each day as she did when she was younger. Often she feels abdominal pain and has a lot of gas. When you ask how long it has been since she noticed this change, she replied, "It has really become a problem only in the past month or so." A couple of weeks ago, she began having episodes of diarrhea and rarely has a formed stool. She plans to ask her physician for "something to get me back on track" during her next doctor's appointment.

As you examine Mrs. Jeffries, you note that her abdomen appears normal upon inspection. You auscultate and hear hyperactive bowel sounds in all four quadrants. Percussion of the abdomen is normal. When you palpate, you feel a large mass in the left lower quadrant; Mrs. Jeffries reports that this area feels tender. You do a rectal examination and palpate a hardened mass within a finger's length of the anus; it is stool.

Answer these questions:

1. Use the correct medical terms to describe these signs:

   feeling of needing to urinate frequently

   inability to start urinary stream

   burning when passing urine

2. Write the S and O of a SOAP nursing note that describes Mrs. Jeffries' urinary problems.

3. Which nursing diagnosis best describes Mrs. Jeffries' urinary problem?
   a. Impairment of urinary elimination: retention
   b. Altered urinary elimination pattern
   c. Incontinence
4. Write a desirable outcome to treat the problem identified in question 3.

5. Write the S and O of a SOAP nursing note that describes Mrs. Jeffries' bowel problems.

6. Which nursing diagnosis describes Mrs. Jeffries' bowel problem?
   a. Alteration in bowel elimination: constipation
   b. Alteration in bowel elimination: diarrhea
   c. Alteration in bowel elimination: bowel incontinence
7. Write a desirable outcome to treat the problem identified in question 6.

8. Suggest at least three nursing actions to achieve the desirable outcome:

9. Mrs. Jeffries indicated that she had frequent gas. Suggest some nursing actions to help her cope with this problem.

Unit VIII SELF-TESTS

CHAPTER 34 ASSESSING RESPIRATORY FUNCTION

1. Trace the pathway of a molecule of oxygen from its entry into the nose of the person, through each portion of the respiratory system, until it reaches a red blood cell.

2. Describe the function of these parts of the respiratory system:

   nasal turbinates

   nasal cilia

   epiglottis

   olfactory receptors

   surfactant

   alveolar-capillary membrane

3. Describe the normal appearance of these parts of the respiratory system:

   nasal mucosa

   posterior pharynx

   posterior chest

   spine

   chest expansion

   anterior chest

4. Name the nursing diagnostic category of these clients:

   a. Mr. Soong Yung, age 50, reports that he "can't breathe well." Upon examination, you find that he has an enlarged thorax with well-developed accessory muscles. His respirations are rapid with pursed-lip expirations. His mucous membranes are cyanotic.

      His nursing diagnostic category is

   b. Robbie Andrews, age 27 months, has a harsh respiratory stridor, flaring nares, and circumoral cyanosis. His father reports that he has coughed sputum for 24 hours.

      His nursing diagnostic category is

c. Mrs. Stalk, age 74, has been hospitalized for several days because of a respiratory infection. She has become confused and restless in the past 12 hours and is no longer coughing as productively as before the confusion began.

Her nursing diagnostic category is

CHAPTER 35 PROVIDING PULMONARY PHYSIOTHERAPY

1. Explain what is meant by the term *pulmonary hygiene*. What two factors determine its effectiveness?

2. Describe the function of

   cough

   mucociliary transport system

   mucus

3. What is sputum? What characteristics of sputum are examined?

4. Explain how these breathing exercises improve ventilation:

   deep breathing

   pursed-lip breathing

   abdominal breathing

5. Identify the pulmonary physiotherapy technique described:

   ______________________ is a method of voluntarily using a cough to clear airways before secretions accumulate.

   ______________________ uses an instrument to monitor ventilation.

   ______________________ and ______________________ mobilize secretions by loosening retained secretions in airways.

   ______________________ places the client in various positions to facilitate drainage of secretions through gravity.

CHAPTER 36 ADMINISTERING OXYGEN

1. Match the terms in Column I with their definitions in Column II.

I. Term	II. Definition
____ oxidation	A. Lack of oxygen
____ combustion	B. Rapid combination of oxygen with another substance
____ spontaneous combustion	C. Dusky or bluish skin color that happens when oxygen content of blood is reduced
____ hypercapnea	D. Low oxygen tension in the blood
____ hypoxemia	E. Rapid combination process of oxygen with other substances that produces intense heat and flames
____ hypoxia	F. Above-normal carbon dioxide blood levels
____ cyanosis	G. The union or combination of oxygen and another substance

2. What is the chemical stimuli for respiration?

3. What causes oxygen-induced hypoventilation?

4. What causes oxygen toxicity? Identify the clinical signs and symptoms of oxygen toxicity.

5. Mrs. Antonio, age 68, has a chronic lung condition. Upon examination, you find that she is confused, sleepy, and has cyanotic mucous membranes. Her respiratory rate is 12 per minute. Her latest blood gas studies show that her pCO_2 is elevated and her pO_2 is depressed. Her nursing diagnostic category is probably

6. The physician orders oxygen 2 L/m by nasal catheter. Prior to initiating this therapy, what safety precautions will you take?

7. Mr. Stanley, age 73, also receives oxygen because of a chronic lung condition. He wears a nasal cannula. What comfort measures are necessary because of this oxygen delivery system?

8. Brian Walton, age 23, has carbon monoxide poisoning. The physician orders a high concentration of oxygen, 90 percent, via a nonrebreather mask. Why does Brian have a potential for injury while this mask is in use, requiring constant vigilance by the nurse?

CHAPTER 37 MANAGING THE CLIENT WITH A CHEST TUBE

1. Define each of these terms:

   pneumothorax

   open pneumothorax

   closed pneumothorax

   spontaneous pneumothorax

   tension pneumothorax

   hemopneumothorax

2. Fill in the blanks:
   The chest tube is connected to a water seal drainage system to prevent reentry of ________________ and ________________ into the chest. The system also acts as a ________________ for fluid removed from the chest. A gravity drainage system is used if the pressure in the chest is ________________ than the pressure in the collection chamber. Reentry of air is prevented by placing the drainage tube ________________. If the pressure in the chest is greater than the pressure in the collection chamber, ________________ is necessary.

3. Joe Hooper, age 28, has a spontaneous pneumothorax confirmed by x-ray. The physician has inserted a chest tube that is connected to water seal drainage. What *client* assessments must you make following this procedure? What *equipment* assessments must you make?

CHAPTER 38 MAINTAINING AN AIRWAY

1. Identify three causes of airway obstruction:

   1)

   2)

   3)

2. Define these terms:

   patent airway

   intubation

   extubation

   tracheostomy

3. Explain why sterile equipment is used for airway suctioning.

4. When assessing the client to determine if he requires airway suctioning, what signs suggest secretions in the airway?

5. The nurse is suctioning Mrs. Boyer's tracheostomy airway. Listed, out of order, are five major steps in performing this technique. Label the steps as 1 through 5 on the blank line provided.

   _____ Introduce the suction catheter into the tracheostomy tube opening and insert until resistance is felt.

   _____ Immerse catheter in water and apply suction to remove secretions in the catheter.

   _____ Rotate and withdraw catheter smoothly within 10–15 seconds.

   _____ Instill normal saline in the tracheostomy opening as the client inspires.

   _____ Attach the sterile catheter to the suction source.

6. Explain the function of these tracheostomy parts:

   outer cannula

   inner cannula

obturator

cuff

7. Mr. Casey, age 69, just had a tracheostomy done because of severe pulmonary infection. He has awakened from the anesthesia and is trying to talk. What will you tell him about his inability to talk? Describe your instructions to him about how to communicate.

CHAPTER 39 ASSESSING CARDIOVASCULAR FUNCTION

1. Indicate the normal values:

   blood pH

   percentage of formed blood elements

   erythrocytes per cubic millimeters of blood

   leukocytes per cu mm of blood

   thrombocytes per cu mm of blood

2. What is the primary function of

   leukocytes

   erythrocytes

   thrombocytes

3. Trace the pathway of a red blood cell from the inferior vena cava, through the heart chambers, valves, pulmonary arteries, and veins, to the aorta.

4. What makes these sounds?

   S_1

   S_2

   S_3 (ventricular gallop)

   S_4 (atrial gallop)

   murmur

5. Identify the nursing diagnosis for these clients:

   a. Mr. Perkins, age 55, reports that he has cramplike pains in both of his calves. Upon examination, you find that he has no pedal pulse in his right leg and a weak pedal pulse in his left leg. The skin is very pale and cool to the touch.

      His nursing diagnostic category is

   b. Mrs. Cohen, age 83, reports that she is very weak and feels tired all the time. Upon examination, you find that she has distended jugular veins, edema in her ankles and feet, and cyanotic mucous membranes.

      Her nursing diagnostic category is

c. Mr. Consoli, age 76, had arterial blood gases taken one hour ago that indicated hypoxia. Since yesterday, he has been sleeping more than usual and has been very confused when awakened.

His nursing diagnostic category is

CHAPTER 40 PROVIDING CARDIOPULMONARY RESUSCITATION

1. Describe the signs of a cardiac arrest.

2. Describe the signs of a respiratory or pulmonary arrest.

3. Identify the two efforts that comprise basic life support as described by the American Heart Association.

4. What does advanced cardiac life support comprise?

5. Define these terms:

   resuscitation

   defrillation

   cardiac tamponade

6. Briefly state the ABC's of basic life support:

   A.

   B.

   C.

Unit VIII CASE STUDY

MANAGEMENT OF OXYGENATION

Joseph Fettini, age 58, was hospitalized today to treat his respiratory problems. In your initial nursing history, you learned that Mr. Fettini smoked for 40 years. For the past five to six years, he has had a persistent cough productive of large amounts of sputum, which has become worse in recent months. Two years ago he sought medical advice and treatment because he was short of breath most of the time and concerned about the persistent cough. Mr. Fettini was told he has chronic obstructive pulmonary disease, a progressive degenerative disorder of the lungs in which the airways are structurally obstructed or clogged with accumulated secretions. His physician advised him to stop smoking (which he did) and prescribed oxygen therapy and a bronchodilator, a medication that opens the airways. Mr. Fettini reported that his breathing improved quite a bit with the therapy. After four weeks of treatment, he no longer needed oxygen and he was able to continue his employment as a truck driver. One week ago, Mr. Fettini "caught a cold." He had a sore throat, "runny" nose, generalized aches and pains, and his cough became worse. Occasionally he noticed blood in the large amount of expectorated sputum. This morning, he felt feverish and decided to see his physician. A chest x-ray showed that he had pneumonia, a lung infection, and his physician recommended hospitalization for treatment.

Currently, Mr. Fettini reports that he feels very tired and doesn't have enough energy to walk to the bathroom. He reports that he feels pain in his chest when he inhales; the pain is worse on his right side just above his waist. He has the most difficulty breathing lying down but says, "I just can't catch my breath even when sitting straight up." Upon examination, you note that his respiratory rate is 26; he doesn't seem to inhale deeply but guards as if in pain. His heart rate is 94; his blood pressure is 154/88. Listening to his lungs, you hear a fine crackling or bubbling sound in the left chest; it is more defined on inspiration. You hear a louder gurgling or bubbling sound in the upper right chest that is louder during expiration. You can barely hear any sounds in the lower right chest. His color is dusky; his lips look deep purplish-red.

The physician's orders are as follows. (Medication orders are not included.)

Bedrest with bathroom privileges
Monitor vital signs every 4 hours
Oxygen therapy via nasal cannula at 2 liters/minute
Percussion, vibration, and postural drainage four times daily

Answer these questions:

1. Use the correct terminology to describe the breath sounds auscultated.

2. Write the subjective and objective portion of a SOAP nurse's note that states the findings of your history and physical examination.

3. List the nursing diagnoses that are present.

4. Which nursing diagnosis represents the most urgent problem of Mr. Fettini? Explain your rationale.

5. Write a desirable outcome for the nursing diagnosis identified in question 4, and list nursing measures for achieving that outcome.

   Outcome

   Measures

6. Mr. Fettini's oxygen cannula is attached to a bubbler on the oxygen flow meter. What is the purpose of the bubbler?

7. List at least three nursing actions necessary to manage Mr. Fettini's oxygen cannula during his therapy.

8. Because respiratory therapists are not available, you will be managing Mr. Fettini's postural drainage exercises. Explain how you will position him to drain the right lower lobes.

9. Because of the secretions accumulated in his airways, you encourage Mr. Fettini to cough effectively to expectorate the sputum. Write the instructions you give him that explain how to cough deeply and splint his abdomen for comfort.

10. Given Mr. Fettini's fatigue and low energy reserves due to inadequate oxygenation, what nursing strategies will you use to conserve Mr. Fettini's strength?

Unit IX SELF-TESTS

CHAPTER 41 PREPARING FOR MEDICATION ADMINISTRATION

1. Match the pharmaceutical preparation in Column I with its description in Column II.

I. Term

_____ capsule
_____ elixir
_____ emulsion
_____ extract
_____ liniment
_____ lozenge
_____ pill
_____ spirit
_____ suppository
_____ syrup
_____ tablet
_____ tincture

II. Definition

A. Alcoholic solution of a volatile substance
B. Alcoholic or water and alcohol solutions prepared from animal or vegetable substances
C. Single-dose unit made by mixing the powdered drug with a liquid and molding into a round or oval shape
D. Concentrated preparations of vegetable or animal substances in water or alcohol
E. Powdered drugs within a gelatin container that dissolve when ingested
F. Powdered medication compressed into a flat, round, or oval preparation that is held in the mouth until it dissolves
G. Sweetened, aromatic solution containing alcohol, sugar, and water
H. Dispersions of equal-sized globules of fat in water or water in fat
I. Mixtures of drugs with oil, soap, water, or alcohol, intended for external application and rubbing
J. Aqueous solution of a sugar that may have a medicinal substance added
K. Mixtures of drugs with some firm base that is molded for insertion or instillation in a body cavity
L. Single-dose units made by compression of powdered drugs into a mold

2. Fill in the blanks:

1 kilogram = _____ gram(s)
1 gram = _____ kilogram(s)
1 liter = _____ milliliter(s)
1 milliliter = _____ liter(s)
1 milliliter = _____ cubic centimeter(s)

1 pound = ____ ounce(s)

1 cup = ____ pint(s)

1 pint = ____ ounce(s)

1 cup = ____ ounce(s)

3. Indicate which two factors determine the method and location of storing medications:

   1)

   2)

4. List all of the parts of a legal medication order that must be present:

5. Explain what these types of medication orders mean:

   standing order

   automatic stop order

   p.r.n. order

   single order

   STAT order

6. Describe how medication is administered with these routes:

   oral

   parenteral

   topical

   instillation

   inhalation

   intravenous

7. List the "five rights" of medication administration:

   1)

   2)

   3)

   4)

   5)

8. Calculate the proper dose in these problems:

   a. The medication order reads: Ferrous sulfate 600 mg p.o. once a day. You have pills that are labeled: Ferrous sulfate 300 mg. How many pills do you give?

   b. The medication order reads: Demerol 75 mg IM prn for pain. You have a vial labeled: Demerol 100 mg per ml. What volume of the drug do you give?

c. The medication order reads: Aspirin 10 grains p.o. q 4 h. You have pills that are labeled: Aspirin 300 mg. How many pills do you give?

d. The medication order reads: Phenobarbital 1/4 grain p.o. q 8 h. You have pills that are labeled: Phenobarbital 30 mg. How many pills do you give?

e. The medication order reads: Ascorbic acid 1 gm p.o. qd. You have pills that are labeled: Ascorbic acid 100 mg. How many pills do you give?

f. The medication order reads: Heparin 5,000 units subcu q 12 h. You have a vial that is labeled: Heparin 10,000 units per milliliter. What volume of the drug do you give?

CHAPTER 42 ADMINISTERING ORAL, TOPICAL, INSTILLED, AND PARENTERAL MEDICATIONS

1. List two advantages and two disadvantages of the oral route of administration:

   Advantages:

   1)

   2)

   Disadvantages:

   1)

   2)

2. List two advantages and two disadvantages of the parenteral route of administration:

   Advantages:

   1)

   2)

   Disadvantages:

   1)

   2)

3. Explain where the medication is placed in these routes:

   topical

   buccal

   sublingual

   instillation

   subcutaneous

   intramuscular

   intradermal

4. Describe:

   ampule

   vial

   prepared disposable injection unit

5. Identify the anatomic landmarks necessary to locate these intramuscular injection sites:

   ventrogluteal

dorsogluteal

deltoid

vastus lateralis

rectus femoris

6. What is the purpose of the Z-track method of intramuscular administration?

7. Select the proper needle gauge and length for these medications:

   a. Susie, age 15, is to receive an intramuscular injection of a viscous antibiotic medication. You will select ______________________________ gauge and ______________________________ needle length.

   b. Mr. Nelson, age 52, is to receive insulin subcutaneously in his arm. Insulin has approximately the same viscosity as water. You will select ______________________________ gauge and ______________________________ needle length.

   c. Mrs. Jessup, age 74, is to receive an iron preparation via a Z-track intramuscular injection. The preparation is slightly heavier than water. You will select ______________________________ gauge and ______________________________ needle length.

   d. Tom Sanders, age 18, is being tested for allergies. He is to receive an antigen intradermally. The preparation is approximately the same viscosity as water. You will select ______________________________ gauge and ______________________________ needle length.

CHAPTER 43 ADMINISTERING INTRAVENOUS MEDICATIONS

1. List two advantages and two disadvantages of intravenous administration.

   Advantages:

   1)

   2)

   Disadvantages:

   1)

   2)

2. Explain these terms:

   primary intravenous administration

   secondary intravenous administration

   intermittent venous access device

   volume control set

   admixture

   bolus

3. Explain two methods of adding medications to a primary infusion container:

   1)

   2)

4. Explain how a volume control set works.

5. Explain how a secondary administration set works.

Unit IX CASE STUDY

MEDICATION ADMINISTRATION

Wendy Bennett, age 29, was admitted to the hospital yesterday because of weakness, fever, frequent urination, and pain and swelling in her left calf. Because Mrs. Bennett has diabetes and gave birth to her second child seven days ago, her physician decided to hospitalize her for diagnostic tests. This morning, her physician concluded that she has a thrombophlebitis (blood clot) in her left lower leg. Further tests determined she has a urinary tract infection. Mrs. Bennett is placed on bedrest.

The medication orders for Mrs. Bennett are as follows:

Regular insulin 10 units subcu q AM
NPH insulin 35 units subcu q AM
Multiple vitamins 2 capsules TID
Calcium carbonate 1.0 Gm po TID with meals
Heparin continuous IV at a rate of 1,000 units/hour
Cefoxitin sodium 1.5 Gm IV q 6 h
Hydromorphone hydrochloride 2 mg IM q 4 h prn for pain

Signed by Dr. J. Mastens

You perform a venipuncture for administering the intravenous drugs, heparin, and cefoxitin. Mrs. Bennett asks you what these drugs are for and why she must have them through an intravenous line rather than orally; you explain that heparin will prevent further clotting and cefoxitin is an antibiotic to treat her urinary infection. You also explain that intravenous administration is more effective and faster, both desirable for her condition.

Answer these questions:

1. Carefully read each of the medication orders. Are they all complete? If not, which one is incomplete? What is missing?

2. In your hospital, clients' meals are served at 0800, 1200, and 1700. Your nursing unit schedules TID medications to be given at 0900, 1300, and 1700. Daily insulin is given at 0700. Medications given q 6 h are scheduled at 0600, 1200, 1800, and 2400. Medications given q 12 h are scheduled at 0600 and 1800. Use this information to make a schedule of the times that Mrs. Bennett receives her regularly scheduled medications between 0600 and 2400.

3. Before you begin preparation of the medications you will administer, you review the five rights of medication administration. List them.

4. The first medication you will administer today is regular insulin and NPH insulin. Each drug comes in a vial. You have insulin syringes, marked U 100, available. Explain how you will draw the two doses in the same syringe.

5. After the insulin is properly prepared in a syringe, you bring it to Mrs. Bennett. What do you always do with the client before administering any drug?

6. Mrs. Bennett states she wishes to receive the insulin in her arm. What angle of insertion will you use?

7. After you give the insulin, Mrs. Bennett asks if she could have "a shot for pain." Looking on the medication administration record, you see that the physician has ordered hydromorphone hydrochloride, which is a narcotic analgesic (pain reliever). How do you determine if she may have it?

8. Because hydromorphone hydrochloride is a narcotic, where is it stored?

9. Hydromorphone hydrochloride is prepared in an ampule labeled, "Hydromorphone hydrochloride 6 mg. in 3 ml." What volume of the drug will you draw into a syringe?

10. The hydromorphone is given IM. It is a clear, watery fluid. What needle size will you select?

11. What would be the ideal site for administering the IM hydromorphone?

12. When preparing to give calcium gluconate, you learn that the medication is prepared in unit doses that are labeled 250 mg. How will you give it?

13. You wish to begin the continuous IV administration of heparin. For intravenous administration, heparin is added to normal saline. You have normal saline 500 ml bags available. You wish to limit Mrs. Bennett's intravenous fluids to 50 ml/hour, and you must ensure administration of heparin 1,000 units/hour. How much heparin will you add to the normal saline bag?

14. You have a continuous intravenous administration set that delivers 60 gtts per ml. To ensure administration of only 50 ml/hour, what is the desired flow rate on the intravenous controller pump?

15. Mrs. Bennett's questions about the medications suggest what nursing diagnosis?

16. Write a desirable client outcome for the nursing diagnosis in question 15.

17. Cefotoxin sodium is a powder in a vial labeled "Cefotoxin sodium 2.0 Gm." The instructions on the vial read, "Add 8.5 ml. sodium chloride and mix until dissolved. Reconstituted drug is 2.0 Gm. in 10 ml. How much of the solution will you need for the 1800 IV dose?

18. The instructions for cefotoxin further read, "For IV administration, add required dose to D_5S 50 cc and administer over 20 minutes." Explain how you will use a secondary administration set to administer this medication.

Unit X SELF-TESTS

CHAPTER 44 MANAGING WOUNDS

1. Explain the differences between these wound types:

   closed and open

   intentional and unintentional

   clean and contaminated

2. Match the wound type in Column I with its description in Column II.

I. Wound	II. Description
_____ incision	A. Skin is separated with irregular edges.
_____ contusion	B. Propelled object pierces the skin or mucous membrane.
_____ abrasion	C. Made intentionally or accidentally with a sharp instrument; skin separates cleanly and in a straight line.
_____ puncture	D. Skin remains intact but underlying tissues and blood vessels are damaged.
_____ laceration	E. Scraping of the skin or tissues
_____ penetration	F. Sharp instrument pierces the skin and underlying tissues.

3. Explain local tissue changes that characterize these stages of wound regeneration.

   inflammatory phase

   proliferative phase

   maturation phase

4. Give an example of the type of wound that heals by

   first intention

   second intention

   third intention

5. Mr. Gomez, age 36, tripped over a broken sidewalk and fell as he was jogging. He scraped the skin over both knees and on the palms of his hands. He rinsed the wounds with clean water within minutes of the injury and has left them undressed. Twelve hours after the injury, the skin is torn away and oozing a sticky clear liquid.

   What type of wound does Mr. Gomez have?

   Was it clean or contaminated?

   What is the exudate called?

Does Mr. Gomez have any risk factors suggesting delayed healing may be a problem? If so, what are they?

What nursing diagnosis does Mr. Gomez have?

6. Mrs. Jensen, age 62, wore new shoes while on a shopping trip. She noticed the shoes felt a little uncomfortable but didn't realize a large blister had formed on her right heel until later when she removed the shoes. The blister broke open and drained. Seven days later, she has a raw, reddened, and draining cavity where the blister was. The drainage is thick and cloudy. Her lower leg is swollen. She has smoked for forty years and has high blood pressure.

   Is Mrs. Jensen's wound accidental or intentional?

   Is the wound open or closed?

   What type of drainage is it?

   Does Mrs. Jensen have risk factors suggesting delayed healing may be a problem? If so, what are they?

   What nursing diagnosis does Mrs. Jensen have?

7. Define:

   hemostasis

   evisceration

   dehiscence

8. Explain the purpose of

   wet-to-dry dressings

   dry sterile dressings

   transparent dressings

   pressure dressings

   wound irrigations

   wound suctioning

9. Indicate where these bandage turns are used:

   circular

   spiral

   spiral reverse

   recurrent

   figure-eight

   spica

10. Indicate the purpose of these binders:

    abdominal or straight

    breast

    scultetus

    single T

    double T

CHAPTER 45 APPLYING HEAT OR COLD

1. Indicate if the following physiologic responses are to heat or cold:

   Increased capillary permeability: heat or cold?

   Increased blood viscosity: heat or cold?

   Enhanced delivery of nutrients to cells: heat or cold?

   Increased tissue metabolism: heat or cold?

   Decreases local sensitivity to pain: heat or cold?

   Relieves muscle tension: heat or cold?

   Limits edema: heat or cold?

2. Give three contraindications to the use of heat:

   1)

   2)

   3)

3. Give three contraindications to the use of cold:

   1)

   2)

   3)

4. Suggest whether a heat or cold application is indicated for these clients and give the rationale:

   a. Mrs. Chung, age 64, has joint pain and stiffness from arthritis. Do you apply heat or cold?

   b. Jack, age 18, has a swollen knee after running a 10 kilometer race. Do you apply heat or cold?

   c. Mr. Arthur, age 42, reports he has aching pains in his shoulders after he raked leaves. Do you apply heat or cold?

   d. Mrs. Conner, age 24, gave birth yesterday. She reports pain and discomfort in the perineum. Do you apply heat or cold?

5. You are to apply a warm moist soak to Mr. Jacob's right arm, where he developed a phlebitis during an intravenous infusion. Explain how you will protect his skin from maceration.

6. Mrs. Sirianni, age 77, has an open, weeping wound on her left outer ankle. You are to use a lamp to apply heat to the area for 20 minutes. Describe the safety precautions you will take.

7. Mr. Stein, age 69, broke his femur two days ago and had surgery to reduce it. He has a heavy pressure dressing on the incision site where you are to apply an ice pack for a half hour; remove for a half hour and replace for another half hour. What safety precautions will you use?

CHAPTER 46 MANAGING DECUBITUS ULCERS

1. Describe the appearance of the skin and lesion during these stages of decubitus ulcer formation:

   Stage I

   Stage II

   Stage III

   Stage IV

2. Explain the difference between friction and shearing force.

3. Name at least five risk factors for decubitus formation:

   1)

   2)

   3)

   4)

   5)

4. Dan Jessel, age 24, has been paralyzed from the waist down because of a spinal cord injury received five years ago. He is slightly underweight for his age, sex, and height. He is incontinent of urine but uses an external catheter; he has a bowel training program. What risk factors are present for skin breakdown?

5. To prevent skin breakdown on Dan, what preventive measures will you take? List at least five.

   1)

   2)

   3)

   4)

   5)

Unit X CASE STUDY

MANAGEMENT OF WOUNDS

Minnie Schwartz, age 66, has many health problems. Three years ago, she had a cerebral vascular accident (a stroke) that caused weakness and paralysis in her left arm and leg. Because she has not been able to walk since that time, she has been in a long-term care facility. Recently she developed an infection in the left shoulder joint that caused severe pain. Her physician transferred her to the hospital for diagnosis and treatment. Tests determined the shoulder joint had an abscess, which is a pocket of purulent exudate (pus). A surgeon made an incision just below the acromion on the back of the shoulder into the abscess to drain the pus; meanwhile, intravenous administration of antibiotic therapy was begun. At the time of Mrs. Schwartz's admission to the hospital, the admitting nurse found a reddened area over her coccyx surrounding an open wound that was draining serous exudate. Another reddened area was found on her left heel; in the center was broken skin and discoloration but no exudate.

Currently Mrs. Schwartz has a dry sterile dressing of thick gauze pads over the incision on her left shoulder that is secured with Montgomery straps and changed q 4 h or more frequently when necessary. Because of the residual paralysis (from the stroke), Mrs. Schwartz's left arm is immobilized in a triangular sling to lessen the weight of her arm pulling on the shoulder wound. The coccyx wound is irrigated twice daily with a solution of half-strength hydrogen peroxide and saline; sterile gauze moistened with povidone-iodine is packed into the open area and covered with sterile 4 × 4 pads. The povidone-iodine soaked gauze is allowed to dry before removal. The left heel wound is covered with a transparent dressing.

As the nurse managing Mrs. Schwartz this morning, you noticed that the intravenous infusion site (for antibiotic therapy) on her right arm is red, painful, and warm to the touch. Further inspection confirms that the infusion is infiltrated. You remove the IV catheter and start another elsewhere. When contacted, the physician instructs you to place a moist warm pack on the reddened arm.

Answer these questions:

1. Because of the presence of multiple wounds, Mrs. Schwartz had a nursing diagnosis of

2. Suggest a desirable outcome for the nursing diagnosis identified in question 1.

3. Mrs. Schwartz's immobility and generalized debilitation are critical factors in the development of her decubitus ulcers. List at least five nursing measures to prevent further decubitus formulation.

4. What is the purpose of the thick absorbent pads secured over the shoulder wound?

5. Briefly explain the critical steps taken when changing the shoulder wound dressing.

6. The wounds on Mrs. Schwartz's coccyx and heel are decubitus ulcers. Which stage of development is the coccyx wound? Which stage of development is the heel wound?

7. Explain the purpose of irrigating the coccyx wound with hydrogen peroxide.

8. Explain the purpose of packing the wound with gauze moistened with povidone-iodine.

9. What is the purpose of the transparent dressing over the left heel wound?

10. Why is moist heat being applied to Mrs. Schwartz's arm?

11. Describe how you will protect Mrs. Schwartz's skin from moisture and her tissues from excessive heat.

Unit XI SELF-TESTS

CHAPTER 47 PREPARING THE CLIENT FOR SURGERY

1. What is the purpose of preoperative assessment of the client?

2. Identify at least three physical factors that are assessed by the nurse preoperatively and explain the purpose of each:

   1)

   2)

   3)

3. Identify at least three psychological factors that are assessed preoperatively and explain the purpose of each:

   1)

   2)

   3)

4. Explain the legal reason for the informed consent; identify the health care provider who is responsible for obtaining it; explain the nurse's role in informed consent.

5. List three purposes of preoperative physical preparation:

   1)

   2)

   3)

6. Identify the nursing diagnoses for these clients who are waiting to have surgery and suggest at least one nursing measure to treat it.

   a. José Perez, age 56, entered the morning of surgery admission unit to have an inguinal hernia repair. Because he will have general anesthesia, he will be admitted to a postoperative nursing care unit after surgery. During the nursing admission history, you learn that Mr. Perez thinks he will be returning home later that day, after he wakes up.

   His nursing diagnosis is

Your nursing measure is

b. Mrs. Stuart, age 41, entered the morning of surgery admission unit to have a modified mastectomy (removal of the breast) because a recent biopsy revealed a malignancy. She asks many questions during her physical preparations. When taking her pulse, you notice that her hands are trembling. She repeatedly mentions being worried about how she will fit into her clothing after surgery.

Her nursing diagnosis is

Your nursing measure is

c. Mr. Ford, age 59, was admitted two days ago because he appeared to have a bowel obstruction. Because his condition became worse, he will be going to surgery shortly for an emergency procedure to relieve the obstruction. He just received a sedative and is waiting for the transport person to arrive. He tells you he feels like he is floating, and he appears sleepy.

His nursing diagnosis is

Your nursing measure is

CHAPTER 48 MANAGING THE POSTOPERATIVE CLIENT

1. Describe behaviors exhibited during Stage 2 and Stage 1 of recovery from anesthesia:

2. List at least eight pieces of information that is reported to the receiving nurse when the surgical client is transferred to the PAR:

   1)

   2)

   3)

   4)

   5)

   6)

   7)

   8)

3. For each of these body systems, suggest one nursing assessment to make during the first two hours following surgery:

   cardiovascular

   respiratory

   gastrointestinal

   integumentary

   metabolic

   renal

4. For each of these body systems, identify a potential nursing diagnosis that may occur postoperatively and suggest one nursing measure to treat that diagnosis:

   immune

   respiratory

   gastrointestinal

   musculoskeletal

   integumentary

   metabolic

   renal

5. Explain the cause of these postoperative complications:

   atelectasis

   hemorrhage

   thrombophlebitis of the leg

   pulmonary embolus

   nausea and vomiting

   urinary retention

   wound infection

Unit XI CASE STUDY

PERIOPERATIVE MANAGEMENT

PART I. BEFORE SURGERY

Gerald Hall, age 45, has polyps (growths) in his colon that have been bleeding occasionally. Because polyps sometimes precede the development of intestinal cancer, his physician has recommended their surgical removal. Mr. Hall is scheduled for surgery tomorrow at 0730.

You are admitting Mr. Hall at 1900 to the preoperative unit and will be preparing his teaching plan. During your nursing history, Mr. Hall tells you that he has been on a clear liquid diet for ten days to decrease the amount of waste material in the intestines. He has also been taking an antibiotic to limit microorganism growth in the intestines. He knows the surgery planned is a resection (removal) of a portion of the large intestine. He has never had surgery before and reports that he doesn't know what will happen. His vital signs are: temperature 98.6°F, pulse 72, respirations 16, and blood pressure 130/68.

The preoperative orders for Mr. Hall are

Soap suds enemas until clear this evening
Clear liquid diet
NPO after midnight
Begin 1000 D_5W at 0600; infuse at 75 ml/hr
Insert indwelling urinary catheter before surgery in AM
Atropine 0.4 mg subcu at 0700 tomorrow

Answer these questions:

1. Your nursing history and Mr. Hall's planned surgery suggest a nursing diagnosis of
2. The desired client outcome for this diagnosis is
3. List the key points you will cover in your preop teaching plan. (Include all those activities done postoperatively to prevent complications.)
4. The purpose of the enemas until clear is

5. The purpose of holding food and fluids after midnight is

6. The purpose of the intravenous infusion is

7. Why is an indwelling catheter being inserted before surgery?

PART II. IMMEDIATELY AFTER SURGERY

After his surgery was completed at 1230, Mr. Hall returns from the PAR at 1445. He is alert and responds appropriately to questions but is sleepy. The PAR nurse reports that he has not received any pain medication. His pulse is 68, respirations are 16, temperature is 98.4°F, and his blood pressure is 122/68. He has an intravenous infusion of D_5W running continuously; 580 ml of solution remains. He has a double-lumen nasogastric tube attached to continuous high suction; it is draining a small amount of greenish-brown fluid with specks. His surgical wound has not been covered with a dressing. The incision is approximately 6 inches long and is approximated with large wire sutures. Inspection shows the wound to be dry. Mr. Hall has an indwelling urinary catheter that is draining straw-colored urine. Both the nasogastric drainage and urinary collecting bag were emptied by the PAR nurse before Mr. Hall was transferred to his own room. Mr. Hall groans as you assess his incision and drainage tubes; he asks if he may have something for pain. (The time of this assessment is 1500.)

The postoperative orders are

NPO
Add 2,000 ml D_5W with 20 mEq KCL to current bag; infuse until 0800 tomorrow.
NG to high constant suction
Irrigate NG prn
Discontinue indwelling catheter
OOB × 1 tonight; begin progressive ambulation tomorrow
Morphine sulfate 10 mg. IM q 3 h prn for pain
Incentive spirometer q 2 h × 2 days

Answer these questions:

8. Write a SOAP note on Mr. Hall's condition upon return from the PAR.

9. Prepare expected outcomes that reflect Mr. Hall's condition, as well as actual and potential problems.

10. The intravenous infusion is regulated by a pump. At what flow rate will you set it?

11. At approximately what time will you add another intravenous bag? (Remember you presently have 580 ml in the bag and will be infusing at the rate determined in question 10.)

12. Prepare a schedule for your nursing actions with Mr. Hall from 1500 until 2300 on this evening of surgery.

13. You removed Mr. Hall's catheter at 1530, as ordered. To follow up, what must you do?

14. At 2000, you notice that Mr. Hall's nasogastric tube doesn't seem to be draining. What will you do?

15. After using the incentive spirometer, Mr. Hall reports he cannot cough because the pain is too severe. What will you do?

16. Mr. Hall refuses to get out of bed when you tell him you plan to help him. What will you do?

Unit XII SELF-TESTS

CHAPTER 49 SUPPORTING THE DYING CLIENT AND THE FAMILY

1. The following behaviors reflect one or more stages of dying, as identified by Dr. Elisabeth Kubler-Ross. Name the stage(s).

   a. Jane Kersey, age 49, has a muscle-wasting disease that is terminal. She is unable to perform activities of daily living because of profound weakness and paralysis; she receives nutrients through total parenteral nutrition because she cannot swallow. Her death seems imminent. Her son, Nelson, age 26, plans to be married in two months. Mrs. Kersey asks you, her nurse, to intensify her passive range of motion exercises so that she will be stronger. She tells you, "I want to be strong enough to sit in a wheelchair for the wedding ceremony."

   Mrs. Kersey demonstrates what stage(s) of dying?

   b. Jake Peterson, age 35, has AIDS. Staying in a hospice, he began refusing to see his many visitors several days ago. He refuses to eat and drinks very little. He will not leave his room, even though he is able to walk with assistance. He has given all of his valued possessions, except his Bible, to his family. Some days he cries for hours without pause; other days he reads his Bible and tells you, the nurse, that he feels "at peace."

   Mr. Peterson demonstrates what stage(s) of dying?

   c. John O'Brien, age 72, sought medical help when he became so short of breath that he couldn't walk more than a short distance. He has constant chest pain and a cough productive of blood-tinged sputum. A chest x-ray showed one large mass in the right upper lobe and several smaller masses through the right and left lungs. His physician has told him that the tumors appear to be cancerous. Mr. O'Brien tells you, the nurse, "The doctor doesn't know what he is talking about. My dad had tuberculosis; his problems were just like mine."

   Mr. O'Brien demonstrates what stage(s) of dying?

   d. Mrs. Tranh, age 37, returned to the hospital because of swelling, pain, and absence of bowel movements for several days. Six months ago, she had a total hysterectomy (removal of the uterus) because of cancer. After exploratory surgery, the physician told her that she has widespread tumors in the abdomen that is a recurrence of the cancer. Now Mrs. Tranh refuses to participate with postoperative nursing measures such as deep breathing, coughing, or walking. She also refuses pain relief measures. She insists on remaining in bed and won't talk with the nursing staff but has called the agency client advocate to report that the nurses are "mistreating" her.

   Mrs. Tranh demonstrates what stage(s) of dying?

2. List at least one physiologic change in each of these body systems that occurs as death approaches:

   respiratory

   circulatory

   metabolic

   musculoskeletal

   gastrointestinal

   renal or urinary

   neurologic

   visual

3. What are the traditional clinical indicators of death?

4. What is the accepted legal definition of death when cardiac and respiratory function are controlled by artificial means?

5. Explain what services are offered to the dying client and his family by these agencies:

   hospice

   home care

   respite care

6. Briefly describe a behavior that suggests these stages of bereavement:

   shock and disbelief

   developing awareness (stage of pain)

   resolution or restitution

CHAPTER 50 PROVIDING POSTMORTEM CARE

1. Describe the changes in body tissues involved with

   rigor mortis

   algor mortis

   livor mortis

   autolysis

2. Explain the purpose of the autopsy:

3. What is the physician's responsibility regarding an autopsy? What is the nurse's responsibility?

4. List at least five actions done as part of postmortem care:

   1)

   2)

   3)

   4)

   5)

Unit XII CASE STUDY

MANAGEMENT OF THE DYING CLIENT

Jason Carr, age 18, has an inoperable brain tumor that is growing rapidly. Only four months ago he was healthy and vigorous, a high school senior planning on entering college next year, and a varsity basketball player. His problems began when he noticed weakness on his left side; soon he was walking with a limp. Next he began to have severe headaches with nausea and vomiting; nothing seemed to relieve the headaches. After several visits to his family physician and a complete diagnostic work-up, Jason and his parents learned about the tumor. He has received radiation therapy to his head, which retarded the tumor's growth briefly. He also received chemotherapy with drugs to retard the tumor's growth. As a side effect of the chemotherapy, Jason's hair fell out. Currently, he is unable to walk because of weakness and paralysis in his lower legs; he is blind in the right eye; his speech is slurred. He is incontinent of urine and stool. He has some weakness in his left arm but still has complete use of his right hand (the right is his dominant side).

After several hospitalizations, Jason and his parents faced the reality of his impending death. Together they decided they preferred that Jason remain at home for what time he has left. Mrs. Carr has taken a leave of absence from her job to be with Jason; she is his primary caregiver. Jason spends much of his time in a wheelchair; Mrs. Carr takes him for walks that seem very special to both of them. Once a week, a home health aide provides respite care. Mrs. Carr shops and sees friends on that day. Jason's younger brother, Steve, age 15, spends most of his after school hours with Jason. They play cards, listen to tapes, or play video games on their home computer.

You are the home care nurse who visits Jason and his family every few days to answer their questions, provide emotional support, and offer respite for Mrs. Carr so that she can spend several hours out of the home. On your most recent visit, you spend time alone with Jason. He wears a baseball cap all the time; he tells you he is embarrassed to appear without it because of his bald head. He reports that he no longer has headaches, which helps him think more clearly. He shows you his diary; he is recording his thoughts and feelings. He also shows you that he has labeled all of his belongings, willing them to his brother and his friends. His diary is willed to his mother. He has put together a photograph album; before he became ill, Jason took a photography course in high school. Now he wishes to preserve some of his work. The photograph album is willed to his father. Jason tells you that he is very sad to leave his family.

Answer these questions:

1. Jason's discomfort with his appearance suggests a nursing diagnosis of
2. Jason's sadness regarding his impending death suggests a nursing diagnosis of
3. Although the inevitable outcome in Jason's future is death, what desirable outcome can you expect for the entire Carr family?

4. What does Jason's behavior regarding his belongings and his diary mean to you?

5. What is the purpose of respite care?

6. Plan some nursing strategies that you can implement to help this family cope with the impending death of its member.

Unit XIII SELF-TESTS

CHAPTER 51 COLLECTING AND TESTING SPECIMENS

1. Explain the difference between gross, microscopic, and chemical examinations of body substances.

2. What is the difference between a smear and a culture?

3. List six nursing responsibilities related to collecting specimens:
   1)
   2)
   3)
   4)
   5)
   6)

4. Fill in the boxes in the following chart with the information on what type of diagnostic tests are done on these substances, why the test is done, and any special client preparations (other than teaching the purpose of the test).

Specimen	Type of Test	Purpose	Special Client Preparation?
nose secretions			client education
sputum			client education

Specimen	Type of Test	Purpose	Special Client Preparation?
gastric secretions			client education
venous blood			client education
capillary blood			client education
arterial blood			client education
wound drainage			client education
midstream urine			client education
stools			client education

CHAPTER 52 ASSISTING WITH DIAGNOSTIC EXAMINATIONS OR PROCEDURES

1. Match the diagnostic test listed in Column I with its purpose in Column II.

I. Diagnostic Test	II. Purpose
_____ vaginal smear	A. Removes fluid from the thorax for analysis.
_____ electrocardiogram	B. Visualizes body tissues at many planes to present a three-dimensional picture.
_____ electroencephalogram	C. Records electrical conduction activity of the heart.
_____ electromyelogram	D. Removes small piece of tissue for gross and microscopic examination.
_____ CAT scan	E. Collects cells for cytologic analysis.
_____ dye contrast studies	F. Records electrical brain wave activity.
_____ tissue biopsy	G. Removes fluid from the abdomen for analysis.
_____ lumbar puncture	H. Records electrical activity generated by muscular contraction.
_____ thoracentesis	I. Visualizes vascular network of a body part.
_____ paracentesis	J. Removes cerebrospinal fluid for examination and analysis.

2. These clients are scheduled for diagnostic procedures:

   a. Mr. G. Martinez, age 69, is having a thoracentesis to remove fluid from an abscess in his lungs. Explain to Mr. Martinez why the procedure is necessary, what he will experience, and what he must do during it.

   b. Linda Curtis, age 25, is having her first vaginal examination and will have cytologic smears taken. Explain to Ms. Curtis how the examination is done and the purpose of cytologic smears.

c. Mr. S. Charles, age 51, is scheduled for an electrocardiogram. Explain to him how the examination is done.

d. Little Jamie Karl, 7 months old, is going to have a lumbar puncture. Explain to his parents how the test is done and what its purpose is.

e. Mrs. Chester, age 60, is scheduled for an abdominal CAT scan. Explain to her how this test will be done.

3. These clients are also scheduled for diagnostic procedures.

   a. Mr. Vogel, age 49, is to have a liver biopsy. What preparations are required for this procedure?

   b. Mrs. Polinski, age 71, is scheduled to have an angiogram of the carotid artery. What preparations are required for this procedure?

   c. Ms. Stein, age 45, is scheduled to have a bone marrow biopsy. What preparations are required for this procedure?

   d. Mr. Hever, age 52, is scheduled for an electroencephalogram. What preparations are required for this procedure?

PERFORMANCE CHECKLISTS

Name ______________________ Date ______________________

Observed by ______________

CHAPTER 3 COMMUNICATING

SKILL 3.1 Communicating with the Client

_____ 1. Assess aspects of self that may affect communication with the client.

_____ 2. Assess the client's ability to communicate.

_____ 3. Identify the relevant nursing diagnosis and plan the expected client outcomes.

_____ 4. Demonstrate acceptance of the client as a person while avoiding reinforcement of unacceptable behaviors:

- Make yourself available to the client, being present and demonstrating interest and concern.
- Remain objective in observations by determining reasons for the client's behaviors.
- Accept expressions of negative feelings and promote verbalization of feelings experienced by the client.

_____ 5. Be consistent in expectations of the client:

- Meet with the client at mutually agreed times.
- Explain any changes in the schedule.

_____ 6. Show respect for the client:

- Listen when the client is speaking and show interest.
- Avoid making value judgments or imposing own values on the client.
- Communicate optimism, hope, and a realistic expectation that the health status of the client will improve.

_____ 7. Develop a bond of trust:

- Avoid making promises that cannot be kept.
- Be truthful, reliable, and responsive to the client's needs.
- Be open, honest, and authentic with the client, providing information as needed or requested.

_____ 8. Demonstrate sensitivity to the client's feelings and needs:

- Avoid negating the client's experience or belittling his feelings.
- Make an effort to gain a perspective from the client's point of view and to understand his feelings.
- Communicate your understanding and acceptance of differences in cultural customs and values.

_____ 9. Express an empathetic, sensitive understanding of the client's feelings and inner experiences.

_____ **10.** Facilitate the client's expression of thoughts and feelings through the use of the following skills of communication:

- Indicate recognition or acknowledgment of the client or of an accomplishment by the client.
- Provide a broad opening statement.
- Use silence but remain attentive and interested, or expectant.
- Indicate acceptance that the nurse is receptive to the client's communication.
- Seek clarification or validation from the client if there is doubt that the communication has been understood.
- Focus or concentrate attention on a point that seems important.
- Share observations to communicate your perceptions about the client.
- Assist the client to put unexpressed feelings into words by attempting to translate words into feelings.
- Indicate that you are emotionally available.
- Suggest collaboration by offering to assist client with a problem.
- Encourage the formulation of a plan of action to promote problem-solving skills.
- Give information when the client needs facts.
- Summarize to provide a review of the pertinent points discussed toward the end of an interaction.

_____ **11.** Avoid blocking communication by maintaining an awareness of the all too common pitfalls:

- Avoid falsely reassuring the client.
- Avoid giving approval that places value judgments.
- Avoid introducing an unrelated topic or changing the subject.
- Avoid interpreting meanings that the client's remarks or behaviors represent at an unconscious level.
- Avoid stereotyped comments.
- Avoid agreeing with the client.
- Avoid rejecting the client's ideas or topics of discussion as unworthy.
- Avoid disapproving of the client's feelings, thoughts, or behaviors as "bad" or "wrong."
- Avoid disagreeing with the client.
- Avoid advising the client what to do or not do.
- Avoid probing with persistent questions.
- Avoid challenging the client.
- Avoid belittling the client's feelings.
- Avoid giving literal responses to abstract or symbolic comments.
- Avoid denial.

_____ **12.** Maintain open lines of communication.

_____ **13.** Reassess the client to determine if the expected outcomes are achieved.

Name ______________________ Date ______________________

Observed by ____________

SKILL 3.2 Interviewing the Client

_____ 1. Assess aspects of self and client that could affect the quality of the interview.

_____ 2. Assess aspects of the environment that would contribute to the success of the interview.

_____ 3. Identify nursing diagnoses and plan the expected client outcomes.

_____ 4. Intervene in immediate needs of client and self, ensuring the comfort of both.

_____ 5. Confirm the privacy of the setting.

_____ 6. Establish the validity of the client as a historian.

_____ 7. Facilitate the communication of the desired information and feelings through incorporation of therapeutic skills of communication with the following guidelines to effective interviewing.

- Begin by introducing yourself and stating the purpose and approximate length of the interview.
- Express warmth and interest in the client as an individual.
- Promote a sense of trust.
- Provide the client the initiative in relating information while giving a clue as to the type of information desired.
- Use questions that are open-ended and indirect.
- Employ minimal verbal activity and maximum listening skills.
- Facilitate the expression of feelings.
- Consider the timing of the questions. Begin with the least threatening of the questions, leaving the more sensitive or painful ones to the end or until later interviews.

_____ 8. Avoid the common but ineffective approaches to interviewing.

- Avoid direct, closed-ended questioning that can be answered by a "yes" or "no."
- Avoid questions that invite specific responses.
- Avoid the task-oriented approach.
- Avoid interjecting and sharing your own experiences.
- Avoid communicating personal values or prejudices.
- Avoid pressuring the client for information of a personal nature.
- Avoid questions that are accusing or condemning in nature.
- Avoid double-barreled questions ("or" questions).
- Avoid the use of questions that needlessly increase anxiety.
- Avoid irrelevant questions.

Name ______________________________ Date ______________

Observed by ____________

CHAPTER 4 TEACHING THE CLIENT

SKILL 4.1 Teaching the Client

_____ 1. Assess the client's knowledge related to the illness or to health care maintenance needs.

_____ 2. Assess the client's readiness to learn.

_____ 3. Assess aspects of the environment that contribute to success of the learning experience.

_____ 4. Identify the nursing diagnosis and plan the expected client outcome.

_____ 5. Ensure knowledge and skills possessed by *self* in relation to needs for the client's health care needs.

- Identify own knowledge and skills.
- Remediate any deficits in own knowledge and skills.

_____ 6. Implement the teaching plan:

- Involve the client and family or significant others in the learning activities.
- Prepare realistic short- and long-term learning goals that address the deficits in knowledge of the client and significant others.
- State measurable criteria for success and share them with the client and family or significant others.
- Employ individualized materials and teaching strategies to meet the unique needs of the learner.
- Arrange alternative approaches for those who do not speak the dominant language, are unable to see or hear well, or have impaired cognitive, memory, or thought processes.

_____ 7. Ensure readiness of the client to learn:

- Clarify the learner's verbalizations of acknowledgment of the illness.
- Confirm the client's perception of the relevance of the information to the needs for maintenance and promotion of health.
- Validate physical and emotional comfort of the learner.
- Provide realistic assurance regarding the capability of the learner to acquire the necessary knowledge and skills.

_____ 8. Confirm the conduciveness of the environment to learning.

- Find a quiet place with adequate lighting and comfortable temperature and seating arrangements.
- Demonstrate warm acceptance of the client and significant others.
- Positively reinforce knowledge and skills acquired by the client and his significant others.
- Provide constructive criticism in situations where knowledge and skills require improvement.

Name ______________________________ Date ______________

Observed by __________

CHAPTER 5 REPORTING AND RECORDING

SKILL 5.1 Recording

A. Entering a note in the written record:

_____ 1. Ensure legality of entry:

- Write date and time of each entry.
- Use ink.
- Complete entry with signature and abbreviated title.
- Leave no blank spaces on the chart lines.
- Make no erasures.
- Add no information after signing the note.

_____ 2. Ensure completeness and promptness.

_____ 3. Use proper grammar and style:

- Write complete phrases but omit the grammatical subject of sentence.
- Punctuate each phrase with a comma or period.
- Spell correctly.
- Use agency-accepted medical abbreviations.

_____ 4. Identify and record relevant assessment data.

_____ 5. Include all pertinent assessment data in an organized pattern.

_____ 6. Use precise descriptors that clearly identify what is being discussed.

_____ 7. Specify exact anatomic locations.

_____ 8. Mention common items for size comparison if unsure of exact dimensions of lesions or area.

_____ 9. Record client's actions or responses, not the nurse's.

_____ 10. Make entries at regular intervals.

_____ 11. Record the following events, noting time and date:

- Initial assessment is completed.
- Client's condition changes.
- Nursing measures are done, such as treatments, assisting with activities of daily living, or teaching activities.
- The physician or another health provider visits.
- Medications are given.
- Nurse leaves the unit.

B. Entering data into a medical information system:

_____ 1. Determine if the system is operating; open system if necessary.

_____ 2. Enter the system in the correct manner.

- Type access code on the keyboard.
- Press "ENTER" or "RETURN" key.

_____ 3. Identify and enter desired submenu:

- Type key of appropriate number or letter.
  OR
- Tap lightpen against appropriate phrase, number, or letter.

_____ 4. Enter desired data, phrase, or information into system.

- Type key of appropriate number or letter.
  OR
- Tap lightpen against appropriate phrase, number, or letter.
  OR
- Enter information in whatever manner the system requires.

_____ 5. Select "Review" when all data are entered.

_____ 6. Read monitor to determine that data entered are correct.

_____ 7. Correct errors according tc system format.

_____ 8. Press "ENTER" or "RETURN" key when satisfied all data are correct.

_____ 9. Sign off in designated manner.

C. Recording data on a flowsheet:

_____ 1. Identify the data requested on the flowsheet.

_____ 2. Assess the client for the required information.

_____ 3. Enter date and time of assessment on the flowsheet.

_____ 4. Write data in the correct slot.

_____ 5. Sign initials or signature in the correct slot.

Name ______________________________ Date ______________

Observed by __________

SKILL 5.2 Reporting

_____ 1. Identify the client by name, room number; state his sex and age.

_____ 2. Identify the client's physician, if this is agency policy.

_____ 3. State the client's medical diagnosis.

_____ 4. State the name and date of any surgeries that client has had.

_____ 5. Describe the client's condition at present; note any changes since previous report:

- new or changed signs/symptoms
- current vital signs
- fluid intake and output
- wound condition
- drainage from body cavities or tubes

_____ 6. Identify any new or changed therapies or medications ordered since the previous shift.

_____ 7. Identify any tests, procedures, or surgeries planned.

_____ 8. Report status of ongoing therapies such as intravenous infusions.

_____ 9. Identify family or social problems that may require nursing attention.

_____ 10. Report any progress toward resolving the client's nursing diagnoses; state any new nursing diagnoses that may have been identified since last report.

_____ 11. Report progress of teaching plan, if relevant.

_____ 12. Conclude and proceed to the next client and repeat this information for him.

Name ______________________________ Date ______________

Observed by ______________

CHAPTER 6 WRITING A NURSING CARE PLAN

SKILL 6.1 Writing a Nursing Care Plan

A. Establishing the problem list:

_____ 1. Obtain the client's nursing history by interviewing the client.

_____ 2. Physically examine the client to clarify his present physical condition and identify any variations from normal.

_____ 3. Review laboratory exam and diagnostic test results; identify data pertinent to nursing management.

_____ 4. Document assessment data in a systematic fashion.

_____ 5. Analyze the data for trends or patterns that suggest a nursing diagnosis. When a diagnosis seems evident, confirm with further assessment data as necessary.

_____ 6. Record identified actual nursing diagnoses on the problem list.

_____ 7. Determine the client's medical diagnosis from the health record or the physician.

_____ 8. Record medical diagnoses on the problem list.

_____ 9. Determine anticipated diagnostic procedures or projected therapies (such as surgery or radiation therapy) from the health record, the physician, or other health care provider.

_____ 10. Decide if anticipated procedures or therapies suggest a potential nursing diagnosis.

_____ 11. Document potential nursing diagnoses on the problem list.

_____ 12. Analyze the problem list to determine which problem is most urgent.

_____ 13. Rank the problems according to priorities on the nursing care plan.

B. Identify the objectives or outcomes:

_____ 1. Ask yourself, "What do I want to do for this client with this problem?"

_____ 2. Ask yourself, "What do I want to happen to the client as a result of my actions?"

For the nursing objective:

_____ 3. Make the actor in the objective "the nurse."

_____ 4. State the activity that the nurse will do to address the client's problem.

_____ 5. Determine how the activity is to be performed in order to be accurate, complete, and safe.

_____ 6. Determine when or in what situation the activity is to be performed or completed.

_____ 7. Reexamine the complete objective and determine if it says what it is intended to say.

_____ 8. Indicate whether the objective is short-term or long-term.

_____ 9. Rank the objectives in order of priority, listing first those objectives that are most urgent for the client's life or safety.

For the client outcome:

_____ 10. Make the actor in the objective "the client."

_____ 11. State the activity that is desirable for the client to do to solve, alter, or prevent his health problem.

_____ 12. Determine how the activity is to be performed in order to be accurate, complete, or safe.

_____ 13. Determine when or in what situation the activity is to be performed or completed.

_____ 14. Reexamine the complete outcome and determine if it says what it is intended to say.

_____ 15. Indicate whether the outcome is short-term or long-term. Or suggest a date by which the outcome is to be achieved.

_____ 16. Rank the outcomes in order of priority, listing first those objectives that are most urgent for the client's life or safety.

C. Determining and implementing the nursing orders:

_____ 1. Identify all nursing strategies that may help the client achieve his desired outcomes.

_____ 2. Identify which measure(s) absolutely must be done in order to achieve the outcome; list it (them) first.

_____ 3. Identify which measure may be deferred or implemented as a last resort; list it last.

_____ 4. Determine which other measures may be deemed helpful but not essential to achieving the outcome; list them in order of increasing complexity.

_____ 5. Reexamine the possible orders; alter as desired.

_____ 6. Add all medical orders to the care plan.

_____ 7. Write the problem, goals, and nursing orders in the appropriate document.

_____ 8. Include the medical orders on the document.

_____ 9. Date and sign the care plan.

_____ 10. Use the orders as a guide for organizing and carrying out nursing actions while managing the client.

D. Evaluating the outcome of the nursing care plan:

_____ 1. Examine the expected outcomes at regularly scheduled intervals.

_____ 2. Compare recent assessments of the client with the criteria of the outcome; determine if the criteria are achieved.

Name ______________________ Date ______________

Observed by ____________

_____ 3. Designate "achieved" or "resolved" next to the desired outcome if the client has achieved it, recording assessment data that document the resolution.

_____ 4. Date and sign name for resolved outcomes.

_____ 5. Designate "pending" or "unresolved" next to the desired outcome if the client has not achieved it according to the criteria.

_____ 6. Date and sign name on the unresolved outcomes indicating that the outcome was evaluated, even though not resolved.

_____ 7. Reassess the client to determine if new data are present that alter the problem; change the problem list if necessary.

_____ 8. Reassess the outcome to determine if it is unrealistic for the client; change the outcome if necessary.

_____ 9. Add new orders to the care plan if other strategies are desirable for achieving the goals.

_____ 10. Date and sign all new entries on the nursing care plan.

Name ______________________________ Date ______________________

Observed by ______________

CHAPTER 7 PROVIDING PHYSICAL AND BIOLOGIC SAFETY

SKILL 7.1 Applying Restraints

A. Vest or jacket restraint:

_____ 1. Assess the client to determine the nursing diagnosis.

_____ 2. Plan the expected outcomes of the application of the restraints and gather the necessary equipment.

_____ 3. Explain to the client that he will be wearing a jacket attached securely to the bed. Explain exactly why he will wear this restraint.

_____ 4. Leave the client's hospital gown in place; ensure that it is clean.

_____ 5. Place the client's arms through the armholes.

_____ 6. Overlap the front bodice pieces.

_____ 7. Thread the straps through the vertical slots or belt loops on the side of the vest.

_____ 8. Smooth the vest in place. Criss-cross the straps over the front of the vest.

When the client is in bed:

_____ 9. Secure the straps to the movable part of the mattress frame of the client's bed, tying with a half-bow knot.

When the client is in a chair:

_____ 9. Cross the straps behind the seat of the chair and secure to the chair's lower legs so that the right strap is tied to the left chair leg and the left strap is tied to the right chair leg.

_____ 10. Ensure that the client's safety is protected.

B. Belt restraint:

_____ 1. Assess the client to determine the nursing diagnosis.

_____ 2. Plan the expected outcomes of the application of the restraints and gather the necessary equipment.

_____ 3. Explain to the client that he will be wearing a belt attached securely to the bed. Explain exactly why he will wear this restraint.

_____ 4. Leave the client's hospital gown in place; ensure that it is clean.

_____ 5. Position the client on his back.

_____ 6. Place the long portion of the belt under the client.

_____ 7. Securely tie the ends of the belt to the movable mattress frame.

_____ 8. Bring the shorter portion of the belt around the client's waist and attach.

_____ 9. Ensure that the client's safety is protected.

C. Wrist or ankle restraint:

_____ 1. Assess the client to determine the nursing diagnosis.

_____ 2. Plan the expected outcomes of the application of the restraints and gather the necessary equipment.

_____ 3. Explain to the client that he will have a strap tied around his wrist or ankle that is attached securely to the bed. Explain exactly why he will wear this restraint.

_____ 4. Leave the client's hospital gown in place; ensure that it is clean.

_____ 5. Wrap padding around the client's wrist or ankle.

_____ 6. Wrap the restraint over the padding.

_____ 7. Draw the tie through the vertical opening on the side of the restraint and pull securely.

_____ 8. Attach the ends of the tie to the movable mattress frame with a half-bow tie.

_____ 9. Ensure that the client's safety is protected.

D. Mitt restraint:

_____ 1. Assess the client to determine the nursing diagnosis.

_____ 2. Plan the expected outcomes of the application of the restraints and gather the necessary equipment.

_____ 3. Explain to the client that his hands will be secured in a mitt. Explain exactly why he will wear this restraint.

_____ 4. Leave the client's hospital gown in place; ensure that it is clean.

_____ 5. Gently curl the client's fingers around a rolled bandage or soft rubber ball.

_____ 6. Pull the mitt around the hand and securely tie the wrist ties.

_____ 7. Attach the ends of the ties to the movable mattress frame with a half-bow tie.

_____ 8. Ensure that the client's safety is protected.

E. Elbow restraint:

_____ 1. Assess the client to determine the nursing diagnosis.

_____ 2. Plan the expected outcomes of the application of the restraints and gather the necessary equipment.

_____ 3. Explain to the client that his elbows will be kept straight with a restraint. Explain exactly why he will wear this restraint.

_____ 4. Leave the client's hospital gown in place; ensure that it is clean.

_____ 5. Inspect the restraint to determine that the rigid parts are intact.

_____ 6. Straighten the client's arm and place his elbow in the center of the restraint.

_____ 7. Wrap the restraint around the arm.

_____ 8. Secure the restraint with the ties, safety pins, or tape.

_____ 9. Ensure that the client's safety is protected.

Name ________________________________ Date ______________________

Observed by ____________

F. Mummy restraint:

_____ 1. Assess the infant client to determine the nursing diagnosis.

_____ 2. Plan the expected outcomes of the application of the restraints and gather the necessary equipment.

_____ 3. Explain the procedure to the client's parents and invite their help, if appropriate.

_____ 4. Lay a blanket or sheet on a flat surface.

_____ 5. Fold down one corner of the blanket so that the tip is on the center.

_____ 6. Place the infant supine on the blanket with his head resting midway on the folded corner.

_____ 7. Fold one corner of the blanket over the infant and tuck it under his body just below the axilla.

_____ 8. Fold the second corner over the infant and tuck it under his body.

_____ 9. Raise the infant and fold the bottom corner of the blanket under his body.

Name ______________________ Date ______________________

Observed by ____________

SKILL 7.4 Providing Protective Asepsis

A. Setting up the isolation room:

_____ 1. Explain to the client that he is to be placed in isolation and explain the reason for it.

_____ 2. Select a single room with these features for the client (if he is to occupy a single room):

- sink in the room
- adjoining private bathroom
- rack or hooks to hang reusable gowns, if required

_____ 3. Stock the room with these supplies:

- single-use antiseptic soap
- paper towels near a sink
- laundry hamper
- waste receptacle lined with plastic trash bags
- bedside supplies such as tissues, client's soap, and other toiletries, water container, and cup
- fresh linen
- client's thermometer, stethoscope, and sphygmomanometer
- receptacle for used needles and syringes

_____ 4. Place these supplies outside the door to the room:

- cart for holding supplies
- clean gowns, masks, and gloves
- large plastic or fabric laundry bags
- large plastic disposable trash bags
- disinfectants as indicated

_____ 5. Post a sign on the room door that indicates what precautions are to be taken.

_____ 6. Post a sign on the room door that directs visitors to inquire at the nurse's station.

_____ 7. Move the client into the room.

_____ 8. Demonstrate the protective measures the client and the family need to take in order to protect themselves. Answer questions and concerns.

B. Donning protective garments:

_____ 1. Remove watch and all other jewelry except plain wedding band.

_____ 2. Place watch in a clear plastic bag if it is to be used in the isolation room.

_____ 3. Wash hands.

_____ 4. Don mask.

_____ 5. Select gown from the isolation cart.

_____ 6. Hold the gown up at the inside neck surface or facing and let the gown unfold downward with the open part at the back facing the nurse.

_____ 7. Slip arms into sleeves one at a time, touching only the neck of the gown.

_____ 8. Pull a sleeve up onto one arm and shoulder, working inside the sleeve with the other hand covered by the gown.

_____ 9. Place the other arm in other sleeve in the same manner.

_____ 10. Place fingers inside the gown neck at the back and adjust the gown to fit comfortably on the shoulders.

_____ 11. Tie the neck ties without touching the hair.

_____ 12. Draw edges of the gown together so that one side overlaps the other and all of the back is covered.

_____ 13. Tie waist belt snugly.

_____ 14. Don clean or sterile gloves.

_____ 15. Gather supplies and watch and enter the isolation unit.

_____ 16. Set watch near where it will be used; position opening of plastic bag so that watch can be readily removed.

C. Removing protective garments:

_____ 1. Remove gloves by peeling them off from the inside out. (When gloves are off, they will be inside-out.)

_____ 2. Remove mask by touching only the ties.

_____ 3. Untie waist ties.

_____ 4. Wash hands.

_____ 5. Untie neckties. Avoid contaminating hands by touching the outside of the gown.

_____ 6. Begin removal of sleeves of gown by placing a forefinger under the cuff of one sleeve.

_____ 7. Pull the sleeve over the hand without touching the outside of the gown.

_____ 8. Work the other sleeve off the arm with the gown-covered second hand.

_____ 9. Slip out of gown without touching the outside or allowing the outside of the gown to touch the nurse's uniform.

_____ 10. Fold the gown inside out without shaking or fanning it.

_____ 11. Roll up the folded gown and deposit it in the dirty laundry bag.

_____ 12. Wash hands.

_____ 13. Open door of room with a paper towel on leaving.

D. Bringing supplies and equipment into the room:

_____ 1. Select disposable eating utensils if possible.

_____ 2. Place the item or supply on the isolation cart outside the room.

_____ 3. Don the isolation garments in the usual manner.

Name ________________________ Date ________________

Observed by ____________

_____ 4. Hold the supplies in the gloved hands and enter the isolation room by pushing open the door with the arms or back.

_____ 5. Discard equipment in the trash receptacle after use.

_____ 6. Exit and remove garments in usual manner.

E. Double-bagging to remove trash and discarded linens from the room:

_____ 1. Dress and enter the isolation room in the usual manner.

_____ 2. Empty waste materials into designated bag (brown paper to plastic) in room.

_____ 3. Seal bag securely. Set up a new bag for continued use.

_____ 4. Direct a "clean person" (second health care worker) outside of the room to hold open a clean bag with the top cuffed over his hands. (If second worker is not available, place a clean bag in a laundry cart with the top cuffed over and ready to receive the sealed laundry bag from inside the room.)

_____ 5. Place the sealed bag carefully inside the clean bag being held by the "clean person," taking care to touch only the inside of the outer bag.

_____ 6. Direct the "clean person" to close, secure, and label the double-bagged package for disposal.

_____ 7. Exit the isolation room in the usual manner.

_____ 8. Remove double-bagged waste material or dirty linen to the appropriate area for prompt disposal.

_____ 9. Wash hands.

F. Removing a specimen from the room:

_____ 1. Bring the correctly labeled specimen container and a clear plastic bag into the isolation room when entering.

_____ 2. Collect the specimen in the usual manner; close it securely, and place it in the plastic bag.

_____ 3. Direct a "clean person" outside of the isolation room to hold open a second, larger clear plastic bag, cuffed over the hands.

_____ 4. Place the specimen bag inside the larger bag, carefully avoiding touching the outside of the bag.

_____ 5. Direct the "clean person" to close, secure, and label the double-bagged specimen.

_____ 6. Exit the isolation room in the usual manner.

_____ 7. Take the double-bagged specimen to the appropriate laboratory as quickly as possible.

G. Transporting the isolated client:

_____ 1. Tell the client that he will be leaving the room. Explain where he will go and why. Describe the procedure to be used in transporting him.

_____ 2. Cover the transport vehicle (wheelchair, gurney), if used, with a clean sheet before taking it into the room.

_____ 3. Help the client to don a mask and cap if he is leaving a strict or respiratory isolation room.

_____ 4. Assist the client into the vehicle.

_____ 5. Place a clean sheet over the client, covering him from shoulders to feet.

_____ 6. Notify persons who will receive the client of the isolation precautions that will be required.

_____ 7. Exit the room with the client.

Name ______________________________ Date ______________

Observed by ____________

CHAPTER 8 HELPING THE CLIENT TO DRESS

SKILL 8.1 Assisting with Dressing

A. Removing and replacing a gown when the arm is immobile:

_____ 1. Explain to the client what is to be done.

_____ 2. Gather the necessary supplies, bring to the bedside, and place near the client.

_____ 3. Wash hands.

_____ 4. Pull the curtains around the client's bed, and close the door to the room.

_____ 5. Raise the bed to a comfortable working level for the nurse.

_____ 6. Lower the side rail on the working side of the bed. Ensure that the opposite side rail is up.

_____ 7. Cover the client's upper body with a towel or bath blanket. If the client is in a chair, unfold and place the clean gown over the soiled one.

_____ 8. Turn the client away from the nurse. If the client is sitting in a chair, instruct him to lean forward.

_____ 9. Untie the neck and back ties. Open the back sides of the gown and slip it toward the client's shoulders.

_____ 10. Position the client on his back. Position self on the side of the client's immobile arm.

_____ 11. Instruct the client to raise his mobile arm, and slip the shoulder and sleeve down the arm until the gown is removed from the client.

_____ 12. Gently grasp the client's immobile arm at the wrist or elbow and slip the shoulder and sleeve down and off the client's arm and hand.

_____ 13. Reposition the client's immobile arm in alignment. Keep the bath blanket or towel over the client's body.

_____ 14. Discard the soiled gown in the laundry hamper or set aside.

_____ 15. Position the fresh gown over the bath blanket or towel on the client's chest.

_____ 16. Grasp the client's immobile arm at the wrist or elbow and direct it through the sleeve of the gown. Slip it up to the client's shoulder.

_____ 17. Instruct the client to slip his mobile arm through the other sleeve, and help slip the gown up the arm and over the shoulder.

_____ 18. Turn the client away from the nurse, and pull the back sides of the gown together and tie the ties.

If the client is in a chair, instruct him to lean forward:

_____ 19. Smooth the gown over the client's body and remove the bath blanket or sheet.

_____ 20. Position client comfortably and attach the call signal within his reach. Open the curtains.

_____ 21. Discard the soiled gown in the laundry, if not already done.

_____ 22. Wash hands.

B. Removing and replacing a gown when the arm has an intravenous tubing:

_____ 1. Explain to the client what will be done.

_____ 2. Place a clean gown within reach of the client's bedside.

_____ 3. Identify the arm with the IV and determine the exact location of the IV site.

_____ 4. Examine the IV bottles. Detach any secondary attachments so that only one bottle remains.

_____ 5. Position self and IV pole on the side of the client where the IV attaches.

_____ 6. Place a towel or bath blanket over the client's upper body.

_____ 7. Untie the client's gown at the back.

_____ 8. Pull gown forward over the client's shoulders and arms. Remove the free arm from the gown sleeve.

_____ 9. Remove sleeve of the gown over the arm with the IV site, taking care not to disturb the IV site. The sleeve will now be around the IV tubing.

_____ 10. Gather the sleeve into a compact bundle around the IV tubing. Reach through this sleeve bundle toward the IV bottle.

_____ 11. Remove the IV bottle from the pole with the other hand. Then grasp the bottle with the hand in the sleeve, and slip the bundled gown over the bottle and remaining tubing. The gown is now free of the client and the IV bottle and tubing.

_____ 12. Replace the bottle on the pole, and set aside the soiled gown.

_____ 13. Unfold the clean gown, and gather in a bundle the sleeve of the gown that will go over the arm with the IV. Insert a hand through the sleeve from the *inside* of the gown.

_____ 14. Remove the IV bottle from the stand, and hold it in the hand that is inserted through the sleeve.

_____ 15. Roll the sleeve over the bottle and tubing, until the sleeve opening is at the IV site.

_____ 16. Pull the sleeve up the arm with the IV, carefully preventing the IV site from being disturbed. The arm with the site is now in the sleeve of the gown.

_____ 17. Hang the IV bottle on the pole.

_____ 18. Help the client to don the other sleeve of the gown.

_____ 19. Pull the shoulders of the gown over the client's shoulders and fasten the back ties. Smooth the gown over the client's body and remove the covering bath blanket or towel.

Name ________________________________ Date ________________

Observed by ____________

_____ 20. Position the client comfortably, and attach the call signal within his reach.

_____ 21. Reassemble the IV secondary bottle, if necessary. Determine that the flow rate is accurate.

_____ 22. Discard soiled gown and wash hands.

C. Removing and replacing pajama bottoms when the leg is immobile:

_____ 1. Explain to the client what is being done.

_____ 2. Gather the necessary supplies, bring to the bedside, and place near the client.

_____ 3. Wash hands.

_____ 4. Pull the curtains around the client's bed and close the door.

_____ 5. Raise the bed to a comfortable working level.

_____ 6. Lower the siderail on the working side of the bed. Ensure that the opposite side rail is up.

_____ 7. Untie the client's pajama tie, and loosen the drawstring belt.

_____ 8. Cover the client's body with a towel or bath blanket.

_____ 9. Instruct the client to flex his mobile leg and push his hips away from the bed. Assist by placing hands under the lumbar area and pushing away from the bed. (If the client is in a chair, instruct the client to anchor his immobile leg next to his mobile leg. Grasp the client's arm on his immobile side and instruct him to stand while assisting him. If the client is weak or unstable, a second health worker can assist.)

_____ 10. Pull the pajamas down toward the client's knees. When the pajamas are below the client's hips, instruct him to rest his hips on the bed again.

_____ 11. Pull the pajamas toward the feet, by rolling and gathering the fabric in the hands.

_____ 12. Grasp the client's immobile leg at the knee and ankle, lift and roll the pajamas off the foot.

_____ 13. Instruct the client to raise his mobile foot, and remove the pajamas.

_____ 14. Discard the soiled pajamas in the laundry hamper or set aside.

_____ 15. Unfold and gather the legs of the clean pajamas toward the waist.

_____ 16. Grasp the client's immobile leg at the knee and ankle, lift and pull the garment over the foot and ankle.

_____ 17. Instruct the client to raise his mobile foot and pull the other part of the garment over that foot and ankle. (If the client is in a chair, instruct the client to anchor his immobile leg next to his mobile leg. Grasp the client's arm on his immobile side and instruct him to stand while assisting him. If the client is weak or unstable, a second health worker can assist.)

_____ 18. Unroll and pull the pajamas toward the client's knees.

_____ 19. Instruct the client to flex his mobile leg and push his hips away from the bed. Assist by placing hands under the lumbar area and pushing away from the bed.

_____ 20. Unroll and pull the pajamas up over the client's hips to the waist. Instruct him to lower his hips.

_____ 21. Pull the drawstring belt and tie comfortably for the client.

_____ 22. Remove the bath blanket or towel.

_____ 23. Position the client comfortably and attach the call signal within his reach. Open the curtains.

_____ 24. Discard the soiled pajamas, if it has not been done.

_____ 25. Wash hands.

If the client is in a chair, he may sit.

D. Donning and removing robe:

_____ 1. Explain to the client what is to be done.

_____ 2. Get the client's robe from its storage place, bring to the bedside, and place near the client.

_____ 3. Wash hands.

_____ 4. Assist the client to a dangling position or to sit in a chair, if he is in bed.

_____ 5. Unfold the robe and hold it by the shoulders, behind the client's back, opening away from the client's back.

_____ 6. Instruct the client to slip his arms into the armholes; slip the robe up to the shoulders. (If the client has an immobile arm, gather the corresponding robe sleeve up to the shoulder. Grasp the arm by the elbow or wrist, and slip the sleeve over the arm, unrolling toward the shoulder. Position the other armhole near the client's mobile arm and direct him to slip his arm into it. Slip the robe over the arm and other shoulder.)

_____ 7. Position the robe over the shoulders and straighten the collar.

_____ 8. Wrap the sides of the robe front around the client. Tie the waist belt.

_____ 9. Proceed with the client's activities.

_____ 10. Untie the waist belt, and separate the sides of the robe front.

_____ 11. Grasp the robe at the shoulders, instruct the client to extend his arms behind him, and slip the robe off the shoulders and arms. (If the client has an immobile arm, instruct the client to extend his mobile arm behind him, and slip robe off the mobile arm and shoulder first. Hold the arm at the wrist, and slip the remainder of the robe from the shoulder and arm.)

_____ 12. Assist the client to his next activity.

E. Removing and replacing elastic stockings:

_____ 1. Explain to the client what is to be done and the purpose of the elastic stockings.

_____ 2. Wash hands.

Name ________________________________ Date ____________________

Observed by ____________

____ 3. Draw the curtains around the bed or close the door.

____ 4. Position the client in the bed or on a chair with his legs elevated parallel to the floor. Drape the client with covers as necessary.

____ 5. Elevate the bed to a comfortable working height, if the client is in bed.

____ 6. Squat to the level of the client's feet and legs, if he is in a chair.

____ 7. Pull the stocking gently outward from the proximal end (thigh) to the foot. Ease it gently over the heel of the foot, tugging the fabric out from the heel to remove it, if necessary.

____ 8. Remove the stocking from the foot. Smooth the stocking until it is flat; hang over a chair or side rail to air. (The elastic stocking is left off the leg for approximately 20–30 minutes to expose the skin to the air for rest. Use this time to provide skin care as needed.)

To replace:

____ 9. Turn the stocking inside out and locate the heel.

____ 10. Raise the client's foot by holding it at the heel or ankle, if the client is sitting in a chair.

____ 11. Slip the stocking over the heel of the foot and smooth in place.

____ 12. Pull the stocking gently over the foot, ankle and up the calf, smoothing the elastic in place.

____ 13. Tug gently toward the upper body when the stocking is completely positioned.

____ 14. Check with the client to determine if the stocking feels uniformly snug and comfortable. Make necessary changes.

____ 15. Position the client comfortably and attach call signal within his reach. Open the curtains and the door.

____ 16. Wash hands.

F. Putting on shoes or slippers:

____ 1. Explain to the client what is to be done.

____ 2. Place the client's shoes or slippers near the client's feet.

____ 3. Place the client in a dangling position if he is in bed, or have him sit in a chair.

____ 4. Hold the shoe or slipper with the dominant hand, and grasp the foot at the heel with the nondominant hand.

____ 5. Slip the shoe or slipper over the client's toes, wiggling the shoe from side to side to direct the foot in place. Slip the heel of the foot into the heel of the shoe.

_____ 6. Ask the client if the fit is comfortable. Adjust as necessary.

_____ 7. Follow the same steps with the other foot.

_____ 8. Wash hands.

_____ 9. Assist the client to his next activity.

Name ______________________________ Date ______________________________

Observed by ______________

SKILL 8.2 Dressing an Infant

A. Changing an infant's diaper:

_____ 1. Assess the infant client to determine the nursing diagnosis.

_____ 2. Plan the expected outcomes of the diapering process and gather the necessary equipment and supplies.

_____ 3. Explain to the infant's parents what will be done (if they are present).

_____ 4. Dampen washcloth with warm water. Bring all equipment to the changing table.

_____ 5. Wash hands.

_____ 6. Fold a fresh diaper, if necessary, and set it aside on the changing table.

_____ 7. Lift the infant from his crib by holding him under his back and under the neck. Place him on the changing table.

_____ 8. Remove the infant's outer clothing and raise the upper clothing from the diaper area. Remove the plastic or rubber pants if present.

_____ 9. Unfasten the safety pins and place them out of the baby's reach but in direct line of the nurse's vision.

_____ 10. Remove the soiled diaper, using any dry corner to wipe feces or urine from the infant's skin. Carefully remove feces from all folds and creases of the infant's body.

_____ 11. Set the soiled diaper aside but out of baby's reach.

_____ 12. Clean the baby's skin with the washcloth and pat dry. Add powder or lotion as desired.

_____ 13. Explain to the infant's parents why cornstarch is preferable to talcum powder, but it must still be used with caution.

_____ 14. Inspect the baby's skin for rashes or breaks.

_____ 15. Hold the baby's feet and ankles with the nondominant hand and lift the baby's lower body from the pad. Place the clean folded diaper in position between the legs. Lower the body back to the pad.

_____ 16. Wrap the front and back of the diaper around the pelvis so that the diaper fits snugly around the thighs and the waist.

_____ 17. Fasten the front and back of the diaper on each side with safety pins or adhesive tabs. Hold hand under the area to be pinned.

_____ 18. Replace plastic or rubber pants if they are not soiled. Replace with clean, fresh pants if they are soiled.

_____ 19. Reposition upper garment and replace outer clothing as necessary.

_____ 20. Place the baby back in his crib and raise the side rails. Provide covering as necessary.

_____ 21. Rinse the soiled diaper in a toilet bowl and discard in the diaper hamper.

_____ 22. Wash hands.

B. Changing the infant's clothing:

_____ 1. Wash hands.

_____ 2. Place the infant on a changing table. Keep him within sight and reach at all times.

_____ 3. Remove and replace all garments in same manner as removing and replacing garments of an adult.

_____ 4. Use one hand to open arm and leg openings while directing the infant's limbs through the openings with the other hand.

_____ 5. Fasten the garments so that they are secure (won't easily be freed) but also loose so that the infant's movements are not restricted.

_____ 6. Remove and replace garments quickly.

Name ____________________ Date ____________

Observed by ____________

CHAPTER 9 ASSESSING AND BATHING THE SKIN

SKILL 9.1 Assessing the Skin

____ 1. Explain to the client that his skin will be examined.

____ 2. Close the door to the room or draw the bedside curtains.

____ 3. Wash hands.

____ 4. Assist the client to undress or uncover the skin area for examination. Examine only one area at a time.

____ 5. Direct the lamp on the exposed skin area.

____ 6. Inspect the skin for color. Note symmetry of body surfaces, color of sclera, conjunctiva, oral mucosa, nailbeds, and palms of hands.

____ 7. Inspect for vascularity and evidence of bleeding or bruising.

____ 8. Inspect bony prominences for pallor or redness.

____ 9. Inspect for moisture: dryness, perspiration, excess oil. Note excess moisture in skin folds.

____ 10. Palpate for temperature by placing the backs of fingers against the skin.

____ 11. Palpate for texture: brush pads of forefingers lightly over the surface noting smoothness or roughness.

____ 12. Palpate for turgor: lightly pinch a fold of skin on the back of the client's hand or forearm between thumb and forefinger; release. Note mobility of skin and speed with which it resumes its shape.

____ 13. Inspect for lesions.

If lesion is observed:

____ 14. Note exact anatomic location.

____ 15. Observe the distribution of the lesion: generalized or localized?

____ 16. Observe the grouping or arrangement of the lesions: linear, clustered, or annular (circular).

____ 17. Note color of lesion.

____ 18. Don disposable gloves if lesion is open or draining.

____ 19. Identify type of lesion if possible by inspecting shape and size; palpate for elevation and consistency.

____ 20. Gently palpate areas that appear edematous. Note location, extent of edema, and tenderness.

____ 21. Press edematous area with two forefingers for 5 seconds; release. Note presence or depth of indentation.

_____ **22.** Discard gloves, if present. Remove lamp.

_____ **23.** Assist client to replace clothing.

_____ **24.** Open curtains or door to room.

_____ **25.** Wash hands.

Name ______________________________ Date ______________________

Observed by ____________

SKILL 9.2 Providing Morning or Evening Care

A. Morning care:

_____ 1. Waken the client and explain what is to happen.

_____ 2. Wash hands.

_____ 3. Gather the necessary equipment and position on the overbed table, next to the client's bed.

_____ 4. Pull the curtains around the client's bed or close the door to the room.

_____ 5. Offer the client the bedpan or urinal. Remove and discard contents.

_____ 6. Position the client in a mid to high Fowler's, and place the overbed table over the client's legs.

_____ 7. Fill the washbasin with warm water and place on the overbed table.

_____ 8. Place mouth care equipment on the overbed table.

_____ 9. Assist the client with face washing and handwashing and mouth care in whatever way necessary. Provide shaving equipment or makeup as requested. Help client to comb or brush his hair.

_____ 10. Remove the overbed table and discard water, replace supplies and equipment when the client has completed care.

_____ 11. Position the client comfortably and attach call signal within reach.

_____ 12. Wash hands.

B. Evening care:

_____ 1. Explain to the client that evening care is to be done.

_____ 2. Draw the curtains around the bed and close the door to the room.

_____ 3. Wash hands.

_____ 4. Place supplies within reach on the overbed or bedside table.

_____ 5. Offer the client the bedpan or urinal, and remove and discard contents.

_____ 6. Loosen the lower bed linens and retuck, making a tight fit. Change the draw sheet as necessary.

_____ 7. Smooth and straighten the top linens. Add a blanket if the client wishes, fanfolding it into place at the foot of the bed if the client doesn't wish to be covered immediately.

_____ 8. Perform whatever hygienic or comfort measures seem necessary for the client. Provide fresh drinking water.

_____ 9. Place the client in a prone or lateral position and perform a back massage.

_____ 10. Position the client comfortably and attach the call signal within his reach.

_____ **11.** Raise siderails on both sides of the bed.

_____ **12.** Replace supplies and discard used linens in the laundry.

_____ **13.** Adjust the lighting according to the client's desires. Leave a night light on.

_____ **14.** Wash hands.

Name ______________________________ Date ______________________

Observed by ____________

SKILL 9.3 Providing the Cleansing Bath

A. Bed bath:

_____ 1. Assess the client and determine the nursing diagnosis.

_____ 2. Plan the expected outcomes for the bath.

_____ 3. Explain to the client what is to be done and arrange the time.

_____ 4. Wash hands and put on clean gloves.

_____ 5. Bring the supplies to the bedside and arrange conveniently.

_____ 6. Close the door to the client's room and pull the bedside curtains.

_____ 7. Offer the bedpan to the client, or help to the commode or bathroom. Empty bedpan or help client return to bed.

_____ 8. Discard gloves, wash hands, and put on fresh clean gloves.

_____ 9. Raise the bed to a convenient working level. Position the head of the bed in mid to high Fowler's, if this is tolerable to the client.

_____ 10. Raise the siderail on the side of the bed opposite the nurse. Lower the siderail on the working side.

_____ 11. Move the client to the side of the bed where the nurse is standing.

_____ 12. Place the bath blanket over the top bed linens and unfold so that the linens are completely covered. Have the client hold the edge of the bath blanket, and gently roll the top bed linens under the bath blanket to the foot of the bed.

_____ 13. Remove the top linens, if the bed is to be changed.

_____ 14. Remove the client's soiled gown and pajamas, keeping the bath blanket in position over the client.

_____ 15. Fill the bath basin with water that it is warm to the hands, approximately 105–110°F (40.5–42°C).

If the client is alert and able to move hands and arms:

_____ 16. Place the basin on the overbed table, and position the table over the client's knees, within his reach.

_____ 17. Place the washcloth in the basin of water. Place one towel on the client's chest.

_____ 18. Encourage the client to wash and dry face and hands. Position the soap dish and wash cloth within reach.

If the client is unable to move his hands and arms:

_____ 16. Place the basin on the overbed table and position the bed adjacent to the bed. Position one towel on the client's chest.

_____ 17. Place the washcloth in the water; gently wring it. Use the corner of the cloth to gently wipe the client's eye from the inner to outer canthus. Use a second corner and repeat with the other eye.

_____ **18.** Fashion a wash mitt over the dominant hand by wrapping the cloth around the fingers and folding the excess cloth toward the palm of the hand.

_____ **19.** Gently wash the client's face, ears, and neck using soap only at the client's request. Pat dry with the towel on the client's chest.

_____ **20.** Place a towel lengthwise under the client's arm farthest from the nurse.

_____ **21.** Rinse the washcloth and replenish soap periodically.

_____ **22.** Wash the client's arm from the distal to proximal areas, using firm but gentle strokes. Dry.

_____ **23.** Wash and dry the axilla.

_____ **24.** Place a towel under the other arm and repeat steps 22 and 23.

_____ **25.** If the client has not washed his hands, position the overbed table over his legs and place his hands in the basin. Gently wash and dry the hands, particularly between the fingers. Note the condition of the nails at this time.

_____ **26.** Place the towel over the client's chest and abdomen. Fold the bath blanket to just above the client's pubic area.

_____ **27.** Wash the chest and abdomen, keeping the towel in position. Dry. Wash and dry carefully under the female client's breasts. Reposition the bath blanket.

_____ **28.** Uncover the leg farthest from the work area and place the towel lengthwise under it.

_____ **29.** Wash the leg from the distal to proximal areas, using long, firm strokes. Dry and cover with the bath blanket.

_____ **30.** Repeat steps 28 and 29 with the other leg.

_____ **31.** Lift and uncover the client's foot farthest from the nurse, and place the water basin under it. Immerse the foot, holding the basin steady. Soak for a brief time.

_____ **32.** Gently wash and dry the foot, particularly between the toes. Examine the toenails at this time.

_____ **33.** Repeat steps 31 and 32 with the other foot.

_____ **34.** Discard the wash water, rinse the wash basin, and fill with fresh, clean water.

_____ **35.** Assist the client into a prone or side-lying position facing away from the nurse, keeping the bath blanket in place over the client.

_____ **36.** Place the towel lengthwise on the bed next to the client's back, and fold the bath blanket to expose the client's back and buttocks.

_____ **37.** Wash the back, using long, firm strokes, working from the shoulders to the buttocks. Dry.

Name ______________________ Date ______________________

Observed by ____________

_____ 38. Wash between the buttocks and gluteal folds. Dry. Give a back rub.

_____ 39. Assist the client to his back and raise the head of the bed to a comfortable position for the client.

If the client is alert and able to wash the perineal area:

_____ 40. Position the wash basin within the client's easy reach, and instruct to complete the bath by washing the perineum.

If the client is unable to bathe himself:

_____ 41. Place a towel over the upper chest and abdomen, fold back the bath blanket to expose the pubic area, and carefully wash the perineum and genitalia. Dry.

_____ 42. Remove the towel and draw the bath blanket over the client's entire body.

Proceed with the occupied bedmaking procedure at this time. If the bed change has already occurred:

_____ 43. Reposition the top bed linens over the bath blanket. Remove the bath blanket from under the covers.

_____ 44. Assist the client to don a clean gown and pajama bottoms, if desired.

_____ 45. Assist the client with shaving, hair care, or nail care at this time. Assist the client with deodorants, powders, lotions, or cosmetics as he desires.

_____ 46. Raise siderail into position.

_____ 47. Tidy the bedside environment. Remove soiled towels and linens from the bedside and discard in laundry. Remove the bath basin, empty, rinse, and replace. Replace toiletries.

_____ 48. Position the call signal within the client's reach.

_____ 49. Open the bedside curtains.

_____ 50. Leave the client comfortable.

_____ 51. Discard gloves and wash hands.

B. Shower or tub bath:

_____ 1. Assess the client and determine the nursing diagnosis.

_____ 2. Plan the expected outcomes for the bath.

_____ 3. Consult with the client on the time for the bath. Arrange for the use of the tub or shower at that time, if that is necessary.

_____ 4. Check that the shower or tub is clean and ready for use.

_____ 5. Gather necessary equipment and supplies that may be needed.

_____ 6. Place an "occupied" sign on the door to the shower or tub, or use some other method to signal that the area is occupied.

_____ 7. Fill the tub with approximately 12–14 inches of water that is 105–110°F, if a tub bath is being done. Keep the door to the room closed.

_____ 8. Place a bathmat adjacent to the tub.

_____ 9. Assist the client to the bathroom in whatever fashion is necessary.

_____ 10. Turn on the shower water supply, and regulate the water so that it is a comfortable temperature.

During the bath or shower:

_____ 11. Provide assistance with the bath according to the needs of the client.

_____ 12. Stay available near the bathroom if the client is bathing without assistance.

_____ 13. Assist the client with dressing if necessary.

_____ 14. Assist the client to his room in whatever fashion is necessary.

_____ 15. Clean the tub or shower according to agency policy.

16. Remove "occupied" sign from the hospital bathroom.

_____ 17. Discard used linens and towels in the laundry.

_____ 18. Wash hands.

Name ______________________________ Date ______________

Observed by ______________

SKILL 9.4 Providing Perineal Care

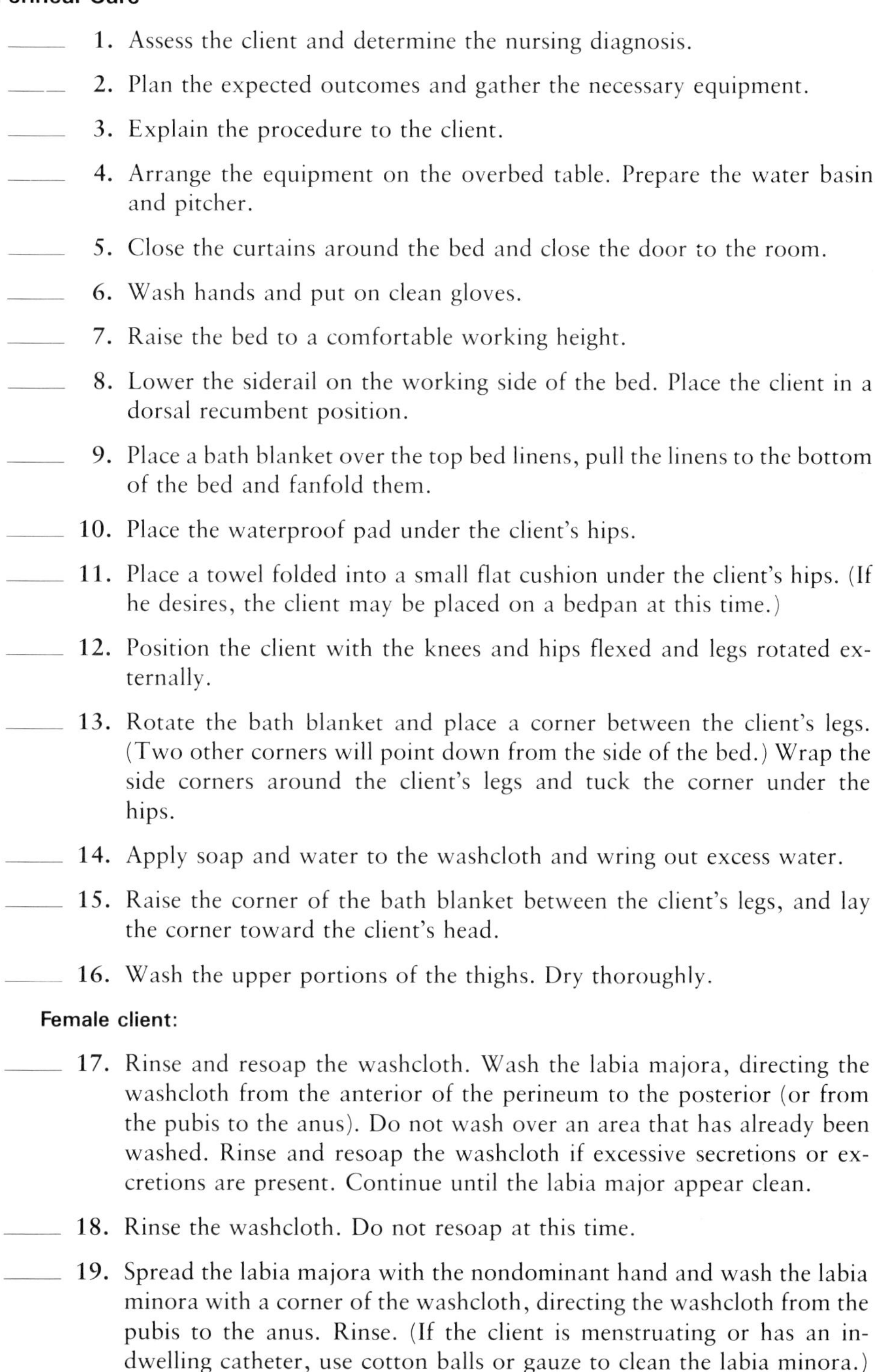

_____ 1. Assess the client and determine the nursing diagnosis.

_____ 2. Plan the expected outcomes and gather the necessary equipment.

_____ 3. Explain the procedure to the client.

_____ 4. Arrange the equipment on the overbed table. Prepare the water basin and pitcher.

_____ 5. Close the curtains around the bed and close the door to the room.

_____ 6. Wash hands and put on clean gloves.

_____ 7. Raise the bed to a comfortable working height.

_____ 8. Lower the siderail on the working side of the bed. Place the client in a dorsal recumbent position.

_____ 9. Place a bath blanket over the top bed linens, pull the linens to the bottom of the bed and fanfold them.

_____ 10. Place the waterproof pad under the client's hips.

_____ 11. Place a towel folded into a small flat cushion under the client's hips. (If he desires, the client may be placed on a bedpan at this time.)

_____ 12. Position the client with the knees and hips flexed and legs rotated externally.

_____ 13. Rotate the bath blanket and place a corner between the client's legs. (Two other corners will point down from the side of the bed.) Wrap the side corners around the client's legs and tuck the corner under the hips.

_____ 14. Apply soap and water to the washcloth and wring out excess water.

_____ 15. Raise the corner of the bath blanket between the client's legs, and lay the corner toward the client's head.

_____ 16. Wash the upper portions of the thighs. Dry thoroughly.

Female client:

_____ 17. Rinse and resoap the washcloth. Wash the labia majora, directing the washcloth from the anterior of the perineum to the posterior (or from the pubis to the anus). Do not wash over an area that has already been washed. Rinse and resoap the washcloth if excessive secretions or excretions are present. Continue until the labia major appear clean.

_____ 18. Rinse the washcloth. Do not resoap at this time.

_____ 19. Spread the labia majora with the nondominant hand and wash the labia minora with a corner of the washcloth, directing the washcloth from the pubis to the anus. Rinse. (If the client is menstruating or has an indwelling catheter, use cotton balls or gauze to clean the labia minora.)

_____ 20. Pour the pitcher of water gently over the perineum at this time, if the client is on the bedpan. Remove the bedpan when the rinse is complete.

_____ 21. Dry the area well with the towel, ensuring that no moisture remains on the tissues. Apply a light dusting of powder or protective cream at this time, if the client desires.

Male client:

_____ 17. Raise the penis and place a towel under it, resting on the scrotum. Grasp the shaft of the penis and retract the foreskin, if present. Wash the glans in a circular fashion, beginning with the urethra and moving outward. Replace foreskin.

_____ 18. Rinse and resoap the washcloth and wash the remainder of the penis using firm, downward strokes. Dry thoroughly.

_____ 19. Rinse, resoap, and wash the scrotum, particularly between all folds of skin. Dry thoroughly.

_____ 20. Pour the pitcher of water gently over the genitalia at this time, if the client is on the bedpan. Remove bedpan and thoroughly dry the genitalia and perineum.

Either male or female client:

_____ 22. Remove the towel pad from under the client's hips and position laterally away from the nurse.

_____ 23. Inspect the area between the buttocks and remove excess stool with tissues, if necessary.

_____ 24. Wash thoroughly between the buttocks, particularly around the anus. Dry thoroughly and apply powder or protective cream if the client desires.

_____ 25. Remove the waterproof pad from under the client's hips. Place the client in a dorsal recumbent position and replace the top covers. Remove the bath blanket.

_____ 26. Position the client comfortably and attach call signal within his reach.

_____ 27. Dispose of towels and washcloths in the laundry. Wash, rinse, and replace equipment in the client's bedside unit.

_____ 28. Discard gloves and wash hands.

Name ______________________________ Date ______________

Observed by ____________

SKILL 9.5 Massaging the Back

_____ 1. Assess the client for the need for massage, and determine the nursing diagnosis.

_____ 2. Determine the expected outcomes and gather supplies and equipment. Place container of massage lotion in a basin of warm water.

_____ 3. Explain to the client that he will receive a back massage.

_____ 4. Gather equipment and place it conveniently at the bedside.

_____ 5. Wash hands.

_____ 6. Draw the curtains around the bed or close the door to the room.

_____ 7. Raise the bed level to a convenient working height.

_____ 8. Lower the siderails on the side of the bed where the nurse will work.

_____ 9. Remove the client's gown, or untie the back ties and slip the back portion of the gown toward the shoulders.

_____ 10. Place the client face down if possible or lying on the side with the back toward the nurse.

_____ 11. Drape the client with the bath blanket or top covers so that the entire back from shoulders to buttocks is exposed to just above the gluteal folds.

_____ 12. Remove the lotion container from the water, apply a moderate amount to the nurse's hands, and smooth the lotion around the entire surface of the palms. If powder is used as the lubricant, apply the powder directly to the back, after telling the client what you are doing.

_____ 13. Tell the client that you are going to apply the lotion to his back.

_____ 14. Smooth the lotion on the back, beginning about the midlumbar region and smoothing it toward the shoulders. Keep one or both hands in contact with the skin surface at all times until the massage is complete.

_____ 15. Begin the massage with *effleurage,* stroking with both of the hands from the buttocks toward the shoulders and back again. Stroke firmly as the hands move from the buttocks toward the shoulder, and lightly as the hands move from the shoulder to the buttocks. Alternate the long strokes with circular strokes. Repeat this pattern 8–10 times.

_____ 16. Change the massage technique to *petrissage,* beginning at the buttocks and kneading the superficial tissues between the fingertips of both hands, moving toward the shoulders. When the hands reach the shoulders, switch to effleurage for the downward stroke, and then repeat petrissage. Repeat this pattern 8–10 times.

_____ 17. Change the massage technique to *friction,* using the palms of the hands to slide the superficial tissues over the underlying tissues. Move from the buttocks toward the shoulders, massage in and out from the midline of the back, until all tissues have been massaged. Switch to effleurage to move back toward the buttocks, and repeat friction toward the shoulders. Repeat this pattern two or three times.

_____ 18. Change the massage technique to *tapotement,* alternating striking the tissues on either side of the back with the ulnar surface of the hand. Move from the buttocks toward the shoulders, switching to effleurage to move back toward the buttocks. Repeat this pattern only once or twice.

_____ 19. Complete the massage by changing the technique to effleurage and stroking the back several more times.

_____ 20. Remove excess lubricant with the towel, if necessary.

_____ 21. Remove bath blanket and replace client's gown and top covers. Open curtains or door.

_____ 22. Position client comfortably with the call signal within reach.

_____ 23. Replace the lubricant in its storage place.

_____ 24. Wash hands.

Name ______________________________ Date ______________________

Observed by ____________

CHAPTER 10 PROVIDING HYGIENE FOR THE MOUTH, EYES, HAIR, AND NAILS

SKILL 10.1 Providing Mouth Care

A. Oral care for the conscious client:

_____ 1. Assess the client and mouth and determine the nursing diagnosis.

_____ 2. Plan the expected outcomes of the procedure and gather the necessary equipment.

_____ 3. Explain to the client what is going to be done.

_____ 4. Place the equipment on the overbed table, within reach of the client. If the client is ambulatory, place the equipment near the client's sink.

_____ 5. Wash hands and put on clean gloves.

_____ 6. Raise the head of the bed so the client is upright.

_____ 7. Raise the client's bed to a comfortable working position.

_____ 8. Place a towel on the client's chest and tuck under the chin.

_____ 9. Pour fresh water into the cup.

If the client is able to brush teeth:

_____ 10. Encourage the client to brush and floss teeth in usual manner. Assist in whatever way is asked for or seems apparent.

_____ 11. Observe the client's hygiene practices and determine if he requires any health teaching.

_____ 12. Remove and dispose of used rinse water. Clean and rinse the emesis basin and return to its storage place. Replace other equipment.

_____ 13. Place the client in a position of comfort. Leave the call signal within his reach.

_____ 14. Remove gloves and wash hands.

If the client is unable to brush teeth independently:

_____ 10. Place dentifrice on the toothbrush.

_____ 11. Wrap a gauze pad around a tongue blade and secure with adhesive tape.

_____ 12. Place emesis basin under client's chin.

_____ 13. Wrap a moistened gauze sponge around the forefinger and middle finger of the nurse's nondominant hand.

_____ 14. Instruct the client to open his mouth.

_____ 15. Insert the tongue blade between the upper and lower teeth, opening the jaws.

_____ 16. Insert gauze-wrapped fingers inside the cheek farthest from the nurse and gently open cheeks and lips.

_____ 17. Dip the toothbrush into the cup of water to moisten.

_____ 18. Brush the upper teeth furthest from the nurse on the inside of the mouth. Hold the brush at a 45° angle from the teeth and brush from the gum margin down to the tip of the teeth in an up-and-down motion. Brush the outside of the teeth in the same manner.

_____ 19. Brush the lower teeth in a similar fashion.

_____ 20. Hold the toothbrush parallel to the tops of the molars and brush both upper and lower molars with a back-and-forth motion.

_____ 21. Remove gauze-wrapped fingers and reposition them inside the cheek nearest the nurse, and gently open the mouth.

_____ 22. Repeat steps 17–20. Remove tongue blade, fingers, and toothbrush.

_____ 23. Position the water cup at the client's mouth and instruct the client to sip some water, rinse, and spit into the emesis basin.

_____ 24. Repeat step 23 until the rinse water is clear.

_____ 25. Repeat the brushing procedure until the mouth and teeth appear clean and the client feels refreshed.

B. Flossing the teeth:

After brushing:

_____ 1. Wrap an end of the floss around each middle finger of the nurse's hand. Stretch the floss taut by pulling tightly with the thumbs.

_____ 2. Insert the taut floss between the upper teeth, beginning at the back of the mouth. Gently slide the floss back and forth, stretched between the teeth, moving from the crowns to the gum line. Continue around the top of the mouth until all interspaces have been flossed. Reposition the floss periodically.

_____ 3. Wrap a fresh length of floss in the same manner as before.

_____ 4. Repeat step 2 with the bottom teeth.

_____ 5. Help the client rinse until the rinse water returns clear.

_____ 6. Wipe around the lips and surrounding face with a washcloth and towel.

_____ 7. Remove and dispose of used rinse water. Clean and rinse the emesis basin and return to its storage place. Replace other equipment.

_____ 8. Place the client in a position of comfort. Leave call signal within his reach.

_____ 9. Remove gloves and wash hands.

C. Mouth care for the client with dentures:

_____ 1. Assess the client and mouth and determine the nursing diagnosis.

_____ 2. Plan the expected outcomes of the procedure and gather the necessary equipment.

_____ 3. Explain to the client what is going to be done.

_____ 4. Place the equipment on the overbed table, within reach of the client. If the client is ambulatory, place the equipment near the client's sink.

Name ____ Date ____________________

Observed by ____________

_____ 5. Wash hands and put on clean gloves.

_____ 6. Raise the head of the bed until the client is upright.

_____ 7. Raise the client's bed to a comfortable working position for the nurse.

_____ 8. Place a towel on the client's chest and tuck under the chin.

_____ 9. Place the denture cup on the overbed table within the client's reach and ask him to remove his dentures.

If the client cannot remove the dentures:

_____ 10. Grasp the upper denture with a gauze sponge and gently wiggle the denture up and down until the suction is broken and the denture is loose.

_____ 11. Place the denture in the cup.

_____ 12. Repeat steps 10 and 11 with the lower denture.

_____ 13. Encourage the client to brush and rinse his mouth in his usual manner.

If the client cannot complete own oral care:

_____ 14. Wrap a gauze sponge around two tongue blades. Moisten with water or a mouthwash.

_____ 15. Wipe the inside of the mouth on all surfaces with a tongue blade.

_____ 16. Place an emesis basin under the client's chin.

If the client can rinse mouth:

_____ 17. Give the client a cup of fresh water. Ask him to rinse mouth and spit into the basin.

If the client cannot rinse mouth:

_____ 14. Place the suction tip under the tongue or between the lower lip and teeth.

_____ 15. Place about 30–50 cc of water in an Asepto syringe and squirt to rinse both sides of the mouth.

_____ 16. Wipe or instruct the client to wipe face and chin dry.

_____ 17. Take the denture cup to a nearby sink. Fill the sink about one-third full of tepid water.

_____ 18. Prepare the toothbrush with a denture cleaning dentifrice.

_____ 19. Remove the denture from the cup over the water. Rinse with tepid water.

_____ 20. Brush the denture on all surfaces with the toothbrush and dentifrice, keeping the denture over the water in the sink at all times.

_____ 21. Rinse the denture with tepid water. Repeat until the denture surface is free of food particles and tissue debris. Rinse again and return the denture to the cup.

_____ 22. Repeat steps 19–21 with the remaining denture.

_____ 23. Return the denture to the client and instruct him to replace them.

If the client cannot replace own dentures:

_____ 24. Prepare the denture with an adhesive cream, if the client so desires, by spreading the cream evenly on the surface of the denture that rests on the gums.

_____ 25. Instruct the client to open mouth; place the denture on the gums. Press gently to create the necessary bond.

_____ 26. Wipe the client's face and hands if necessary.

_____ 27. Position the client comfortably and place the call signal within reach.

_____ 28. Wash hands.

D. Mouth care for the unconscious client:

_____ 1. Assess the client's mouth to determine the nursing diagnosis.

_____ 2. Plan the expected outcomes and gather the necessary equipment.

_____ 3. Gather the necessary equipment.

_____ 4. Wash hands and put on clean gloves.

_____ 5. Prepare the equipment by pouring fresh water into a cup. Fill the Asepto syringe with 30–50 cc of water. Place dentifrice on the toothbrush. Attach a suction tip to the suction source, if available. Wrap gauze pads around a tongue blade and fasten with adhesive tape.

_____ 6. Position the client on side or abdomen with the head lowered.

_____ 7. Place a towel or absorbent pad under head and neck.

_____ 8. Place the suction tip under the client's tongue or between the cheek and teeth in the lower jaw.
OR
Place a kidney basin against the client's cheek and neck directly under mouth.

_____ 9. Wrap a moistened gauze sponge around the forefinger and middle finger of the nondominant hand.

_____ 10. Insert the tongue blade between the upper and lower teeth, and gently open the jaws.

_____ 11. Insert gauze-wrapped fingers inside the cheek farthest from the nurse, and gently pull the cheek and lips to the side.

_____ 12. Dip the toothbrush in the water to moisten.

_____ 13. Brush the upper teeth farthest from the nurse on the inside of the gums. Hold the brush at a 45° angle from the teeth, and brush from the gum margin down to the tip of the teeth in an up-and-down rotation. Brush the outside of the teeth in the same manner.

_____ 14. Brush the lower teeth as in step 13.

_____ 15. Hold the toothbrush parallel to the tops of the teeth, and brush both upper and lower molars with a back-and-forth motion.

_____ 16. Remove gauze-wrapped fingers and, repositioning them inside the cheek nearest the nurse, gently open the client's cheek and lips.

Name ______________________ Date ______________

Observed by ____________

_____ 17. Repeat steps 12–15 and remove tongue blade and toothbrush.

_____ 18. Rinse the client's mouth by injecting about 10 cc of rinse water from the Asepto syringe into each side of the mouth. Allow the rinse water to flow to the suction tip or into the emesis basin.

_____ 19. Repeat step 18 until the mouth is clear of dentifrice.

_____ 20. Continue holding the client's mouth open with tongue blade and fingers, and clean all tissues of the mouth and tongue with a moistened gauze sponge or washcloth. (A tongue blade wrapped with gauze and moistened may also be used for this.)

_____ 21. Rinse again with the Asepto syringe as necessary.

_____ 22. Remove emesis basin and dry the mouth and chin with a towel.

_____ 23. Apply a water-soluble lubricant to the client's lips.

_____ 24. Remove towel or absorbent pad from under the client's head and neck.

_____ 25. Position the client in proper alignment but with head and mouth facing toward the bed for at least 20 minutes following the procedure.

_____ 26. Remove gloves and wash hands.

Name ______________________________ Date ______________________

Observed by ____________

SKILL 10.2 Providing Eye Care

A. Removing, cleaning, and replacing eyeglasses:

_____ 1. Wash hands.

_____ 2. Ask the client to remove glasses. If he is unable to do so, explain to the client that the nurse will remove them.

_____ 3. Grasp the earpieces above the ears. Lift the frame up and out from the ears. Pull down and away from the client's face.

_____ 4. Inspect the lenses.

_____ 5. Wash and rinse the lenses with warm water or cleansing solution. Carefully hold the glasses by the earpieces and do not twist the frame or drop the eyeglasses.

_____ 6. Dry the lenses with a soft cloth or tissue. Do not touch the lenses with fingers or thumbs.

_____ 7. Fold the frame and place eyeglasses in their case; then set it aside in a safe place, usually the drawer in the bedside table.

_____ 8. Remove the eyeglasses from its case and unfold the frames to replace the eyeglasses on the client.

_____ 9. Hold the frames by the earpieces.

_____ 10. Direct the earpieces just above each ear until in the correct position and the nose piece of the frame sits on the bridge of the client's nose.

_____ 11. Determine if the glasses are in the correct position by examining the client's face. Ask the client if the glasses are comfortably in place.

B. Removing, cleaning, and replacing contact lenses:

_____ 1. Ask the client to remove lenses. If he is unable to do so, wash hands and remove them this way:

_____ 2. Separate the upper and lower lids of the eye with thumbs until the lens edges are identified.

_____ 3. Gently push the upper lid to the top edge of the lens. Hold the upper lid in place by gently pressing against the upper bony orbit.

_____ 4. Gently push the lower lid toward the lower edge of the lens. Slip the lens off the eye by pressing gently against it, maneuvering until the lens is freed.

_____ 5. Catch the lens with the hand or the towel. Place in the correct storage container.

_____ 6. Repeat steps 2–5 to remove and store the other lens.

_____ 7. Take the lens container to a nearby sink. Close the drain on the sink and fill with about 3 inches of tap water.

_____ 8. Hold one lens carefully between the thumb and forefinger over the water. Gently squeeze lens cleaner from its bottle onto each side of the lens. Spread the lens cleaner evenly with a finger.

_____ 9. Rinse the lens gently with tap water or distilled water. Replace in container.

_____ 10. Repeat steps 7–9 with the second lens.

_____ 11. Remove one contact lens from case and hold between the thumb and forefinger.

_____ 12. Apply a drop of lens-wetting solution to the inside of the lens.

_____ 13. Hold the outside of the lens on the tip of the index finger, and place gently over the iris and pupil.

_____ 14. Ask the client if the lens is in position.

_____ 15. Repeat steps 11–14 for the remaining contact lens.

C. Cleaning the eyes:

_____ 1. Encourage the client to wash eyes. If this is not possible, explain the procedure to the client.

_____ 2. Bring the equipment to the bedside and place it on the overbed table. Position table adjacent to the bed.

_____ 3. Wash hands.

_____ 4. Raise the bed level to a comfortable working height.

_____ 5. Position the client upright. Place a pillow behind the client's shoulders so that neck is hyperextended and eyes face upward.

_____ 6. Place the towel on the client's upper chest and under chin.

_____ 7. Pour a small amount of water in the basin.

_____ 8. Dip a corner of the washcloth, or a cotton ball, or a gauze sponge into the water. Squeeze to remove the excess water.

_____ 9. Gently wipe the eye from the inner to outer canthus with the dampened cloth or cotton ball.

_____ 10. Gently wipe the second eye in the same manner using a fresh cotton ball or different corner of the wash cloth.

If crusts or exudates are present:

_____ 11. Moisten a gauze sponge and position over the closed eyes. Leave in place until the crusts are softened. Repeat steps 8–10.

If the client is comatose:

_____ 12. Raise the eyelid to instill artificial tears, if ordered by the physician. Repeat every 3–4 hours.

_____ 13. Close the eyelids. Place an eye pad over the eyes and tape in position.

_____ 14. Leave the client in a position of comfort.

_____ 15. Wash hands.

Name ______________________ Date ______________

Observed by ______________

SKILL 10.3 Providing Hair Care

A. To comb or brush the client's hair, the nurse will:

_____ 1. Assess the client and determine the nursing diagnosis relevant to providing hair care.

_____ 2. Plan the expected outcomes.

_____ 3. Explain to the client what is to be done.

_____ 4. Gather the equipment and wash hands.

_____ 5. Position the client so that he is sitting upright in a chair or in bed. Place a mirror before the client so that he can see his image.

_____ 6. Place a clean towel around the client's shoulders.

If the hair is straight or slightly curly:

_____ 7. Comb or brush the hair from the scalp to the ends in sections around the head. Gently stroke the teeth of the comb or bristles of the brush against the scalp.

_____ 8. Arrange the hair in a fashion that is pleasing and attractive to the client. Use combs, barrettes, pins, or elastic bands to securely position long hair.

_____ 9. Braid the hair in one or two braids if the hair is long and the client is in bed most of the time.

If the hair is tight and curly:

_____ 7. Remove tangles or knots by using the fingers to lift and free the strands of hair. Insert the fingers in the hair and spread the fingers apart.

_____ 8. Divide the hair into sections. Working one section at a time, use a wide-tooth comb or pick to free the remaining tangles by beginning at the ends and working toward the scalp.

_____ 9. Brush the hair from the scalp to the ends. Shape and style the hair according to the wishes of the client.

For all clients:

_____ 10. Apply hair products according to the client's wishes.

_____ 11. Remove the towel from the client's shoulders. Discard in the laundry.

_____ 12. Remove hair that has collected in the comb, brush, or pick. Discard. Place the hair equipment in the client's bed unit.

_____ 13. Place the client in a position of comfort and attach call signal within his reach.

_____ 14. Wash hands.

B. To shampoo the client's hair, the nurse will:

_____ 1. Assess the client and determine the nursing diagnosis relevant to shampooing the hair.

_____ 2. Plan the expected outcomes of the shampoo.

_____ 3. Explain to the client what is to be done.

_____ 4. Gather the necessary equipment and wash hands.

If the client is bathing in a tub or shower:

_____ 5. Test the water temperature by feeling with the back of the hand.

_____ 6. Provide the client with a washcloth to cover his eyes.

_____ 7. Rinse the hair with clean water after the bath has been completed.

Proceed to step 11.

If the client can sit up in a chair:

_____ 5. Position a chair facing away from a bathroom sink.

_____ 6. Assist the client to sit in the chair. Place a towel around his shoulders.

_____ 7. Assist the client to hyperextend his head and neck back to the rim of the sink. Place a folded washcloth between his neck and the sink rim. Provide the client with a washcloth to cover his eyes.

_____ 8. Wet the hair thoroughly.

Proceed to step 11.

If the client is on a stretcher:

_____ 5. Position the stretcher so that the head end is next to a sink.

_____ 6. Position the client so that his head extends over the end of the stretcher at his neck.

_____ 7. Place a waterproof pad under the client's neck and shoulders. Place a towel around his shoulders.

_____ 8. Check the water temperature and wet the hair thoroughly using a hand-held spray nozzle or a pitcher.

Proceed to step 11.

If the client is in bed:

_____ 5. Position the bed in a flat position; raise it to a good working height. Position the client toward the nurse. Remove the pillow.

_____ 6. Place a waterproof pad under the client's head, neck, and shoulders.

_____ 7. Place the client's head on the shampoo tray. Fold a washcloth in four parts and position it between the client's neck and the rim of the shampoo tray. Provide the client with a washcloth to cover his eyes.

_____ 8. Place a waste receptacle under the drain of the tray.

_____ 9. Fill the pitcher with water at about 105°F.

_____ 10. Wet the client's hair. Use fingers to massage the water through the hair to ensure that it is thoroughly wet.

Name ______________________ Date ______________

Observed by ____________

For all clients:

_____ 11. Apply a small amount of shampoo to the palm. Rub hands together to work up a lather.

_____ 12. Lather the client's hair. Massage the scalp lightly, moving the tips of the fingers in a circular fashion around all parts of the head.

_____ 13. Squeeze excess shampoo out of the hair. Rinse with clean water.

_____ 14. Repeat steps 9–11.

_____ 15. Wrap a large bath towel around the client's head. If he is in bed, remove the shampoo board. Vigorously dry the hair by massaging with the towel.

_____ 16. Place another towel around the client's shoulders. Remove towel from the head and discard it for laundering.

_____ 17. Comb the hair to remove tangles. Dry it naturally or with a hairdryer.

_____ 18. Comb and arrange the hair as the client desires.

_____ 19. Remove towel from the client's shoulders and remove waterproof pad from the bed, discarding both for laundering.

_____ 20. Wash hands.

C. Suggested alterations for shampooing the hair in the home:

_____ 1. Shampoo the client's hair while client is in the bathtub or shower, if possible.

If client must remain in bed:

_____ 2. Find a large piece of plastic (such as old shower curtain, plastic garbage bag, or dry cleaning bag).

_____ 3. Position client on the back with head hanging below the shoulders.

_____ 4. Tuck one end of the plastic under the head.

_____ 5. Hang opposite end of plastic over end of the bed.

_____ 6. Tuck end of plastic into a large basin or bucket on the floor.

_____ 7. Roll the edges of the plastic into a trough.

_____ 8. Position a towel under the plastic behind the client's neck.

_____ 9. Implement the shampoo using the techniques or following the principles recommended by the clinical agency.

Name ______________________ Date ______________

Observed by ____________

SKILL 10.4 Shaving the Client

A. Shaving the beard:

_____ 1. Assess the client to determine the nursing diagnosis.

_____ 2. Determine the expected client outcomes.

_____ 3. Explain the procedure to the client.

_____ 4. Gather supplies and equipment and position on the overbed table or conveniently near the client.

_____ 5. Wash hands.

_____ 6. Place the client upright with a mirror placed so he can see his image.

_____ 7. Raise bed level to a convenient working height if client is in bed.

_____ 8. Drape a towel around the client's shoulders beneath his chin.

If using an electric razor:

_____ 9. Inspect the cord on the razor to determine that it is intact. Plug it into an outlet.

_____ 10. Shave all planes of the cheeks, upper lip, chin, and neck, moving the head of the razor back and forth over the hair growth. Gently hold the skin taut over the areas while shaving.

Go to step 12.

If using a safety razor:

_____ 9. Evenly apply shaving lather, cream, or soap over the hair growth areas. A damp, hot towel may be applied if the hair growth is particularly tough or long, or if the client prefers.

_____ 10. Hold the skin taut and shave all planes of the cheeks, upper lip, chin, and neck, pulling the razor blade lightly but firmly with direction of hair growth.

_____ 11. Rinse the razor and blade periodically in the water basin.

Whether shaving with an electric or safety razor:

_____ 12. Rinse and dry the shaved areas with a warm wet washcloth or towel.

_____ 13. Apply aftershave lotion or cream, according to the client's wishes.

_____ 14. Remove the towel from the client's shoulders, and discard in laundry.

_____ 15. Place the client in a comfortable position and leave the call signal within reach.

_____ 16. Clean and replace the razor and other supplies.

_____ 17. Wash hands.

B. Shaving the underarms or legs:

_____ 1. Determine how the client wishes shave to be done.

_____ 2. Gather the necessary equipment and position conveniently near the client.

_____ 3. Wash hands.

_____ 4. Position and drape the client in a manner convenient for the procedure. Protect the bed with a waterproof pad or towel if the procedure is being done in bed.

If using an electric razor:

_____ 5. Inspect the cord on the razor to determine that it is intact. Plug it into an outlet.

_____ 6. Shave all surfaces that the client desires in the direction against the hair growth.

If using a safety razor:

_____ 5. Apply shaving lather, cream, or soap evenly over the areas to be shaved.

_____ 6. Shave all surfaces that the client desires in direction against the hair growth. Periodically rinse razor in water.

Whether shaving with an electric or safety razor:

_____ 7. Rinse the entire shaved area with warm water and dry.

_____ 8. Apply deodorant, powder, or lotion according to the client's preferences.

_____ 9. Remove towels, pads, and equipment. Dispose in laundry.

_____ 10. Place the client in a position of comfort and attach call signal within the client's reach.

_____ 11. Clean and replace equipment.

_____ 12. Wash hands.

Name ______________________________ Date ______________

Observed by ____________

SKILL 10.5 Providing Nail Care

_____ 1. Assess the client's nails and determine the nursing diagnosis.

_____ 2. Plan the expected outcomes of the nail care.

_____ 3. Explain to the client what is to be done.

_____ 4. Gather the equipment and arrange it conveniently near the client.

_____ 5. Wash hands.

_____ 6. Fill the basin half full with water about 105°F. Set it on the client's overbed table if the fingernails are being cleaned, or on the floor near the client's feet if the toenails are being cleaned.

If the fingernails are being cleaned and trimmed:

_____ 7. Instruct the client to soak his hand in the basin for about 15–20 minutes. Warm the water after 10 minutes, if desired.

If the toenails are being cleaned and trimmed (the nurse may prefer to wear clean gloves while cleaning and trimming the toenails):

_____ 8. Place a waterproof pad under the client's feet, and place the client's foot in the basin for about 15–20 minutes.

_____ 9. Remove the hand or foot and dry thoroughly, particularly between the fingers and the toes. Place the other hand or foot in the basin.

_____ 10. Push the cuticles back gently with the towel. Repeat, using the blunt end of the orange stick, until the cuticles are neatly pushed back.

_____ 11. Scrape gently under the nails with the orange stick or file. Remove all accumulations, and wipe the stick or file on a tissue. Continue until all nails are cleaned.

_____ 12. Repeat steps 7 and 8 with the other hand or foot.

_____ 13. Remove the basin and set aside.

_____ 14. Clip or trim the nails straight across with the clippers or scissors. Carefully avoid cutting the surrounding tissues.

_____ 15. File and shape the fingernails with the emergy board or file. Smooth the cut edges of the toenails.

_____ 16. Apply lotion to the dry areas of both the feet and the hands.

_____ 17. Position the client comfortably and place the call signal within his reach.

_____ 18. Empty and clean the basin and replace in the client's bed unit. Discard towels in the laundry. Dispose of waterproof pad and other equipment.

_____ 19. Wash hands.

Name ______________________________ Date ______________________

Observed by ____________

CHAPTER 11 USING TECHNIQUES OF PHYSICAL EXAMINATION

SKILL 11.1 Using Techniques of Physical Examination

A. Preparation:

_____ 1. Explain to the client what will happen during the examination. Answer questions and assure the client of his privacy.

_____ 2. Close the door to the examination room or client's room or draw the curtains around his bed.

_____ 3. Wash hands.

_____ 4. Expose the body area to be examined. Drape the remainder of the body as necessary.

_____ 5. Direct lighting on the exposed area.

_____ 6. Place the client in the desired position.

B. Inspection:

_____ 7. Inspect the general shape or form of the body area. Compare to the opposite side of the body.

_____ 8. Observe for abnormalities.

_____ 9. Repeat inspection to verify the findings.

_____ 10. Move to the next skill.

C. Palpation:

_____ 11. Rub your hands together to warm them.

_____ 12. Ask the client to take a deep breath if palpation may cause anxiety or pain.

_____ 13. Use your fingertips to feel or probe a body part. Use gentle pressure.

_____ 14. Lift the fingers completely away from the skin when moving to another body part.

_____ 15. Examine the body part last that may be tender or painful.

_____ 16. Note unusual or abnormal characteristics.

If a lump, nodule, or tumor is located:

_____ 17. Feel for the size, shape, and consistency; attempt to move it with the fingers.

_____ 18. Palpate again to confirm findings. Perform percussion.

D. Percussion:

_____ 19. Place the middle finger (the *pleximeter*) of your nondominant hand on the area to be percussed. Hold the remaining fingers, thumb, and palm away from the client's body.

_____ 20. Flex the dominant wrist briskly and rhythmically, tapping the distal joint of the pleximeter with the tip of the middle finger (the *plexor* or hammer).

_____ 21. Tap two or three times in rapid succession; pause; tap again or move to an area opposite the body from the first area.

_____ 22. Listen carefully for characteristics and qualities of the sounds.

_____ 23. Tap, listen, and compare the sounds in body parts opposite each other.

_____ 24. Move to the next technique.

E. Auscultation:

_____ 25. Cleanse the eartips and chestpiece of the stethoscope with an antiseptic swab.

_____ 26. Place the eartips into your ears, with the curve of the binaurals pointing slightly posterior to the ears.

_____ 27. Tap lightly on the diaphragm of the stethoscope. Rotate the chestpiece if noise is not heard.

_____ 28. Place the flat surface of the diaphragm against the palm and enfold it with the hand for a few seconds.

_____ 29. Tell the client that you will be placing the stethoscope against his body.

_____ 30. Place the flat surface of the diaphragm on the client's body surface and listen.

_____ 31. Note the sound's characteristics and qualities.

_____ 32. Move the diaphragm systematically over the body area, comparing sounds.

F. Conclusion:

_____ 33. Replace the client's clothing or bedcovers.

_____ 34. Reposition the client comfortably.

_____ 35. Open the curtains or door to the room.

_____ 36. Discuss the results of the examination with the client; answer his questions.

_____ 37. Wash hands.

Name ______________________ Date ______________

Observed by ____________

CHAPTER 12 ASSESSING THE VITAL SIGNS

SKILL 12.1 Assessing Temperature

A. Oral temperature:

_____ 1. Assess the client to identify signs or symptoms suggestive of temperature alteration.

_____ 2. Plan the nursing objectives and expected outcomes.

_____ 3. Explain to the client that his temperature is to be measured.

_____ 4. Wash hands.

Before inserting an electronic thermometer:

_____ 5. Remove the thermometer from its base and check to see that it is fully charged.

_____ 6. Place a cover on the probe.

Before inserting a glass thermometer:

_____ 7. Hold the thermometer at the end opposite (distal) the bulb and rinse in cold water.

_____ 8. Wipe the thermometer from the bulb end to the fingers with a clean paper towel.

_____ 9. Holding the thermometer horizontal at eye level, rotate it until the scale is visible and read the mercury.

_____ 10. Grasp the distal end securely and shake the thermometer downward with a brisk flick of the wrist. Read the scale and repeat until the desired temperature is reached.

When using either thermometer:

_____ 11. Instruct the client to open his mouth and hold his tongue against the upper teeth.

_____ 12. Insert the thermometer gently under the tongue between the frenulum and lower gum.

_____ 13. Instruct the client to close his mouth and hold the thermometer in place between his lips.

When using an electronic thermometer:

_____ 14. Watch the digital panel to make sure the thermometer is recording the temperature.

_____ 15. Leave the probe in place until the portable unit signals that the maximum body temperature has been reached.

_____ 16. Check the digital panel and note the temperature.

_____ 17. Grasp the distal end of the probe and instruct the client to open his mouth; remove the probe.

_____ 18. Eject the probe cover into a wastebasket.

When using a glass thermometer:

_____ 14. Leave the thermometer in place for 3–11 minutes, according to agency guidelines.

_____ 15. Hold the distal tip and instruct the client to open his mouth; remove the thermometer.

_____ 16. Wipe the thermometer with a tissue, moving from the distal to bulb end. Discard tissue in wastebasket.

_____ 17. Read the thermometer and record immediately.

_____ 18. Wash the thermometer with cool soapy water and rinse with cool water. Dry with a paper towel and replace in the storage container.

After using either thermometer:

_____ 18. Tell the client his temperature reading.

_____ 19. Wash hands.

B. Rectal temperature:

_____ 1. Assess the client to identify signs or symptoms suggestive of temperature alteration.

_____ 2. Plan the nursing objectives and expected outcomes.

_____ 3. Explain to the client that his temperature is to be measured.

_____ 4. Wash hands.

Before inserting an electronic thermometer:

_____ 5. Remove the portable thermometer from its base; check to make sure the unit is charged.

_____ 6. Place a probe cover on the probe.

Before inserting a glass thermometer:

_____ 5. Hold the thermometer at the end opposite the bulb and rinse in cold water.

_____ 6. Wipe the thermometer from the fingers to the bulb end with a clean paper towel.

_____ 7. Holding the thermometer horizontal at eye level, rotate it until the scale is visible and read the mercury.

_____ 8. Grasp the distal end securely and shake the thermometer downward with a brisk flick of the wrist until the desired temperature is reached.

When using either thermometer:

_____ 9. Don clean disposable gloves.

_____ 10. Apply a lubricant to the bulb end of the thermometer. Place near the client.

_____ 11. Close the curtains around the hospital client's bed unit or close the door to his room. Lower siderails.

Name ______ Date ______

Observed by ______

_____ 12. Assist the client into a lateral position with his upper leg flexed or in Sims' position.

_____ 13. Lower the client's pajama bottoms and arrange bed linens to expose the buttocks only.

_____ 14. Lift the client's upper buttocks gently with the nondominant hand.

_____ 15. Touch the tip of the thermometer to the client's anus, telling him what you are doing. Ask him to take a deep breath.

_____ 16. Insert the thermometer gently into the anus, pointing it toward the client's umbilicus, guiding it along the wall of the rectum. Insert up to approximately 3 inches in adults; about $\frac{1}{2}$ inch in infants.

When using an electronic thermometer:

_____ 17. Watch the digital panel until the portable unit signals that the maximum body temperature is reached.

_____ 18. Remove the thermometer gently.

_____ 19. Note the recording on the digital panel.

_____ 20. Eject the probe cover into a wastebasket.

When using a glass thermometer:

_____ 17. Hold the thermometer in place for 2–4 minutes, according to agency guidelines.

_____ 18. Remove the thermometer gently.

_____ 19. Wipe the thermometer from fingers to bulb with a clean tissue, rotating the tissue around the cylinder; discard tissue.

_____ 20. Read the thermometer and set it aside.

After using either thermometer:

_____ 21. Inform the client of his temperature.

_____ 22. Record the temperature immediately.

_____ 23. Remove residual lubricant from the anal area of the client with a tissue; discard. Or hand a tissue to the client for him to do this.

_____ 24. Reposition the client's pajamas and replace the bedcovers. Raise the siderails.

After using a glass thermometer:

_____ 25. Wash the thermometer with cool soapy water and rinse with cool water; dry with a paper towel.

_____ 26. Replace the thermometer in the storage container.

When using either thermometer:

_____ 27. Discard gloves and wash hands.

_____ 28. Open curtains or the door to the room.

C. Axillary temperature:

_____ 1. Assess the client to identify signs or symptoms suggestive of temperature alteration.

_____ 2. Plan the nursing objectives and expected outcomes.

_____ 3. Explain to the client that his temperature is to be measured.

_____ 4. Wash hands.

Before inserting an electronic thermometer:

_____ 5. Remove the portable thermometer unit from its base. Check to make sure the unit is charged.

_____ 6. Place a probe cover on the probe.

Before inserting a glass thermometer:

_____ 5. Hold the thermometer at the end opposite the bulb and rinse in cold water.

_____ 6. Wipe the thermometer from the fingers to the bulb end with a clean paper towel.

_____ 7. Holding the thermometer horizontal at eye level, rotate it until the scale is visible and read the mercury.

_____ 8. Grasp the distal end securely and shake the thermometer downward with a brisk flick of the wrist until the desired temperature is reached.

When using either thermometer:

_____ 9. Draw the curtain around the client's bed or close the door to his room.

_____ 10. Position the client supine or sitting.

_____ 11. Remove the client's gown or clothing from his arm and shoulder.

_____ 12. Raise the client's arm and gently dry the axilla with a towel.

_____ 13. Place the bulb or probe tip into the center of the axilla. Hold in place.

_____ 14. Lower the client's arm over the thermometer and place the arm across his chest.

_____ 15. Hold the electronic thermometer in place until the maximum temperature is recorded; hold the glass thermometer in place for 10 minutes.

_____ 16. Raise the client's arm and remove thermometer. Replace clothing.

After using an electronic thermometer:

_____ 17. Note the recording on the digital panel and record immediately.

_____ 18. Eject the probe cover into a wastebasket.

After using a glass thermometer:

_____ 17. Wipe the thermometer with a tissue, moving from the distal to bulb end. Discard tissue in wastebasket.

_____ 18. Read the thermometer and record immediately.

Name ____________________ Date ____________________

Observed by ____________

_____ 19. Wash the thermometer with cool soapy water and rinse with cool water. Dry with a paper towel and replace in the storage container.

After using either thermometer:

_____ 20. Inform the client of his temperature.

_____ 21. Position the client as he desires; open bedside curtains or the door to his room.

_____ 22. Wash hands.

Name ____________________ Date ____________________

Observed by ____________

SKILL 12.2 Assessing the Pulse

A. Assessing the apical pulse:

_____ 1. Assess the client to identify factors relating to the pulse rate, rhythm, quality, or how the pulse is to be monitored.

_____ 2. Plan the method of monitoring and prepare the necessary equipment.

_____ 3. Explain to the client that his pulse will be assessed.

_____ 4. Wash hands.

_____ 5. Clean the earpieces and diaphragm of the stethoscope with an antiseptic swab.

_____ 6. Assist the client to a supine or low Fowler's position.

_____ 7. Draw the curtains around the client's bed or close the door to his room.

_____ 8. Adjust the top bed linens and the client's gown so that his left chest is exposed.

_____ 9. Rub the bell or diaphragm of the stethoscope with the palm of your hand.

_____ 10. Place earpieces in your ears.

_____ 11. Place the stethoscope bell on the fourth or fifth intercostal space in the left midclavicular area of the client's chest.

_____ 12. Listen for a "rubb-dubb" sound. Move the bell until it is located.

_____ 13. Listen for the rhythm of the heart beat.

_____ 14. Look at the watch dial. Note the location of the second hand and start counting beats, "zero, one, two . . . " until the 60 seconds have passed.

_____ 15. Remove the stethoscope and replace the client's clothing and bed linens.

_____ 16. Tell the client his pulse rate.

_____ 17. Record the apical rate immediately.

_____ 18. Wash hands. Clean stethoscope earpieces and bell or diaphragm.

B. Assessing the radial pulse:

_____ 1. Assess the client to identify factors relating to the pulse rate, rhythm, quality, or how the pulse is to be monitored.

_____ 2. Plan the method of monitoring and prepare the necessary equipment.

_____ 3. Explain to the client that his pulse will be assessed.

_____ 4. Wash hands.

_____ 5. Position the supine client with his arm across his chest, palm down. Position the sitting client with his arm on his lap, palm down.

_____ 6. Place the first three fingers of your dominant hand on the client's radial artery, located just below his thumb between the radius and tendons.

_____ 7. Locate the pulsating radial artery. Feel the sensations for a few seconds, noting the rhythm and quality of the pulse.

_____ 8. Look at the watch dial. Note the location of the second hand and start counting beats, "zero, one, two . . . " until 15, 30, or 60 seconds have passed.

_____ 9. Multiply the count by 4 if the pulse was monitored for 15 seconds; multiply the count by 2 if the pulse was monitored for 30 seconds.

_____ 10. Tell the client his pulse rate. Return him to a comfortable position.

_____ 11. Record the pulse rate, rhythm, and quality immediately.

_____ 12. Wash hands.

C. Determining if an apical-radial deficit is present:

_____ 1. Listen to the heart sounds apically and palpate the radial pulse simultaneously. Determine whether pulse and beat are synchronous.

D. Measuring an apical-radial deficit:

_____ 1. Explain to the client that one nurse is counting his heart beats while the second nurse counts his radial pulse. Explain that this is done to monitor for abnormalities.

_____ 2. Prepare to monitor the apical pulse as in steps 4–13 in "Assessing the apical pulse."

_____ 3. Direct the second nurse to locate and prepare to count the radial pulse as in steps 5–7 in "Assessing the radial pulse."

_____ 4. Look at the watch dial. Note the location of the second hand and signal to the second nurse to begin counting at "zero, one, two . . . "

_____ 5. Count the remaining 60 seconds silently as the second nurse counts the radial pulse silently.

_____ 6. Say, "Stop," when exactly 60 seconds have passed.

_____ 7. Reposition the client comfortably.

_____ 8. Record the apical and radial rates immediately. Note any deficits.

_____ 9. Wash hands.

Name ______________________________ Date ______________________

Observed by ____________

SKILL 12.3 Assessing Respirations

_____ 1. Assess the client to identify factors relating to the respiratory rate, rhythm, and quality.

_____ 2. Avoid explaining the observation to the client.

_____ 3. Wash hands.

_____ 4. Position the client's wrist over his chest and hold his wrist as if measuring pulse rate.

_____ 5. Hold the client's wrist and pretend to count his pulse rate.
OR
Place your hand on the client's chest to feel the chest rise and fall with every inspiration and expiration.

_____ 6. Observe the client's chest as it rises and falls with inspiration and expiration.

_____ 7. Note the depth, pattern, or quality.

_____ 8. Look at the watch dial. Note the location of the second hand and begin counting the full respiration cycle, "one two, three . . . " or 30 seconds if depth and pattern appear normal or for a full 60 seconds if the client is a young child or has observable abnormalities of depth, pattern, or quality.

_____ 9. Proceed with monitoring the pulse rate.

_____ 10. Record both respiratory and pulse rates immediately. Discuss with the client as seems necessary.

_____ 11. Wash hands.

Name ______________________________ Date ______________

Observed by ____________

SKILL 12.4 Measuring Blood Pressure

A. Measuring blood pressure by auscultation of the brachial artery:

____ 1. Assess the client to determine factors that may affect blood pressure reading.

____ 2. Plan the expected outcomes.

____ 3. Explain to the client that you are going to measure his blood pressure. Answer his questions.

____ 4. Wash hands.

____ 5. Position the client who is sitting with his arm resting on his lap or arm rest with the upper arm at heart level, palms up.
OR
Position the client supine with his arm resting at his side, with the upper arm at heart level, palm up.

____ 6. Check the mercury level (or needle of the dial) to ensure it is at zero.

____ 7. Measure the cuff width against the client's arm to ensure accurate fit.

____ 8. Position yourself within 3 feet of the sphygmomanometer so that the mercury meniscus is at eye level (or the dial of the aneroid manometer is directly in front of the eyes).

____ 9. Palpate the brachial artery pulse.

____ 10. Expel any air in the inflation bladder of the cuff by releasing the valve lock.

____ 11. Wrap the cuff evenly and snugly around the client's upper arm, centering the arrow on the cuff over the brachial artery and placing the lower edge of the cuff about 1 inch above the antecubital fossa.

____ 12. Secure by fastening the Velcro or tucking the end of the wrap under the cuff.

____ 13. Ensure that the connecting tubings are free of each other.

____ 14. Place earpieces of the stethoscope in your ears.

____ 15. Palpate the brachial artery while holding the bell or diaphragm in the palm of your nondominant hand.

____ 16. Hold the hand pump in the dominant hand and tighten the valve lock with the thumb.

____ 17. Inflate the cuff briskly with a pumping action while palpating the artery. Watch the mercury level (or needle of the dial).

____ 18. Note when the brachial pulse disappears; remove your fingers and place bell or diaphragm on the artery immediately.

____ 19. Stop inflating the cuff when the mercury rises 30 mm above the point where the pulse disappeared.

_____ 20. Slowly loosen the valve lock and deflate the cuff.

_____ 21. Listen and watch the mercury level drop; when you hear the first two "tap tap" sounds, note the systolic measurement.

_____ 22. Listen for the change in the Korotkoff's sounds.

_____ 23. When the sounds disappear, note the diastolic measurement.

_____ 24. Open the valve lock completely after noting the diastolic pressure.

_____ 25. Remove the cuff.

_____ 26. Inform the client of his blood pressure reading.

_____ 27. Reposition the client comfortably.

_____ 28. Record the reading immediately.

_____ 29. Wash hands and clean stethoscope.

B. Measuring blood pressure by palpation:

_____ 1. Assess the client to determine factors that may affect the blood pressure reading.

_____ 2. Plan the expected outcomes.

_____ 3. Explain to the client that you are going to measure his blood pressure. Answer his questions.

_____ 4. Wash hands.

_____ 5. Position the client who is sitting with his arm resting on his lap or the arm rest of a chair with the upper arm at heart level, palms up.
OR
Position the client supine with his arm resting at his side, with the upper arm at heart level, palm up.

_____ 6. Check the mercury level (or needle of the dial) to ensure it is at zero.

_____ 7. Measure the cuff width against the client's arm to ensure accurate fit.

_____ 8. Position yourself within 3 feet of the sphygmomanometer so that the mercury meniscus is at eye level (or the dial of the aneroid manometer is directly in front of the eyes).

_____ 9. Palpate the brachial artery pulse.

_____ 10. Expel any air in the inflation bladder of the cuff by releasing the valve lock.

_____ 11. Wrap the cuff evenly and snugly around the client's upper arm, centering the arrow on the cuff over the brachial artery and placing the lower edge of the cuff about 1 inch above the antecubital fossa.

_____ 12. Secure by fastening the Velcro or tucking the end of the wrap under the cuff.

_____ 13. Palpate the brachial artery again.

_____ 14. Hold the hand pump in your dominant hand and tighten the valve lock with the thumb.

_____ 15. Inflate the cuff briskly with a pumping action while palpating the artery. Watch the mercury level (or needle of the dial).

_____ 16. Note when the brachial pulse disappears.

Name ______________________ Date ______________

Observed by ________

_____ 17. Stop inflating the cuff when the mercury rises 30 mm above the point where the pulse disappeared.

_____ 18. Slowly loosen the valve lock and deflate the cuff.

_____ 19. Palpate and watch the mercury level drop; when you feel the first two consecutive pulsations, note the systolic measurement.

_____ 20. Continue to deflate the cuff, noting any change in the character of the palpation.

_____ 21. Open the valve lock completely after the mercury has fallen 35–40 mm.

_____ 22. Remove the cuff.

_____ 23. Inform the client of his blood pressure reading.

_____ 24. Reposition the client comfortably.

_____ 25. Record the reading immediately.

_____ 26. Wash hands and clean stethoscope.

C. Measuring blood pressure by auscultation of the popliteal artery:

_____ 1. Assess the client to determine factors that may affect blood pressure reading.

_____ 2. Plan the expected outcomes.

_____ 3. Explain to the client that you are going to measure his blood pressure. Answer his questions.

_____ 4. Wash hands.

_____ 5. Select a wide cuff to connect to the sphygmomanometer.

_____ 6. Check the mercury level (or needle of the dial) to ensure it is at zero.

_____ 7. Measure the cuff width against the client's leg to ensure accurate fit.

_____ 8. Assist the client to a prone position.

_____ 9. Remove constricting clothing from the leg.

_____ 10. Locate the popliteal pulse behind the knee.

_____ 11. Position yourself within 3 feet of sphygmomanometer so that the mercury meniscus is at eye level (or the dial of the aneroid manometer is directly in front of the eyes).

_____ 12. Expel any air in the inflation bladder of the cuff by releasing the valve lock.

_____ 13. Wrap the cuff evenly and snugly around the client's thigh, centering the arrow on the cuff over the popliteal artery and placing the lower edge of the cuff about 1 inch above the popliteal fossa.

_____ 14. Ensure that the connecting tubings are free of each other.

_____ **15.** Place earpieces of the stethoscope in the ears.

_____ **16.** Palpate the popliteal artery while holding the bell or diaphragm in the palm of the nondominant hand.

_____ **17.** Hold the hand pump in the dominant hand and tighten the valve lock with the thumb.

_____ **18.** Inflate the cuff briskly with a pumping action while palpating the artery. Watch the mercury level (or needle of the dial).

_____ **19.** When the popliteal pulse disappears, remove your fingers and place bell or diaphragm on the artery immediately.

_____ **20.** Stop inflating the cuff when the mercury rises 30 mm above the point where the pulse disappeared.

_____ **21.** Slowly loosen the valve lock and deflate the cuff.

_____ **22.** Listen and watch the mercury level drop; when you hear the first two "tap tap" sounds, note the systolic measurement.

_____ **23.** Listen for the change in the Korotkoff's sounds.

_____ **24.** When the sounds disappear, note the diastolic measurement.

_____ **25.** Open the valve lock completely after noting the diastolic pressure.

_____ **26.** Remove the cuff.

_____ **27.** Inform the client of his blood pressure reading.

_____ **28.** Reposition the client comfortably.

_____ **29.** Record the reading immediately.

_____ **30.** Wash hands and clean stethoscope.

Name ______________________________ Date ______________

Observed by ____________

CHAPTER 13 MEASURING WEIGHT AND HEIGHT

SKILL 13.1 Measuring Weight

A. Measuring weight on a standard scale:

_____ 1. Assess the client for factors that may affect weight.

_____ 2. Plan the nursing objectives and expected outcomes.

_____ 3. Explain to the client that he will be weighed. Explain the purpose.

_____ 4. Bring the scale to the client's bedside if appropriate.

_____ 5. Check the scale balance; adjust as necessary.

_____ 6. Draw the bedside curtains or close the room door.

_____ 7. Ask the client to void if his bladder is full. Assist as necessary.

_____ 8. Assist the client to remove as many clothes as possible.

_____ 9. Place the scale next to a wall or a rigid chair back.

_____ 10. Place a clean paper towel on the foot platform.

_____ 11. Help the client to step onto the center of the foot platform.

_____ 12. Adjust the weights on the balance beam until the beam is level. Note the weight demarcation and record it immediately.

_____ 13. Assist the client to a comfortable position in bed or a chair.

_____ 14. Inform the client if weight gain or loss has occurred.

_____ 15. Return the scale weights to their neutral position at 0.

B. Measuring weight on a chair or bed scale:

_____ 1. Assess the client for factors that may affect weight.

_____ 2. Plan the nursing objectives and expected outcomes.

_____ 3. Explain to the client that he will be weighed. Explain the purpose.

_____ 4. Bring the scale to the client's bedside if appropriate.

_____ 5. Check the scale balance; adjust as necessary.

_____ 6. Draw the bedside curtains or close the room door.

_____ 7. Ask the client to void if his bladder is full. Assist as necessary.

_____ 8. Assist the client to remove as many clothes as possible.

_____ 9. Place a clean drawsheet over the seat of the chair scale.
OR
Place a clean turning sheet under client if he does not have one.

_____ 10. Transfer the client to the chair or bed scale.

_____ 11. Adjust the weights on the balance beam until the beam is level. Note the weight demarcation and record immediately.

_____ 12. Transfer the client back into bed. Assist him to a comfortable position.

_____ 13. Inform the client if weight gain or loss has occurred.

_____ 14. Return the scale weights to their neutral position at 0.

C. Weighing an infant:

_____ 1. Assess the client for factors that may affect weight.

_____ 2. Plan the nursing objectives and expected outcomes.

_____ 3. Wash hands.

_____ 4. Place a protective covering on the scale tray.

_____ 5. Determine if the scale is balanced; if not, correct the balance.

_____ 6. Remove all clothing from the infant.

_____ 7. Place the infant on the scale tray, holding him in place with one hand.

_____ 8. Adjust the balance beam weights with the free hand until it is nearly balanced; remove hand from infant briefly to check that beam is balanced.

_____ 9. Note the weight demarcation line.

_____ 10. Remove the infant from the scale tray; dress and replace him in his crib or in the arms of his parent or another health worker.

_____ 11. Record the weight immediately.

_____ 12. Inform the infant's parent, if present, about the weight.

_____ 13. Remove the protector from scale.

_____ 14. Return the scale weights to their neutral position at 0.

_____ 15. Wash hands.

Name ______________________ Date ______________

Observed by __________

SKILL 13.2 Measuring Height

A. Measuring height with a floor scale measuring device:

_____ 1. Assess the client for factors that may affect height.

_____ 2. Plan the nursing objectives and expected outcomes.

_____ 3. Explain to the client that his height will be measured. Explain the reason.

_____ 4. Instruct the client to remove his shoes or slippers.

_____ 5. Raise the headbar of the floor scale well above the client's head. Extend it to a right angle from the measuring bar.

_____ 6. Instruct the client to stand on the scale foot platform with his body erect against the measuring bar.

_____ 7. Lower the headbar to the highest point on the client's head.

_____ 8. Examine the demarcations on the vertical bar for the exact height. Note and record the height immediately.

_____ 9. Raise the headbar and help the client step off the scale foot platform.

_____ 10. Assist the client to a comfortable bed or chair position.

_____ 11. Tell the client his height.

_____ 12. Lower the headbar and remove scale.

B. Measuring an infant's length:

_____ 1. Assess the client for factors that may affect height.

_____ 2. Plan the nursing objectives and expected outcomes.

_____ 3. Wash hands.

_____ 4. Place a clean paper towel on the flat surface next to the measuring scale.

_____ 5. Place the infant on the surface so that the soles of his feet are flat against the upright measuring structure at zero.

_____ 6. Hold the infant's knees extended and position the top of his head against the measuring device with his face pointing upward.

_____ 7. Note the demarcation on the scale closest to the infant's head.

_____ 8. Remove the infant and place him safely in his bed or with his parent or another health worker.

_____ 9. Record the length immediately.

_____ 10. Tell the client's parents, if present, his length. Wash hands.

Name ______________________ Date ______________

Observed by __________

CHAPTER 14 ADMISSION, TRANSFER, AND DISCHARGE

SKILL 14.1 Admitting the Client

_____ 1. Prepare the client's room or bed unit:

- Open a closed bed.
- Place the bed in its lowest position.
- Check for the presence of unit supplies.
- Equip the unit with any other required supplies.

_____ 2. Introduce yourself to the client and his family when they arrive. Demonstrate both interest and concern for their well-being.

_____ 3. Take the client and his family to the assigned unit.

_____ 4. Ask if the client has any immediate needs; respond to requests immediately.

_____ 5. Introduce client to other clients in the room.

_____ 6. Orient the client to the room and its facilities.

- Show him the bathroom.
- Show him where he may store his clothing or other personal belongings.
- Demonstrate how to control the bed.
- Explain how to work any other bedside equipment that he will use (such as the overbed table).
- Demonstrate how the call signal works.
- Explain how to use the telephone, television, or radio.

_____ 7. Orient the client to the hospital or agency.

- Indicate time of visiting hours.
- Tell him the name of the charge nurse and how to contact her.
- Indicate when meals are served.
- Describe other hospital areas that he may use: lounges, coffee shops, chapel.
- Explain how to obtain a television or radio.
- Explain agency's smoking policy.
- Give him any pamphlets or written materials that explain hospital policies or procedures.

_____ 8. Give the client information about the agency's Patient Bill of Rights and Responsibilities.

_____ 9. Instruct the client to don his own bed clothing or provide a hospital gown. Assist as necessary. If the client is able to undress, provide privacy.

_____ 10. Perform agency's required physical assessments when client is in bed clothing. Usually these are

- vital signs
- height and weight

_____ 11. Interview the client using the agency's admission criteria. These data include

- reason for hospitalization
- brief medical and surgical history
- history of allergies
- present medications or treatments

_____ 12. If client has brought any medications with him, instruct him or the family to take them home, or arrange to store medications in hospital pharmacy.

_____ 13. Inform the client that a urine specimen is required. Provide him with a collecting container and give any necessary instructions.

_____ 14. Inform the client that blood tests, x-rays, or other tests will be performed within a short period of time. Explain the reasons.

_____ 15. Pause to reflect on the admission process with the client; ask if he or his family have questions. Provide answers as completely as possible.

_____ 16. Document admission data immediately; post allergy alerts (if needed) on the chart and Kardex.

_____ 17. Interview the client for the nursing history when other tasks are complete or as time permits.

_____ 18. Perform further physical assessments as needed.

_____ 19. Document all findings in the medical record following agency guidelines.

_____ 20. Implement the physician's orders as soon as they are written.

Name ______________________ Date ______________

Observed by __________

SKILL 14.2 Transferring the Client

A. Intra-agency transfer:

_____ 1. Inform the client of the transfer and explain the reasons. Include the exact room number and telephone number. Provide an opportunity for questions or verbalizing concerns from the client. Inform the client's family as needed.

_____ 2. Check the medical record to ensure that current documentation is complete.

_____ 3. Gather together the following and load all but the records on a utility cart:

- all of the client's personal belongings
- the client's medical records, including the Kardex card, old charts, and medication administration record if kept separate from the medical record
- the client's supplies and equipment that have been charged to him
- bedside unit supplies

_____ 4. Check with the receiving unit to ensure they are prepared for the client's arrival. Determine, if possible, the receiving room.

_____ 5. Record time, method of transfer, and receiving unit in the medical record.

_____ 6. Help the client to transfer to a wheelchair or stretcher.

_____ 7. Transport client and supplies to receiving unit. Carry his records. Monitor his condition frequently if he is unstable.

_____ 8. Deposit medical records, Kardex, medication administration records, and medications at the receiving nurses' station.

_____ 9. Introduce the client to the receiving nurse upon arrival. Together, transport client to his new location.

_____ 10. Help the client to get into his new bed; help unpack his belongings.

_____ 11. Report pertinent information to the receiving nurse.

_____ 12. Return to unit and notify appropriate agency departments that the transfer is complete.

_____ 13. Strip the bed and arrange for cleaning the client's vacated bed unit.

B. Interagency transfer:

_____ 1. Inform the client of the transfer and explain the reasons. Provide an opportunity for questions or verbalizing concerns from the client. Inform his family if he cannot.

_____ 2. Prepare a referral document as required by the receiving agency. Telephone the receiving charge nurse if you have questions or particular concerns.

_____ 3. Arrange a method of transportation from one agency to the other:

- ambulance
- taxi
- family's or friend's private automobile

_____ 4. Check the medical record to ensure that current documentation is complete.

_____ 5. Arrange for copies of the medical record to accompany the client.

_____ 6. Gather and pack the following:

- all of the client's personal belongings
- the client's supplies and equipment that have been charged to him

_____ 7. Telephone the receiving agency to ensure that the nursing staff is ready to receive the client.

_____ 8. Assess the client for potential or actual problems that could harm him during the transfer. Intervene as necessary.

_____ 9. Perform discharge tasks required by the agency.

_____ 10. Help the client to transfer to a wheelchair or stretcher.

_____ 11. Accompany the client to the transporting vehicle.

Name ______________________________ Date ______________________

Observed by ____________

SKILL 14.3 Discharging the Client

Prior to discharge:

_____ 1. Arrange conferences with the client and his caregivers to plan arrangements and answer questions.

_____ 2. Demonstrate therapies that the client or his caregiver will perform at home.

_____ 3. Teach the client and his caregivers about medication effects and administration.

_____ 4. Prepare appropriate referral forms if necessary.

On the day of discharge:

_____ 5. Check the physician's orders for completeness; check for medications or therapies ordered and follow-up care instructions.

_____ 6. Check with the client to determine when his transportation will arrive.

_____ 7. Encourage the client and his caregivers to ask questions regarding his discharge.

_____ 8. Explain all discharge instructions prepared by the physician.

_____ 9. Confirm follow-up arrangements with other health care agencies, if necessary.

_____ 10. Assist the client with dressing and with packing his belongings and supplies as he wishes.

_____ 11. Check drawers, closets, and valuables storage areas to be sure all of the client's belongings are packed.

_____ 12. Load the client's belongings on a utility cart.

_____ 13. Arrange for the client and his family to visit the agency business office to finalize payment arrangements.

_____ 14. Transfer client to a wheelchair or stretcher.

_____ 15. Escort client and his family to the transportation vehicle. Help transfer both the client and his belongings. Leave only when the client is safely in the vehicle.

_____ 16. Upon returning to the nursing unit, notify the appropriate agency department that the client has left.

_____ 17. Strip the client's bed and arrange for cleaning the bed unit.

Name ______________________ Date ______________

Observed by ____________

CHAPTER 15 ASSESSING MUSCULOSKELETAL FUNCTION

SKILL 15.1 Assessing Musculoskeletal Function

_____ 1. Explain to the client that his body posture, form, muscles, and bones will be examined to help determine the nursing assistance required.

_____ 2. Wash hands.

_____ 3. Ask the client to walk from chair or bed to the door of the room and back. Ask him to remain standing.

_____ 4. Observe the client's general appearance. Note body proportions, posture, symmetry of body parts, and the client's ease when moving.

_____ 5. Ask the client to don a hospital gown or remove all of clothing except undergarments. Close the bed curtains or the door to the room.

_____ 6. Inspect the spine, observing for normal curvature, symmetry of muscles, uniform shoulder height.

_____ 7. Note abnormalities in lateral curvature or exaggerated cervical, thoracic, or lumbar curvature of the spine.

_____ 8. Inspect the client's legs for symmetry or deformities.

_____ 9. Ask the client to bend the knees slightly and lean the body forward so that his hands hang freely above feet.

_____ 10. Note the symmetry and ease of movements. Note limitations to joint flexibility.

_____ 11. Have the client sit on a chair or on the side of the bed.

_____ 12. Observe for the following during the examination:

- any alteration in the usual joint range of motion (limitations or instability)
- swelling around a joint or bony prominence
- pain or tenderness during palpation or movement
- increased temperature (heat) of skin over joints or bony prominences
- asymmetric joint movements or muscle mass

_____ 13. Place fingertips on the client's temporomandibular joints; palpate for symmetry, heat, swelling.

_____ 14. Ask the client to move his chin up and down, bend the side of his head toward the shoulders and back, open and close jaw, move the jaw from side to side.

_____ 15. Inspect the neck and head for symmetry, abnormal posture, swelling, or areas of redness.

_____ 16. Ask the client to raise and lower his arms, bending the elbows.

_____ 17. Ask the client to clasp his hands behind his neck and bring the elbows forward.

_____ 18. Ask the client to shrug his shoulders.

_____ 19. Ask the client to rotate the wrists.

_____ 20. Hold the client's hands in your hands; spread and straighten the fingers: curl them under toward the palm of his hand.

_____ 21. Inspect the arms, wrists, and hands for swelling, redness, deformities, or muscle wasting.

_____ 22. Take both of the client's hands in yours and instruct him to grip them as tightly as possible.

_____ 23. Ask the client to place both palms of hands against your palms and push as hard as possible.

_____ 24. Ask the client to lie on his back.

_____ 25. Inspect the knees, ankles, and feet for redness, swelling, nodules, symmetry. Palpate for temperature or swelling.

_____ 26. Hold the client's heel in one hand and bend the foot forward toward the lower leg; straighten it.

_____ 27. Hold the client's ankle; rotate the heel laterally and medially.

_____ 28. Bend and straighten the toes.

_____ 29. Repeat with the other foot.

_____ 30. Ask the client to bend his knee and pull it to his chest, using his hands.

_____ 31. Place the foot on the opposite knee. Pull the knee medially and the foot laterally.

_____ 32. Return the leg to a straight position with your hand on the kneecap. Palpate for crepitation.

_____ 33. Repeat with the other leg.

_____ 34. Ask the client to bend his knees and raise his legs again.

_____ 35. Place your palms against the sole of the client's feet; instruct him to push against your hands with both legs. Note the symmetry of movement and strength.

_____ 36. Assist the client to don clothes or leave in privacy for self-dressing.

_____ 37. Return the bed client to a position of comfort.

_____ 38. Open the curtains or door to the room.

_____ 39. Wash hands.

Name ______________________ Date ______________________

Observed by ______________

CHAPTER 16 POSITIONING, MOVING, AND TRANSFERRING THE CLIENT

SKILL 16.1 Using Body Mechanics

_____ **a.** Use a smooth surface to push or pull an object rather than a rough or uneven surface.

_____ **b.** Roll, push, or pull a person or object rather than lift.

_____ **c.** Stand upright when moving and working.

_____ **d.** Before lifting or moving a heavy object, contract the stabilizing muscles.

_____ **e.** Use the entire arm when lifting an object rather than just the hand and wrist.

_____ **f.** Position feet and legs farther apart when using force to push or pull another person or object.

_____ **g.** Face the direction of movement when moving a heavy object.

_____ **h.** When lifting or moving a heavy object, position one foot in front of the other and rock back and forth, shifting your body weight as you move the object.

_____ **i.** Bend the knee and hip joints when pushing or pulling objects.

_____ **j.** Squat, bending the hips and knees, to lift an object. (Avoid leaning over, bending the back and waist.) Keep your back straight and straighten the hips and knees slowly when lifting an object.

_____ **k.** Hold objects close to the body when lifting or carrying.

_____ **l.** Lower the head of the bed when moving the client up in bed.

_____ **m.** Support the weak and unsteady client at all times when walking with him.

_____ **n.** Lean your own body toward an unsteady client who leans toward your body.

Name ________________________________ Date ________________

Observed by ____________

SKILL 16.2 Positioning the Client in Bed

A. Preparation:

_____ 1. Assess the client to determine if he must be repositioned, what supportive aids to use, and identify his nursing diagnosis.

_____ 2. Plan the expected outcomes of repositioning the client.

_____ 3. Explain the purpose of the move to the client.

_____ 4. Wash hands.

_____ 5. Place the bed in a flat position, raised to a working height comfortable for the nurse. Lower the siderails.

_____ 6. Remove the top covers if necessary.

B. Supine or dorsal recumbent position:

_____ 1. Prepare the client and the bed.

_____ 2. Align the client's head and cervical, thoracic, and lumbar spine in a straight line.

_____ 3. Place a pillow under the client's head and shoulders so that the cervical spine remains straight.

_____ 4. Align the client's shoulders perpendicular to the spine.

_____ 5. Bend the client's arms and rest them on his abdomen.

_____ 6. Straighten the client's legs and slightly separate them.

_____ 7. Place a trochanter roll snugly against each lateral thigh.

_____ 8. Place a footboard against the feet so that the foot remains in a 90° angle to the leg.

_____ 9. Ask the client if he is comfortable. Adjust his body accordingly, keeping the body in correct alignment.

_____ 10. Replace top bedcovers and attach the client's call signal. Lower the bed and raise the siderails.

_____ 11. Wash hands.

C. Prone position:

_____ 1. Prepare the client and the bed.

_____ 2. Place the client on his abdomen and turn his head to one side. The neck will rotate.

_____ 3. Position the arms so that they are resting next to the client's sides, slightly bent and with fingers pointing up.
OR
Position the arm that is opposite the direction of the face above the shoulder, with elbow bent and resting on the bed above the head.

_____ 4. Straighten and separate the legs so that feet drop over the end of the bed, positioning the ankles in the functional angle.

_____ 5. Check the body alignment to see that the cervical, thoracic, and lumbar vertebrae are in a straight line.

_____ 6. Replace the top covers, and place the call signal within the client's reach.

_____ 7. Lower the bed and raise the siderails.

_____ 8. Wash hands.

D. Lateral position:

_____ 1. Prepare the client and the bed.

_____ 2. Place the client on his side, with the lower arm on the bed, bent and positioned in front of the chest.

_____ 3. Place a pillow under the side of the client's head so that the neck is in a straight line with the cervical vertebrae.

_____ 4. Bend the client's hips and knees, and place a pillow lengthwise between the lower thighs, knees, lower legs, and feet.

_____ 5. Bend the upper arm and position it on the client's side or place a pillow on the bed in front of the client and position the arm on the pillow.

_____ 6. Ask the client if he is comfortable, and adjust his position as necessary.

_____ 7. Replace top covers and place the call signal within the client's reach.

_____ 8. Raise the siderails and lower the bed.

_____ 9. Wash hands.

E. Fowler's position:

_____ 1. Prepare the client and the bed.

_____ 2. Raise the head of the bed mechanically or electronically to the desired angle.

_____ 3. Place the pillow beneath the client's head and upper shoulders.

_____ 4. Place the arms in a bent, relaxed position on the client's lap or at his side. If the client has no voluntary muscular control of the arm, place the lower arms and hands on a pillow.

_____ 5. Move the legs slightly apart and tuck a trochanter roll next to each lateral thigh, if the client's legs tend to rotate away from the body.

_____ 6. Position a footboard next to the client's feet, so that the ankle stays at a functional angle.

_____ 7. Straighten the client's top covers and place the call signal within the client's reach.

_____ 8. Lower the bed and raise the siderails.

_____ 9. Wash hands.

F. Left Sims' position:

_____ 1. Prepare the client and the bed.

_____ 2. Roll the client to his left side. Place a pillow under his head.

_____ 3. Assist the client to raise his upper body and pull his left arm under his

Name ______________________ Date ______________________

Observed by ____________

body, and position it beside his back on the bed. Simultaneous to this, the upper chest and right shoulder will lean toward the bed.

_____ 4. Place the right arm on a pillow in front of the head and upper chest, elbow bent and fingers pointing toward the pillow.

_____ 5. Place the left leg on a pillow in front of the body, flexed at the knee with the ankle resting in a natural 90° angle.

_____ 6. Ask the client if he feels comfortable. Adjust his position as necessary.

_____ 7. Replace the top covers, and attach the call signal within the client's reach.

_____ 8. Raise the siderails and lower the bed.

_____ 9. Wash hands.

Name ______________________________ Date ______________________

Observed by ______________

SKILL 16.3 Assisting the Client to Move in Bed

A. Preparing for the move:

_____ 1. Assess the client to determine his nursing diagnosis.

_____ 2. Plan the expected outcomes.

_____ 3. Explain to the client that he will be moved toward the head of the bed.

_____ 4. Wash hands.

_____ 5. Lower the head of the bed so that the bed is in a flat, horizontal position, or as near to flat as the client can tolerate.

_____ 6. Raise the bed to a comfortable working height. Lower the siderails on the side of the bed where you are working.

_____ 7. Remove the pillow from under the client's head and shoulders, and place it upright against the headboard.

B. Moving the supine client toward the head of the bed:

_____ 1. Prepare for the move.

_____ 2. Position the client's arms on his chest, one arm folded on the other. If the client is able to use the trapeze, instruct him to grasp the bar of the trapeze.

_____ 3. Turn to face the head of the bed, and stand with your feet about 2 feet apart, one foot in front of the other.

_____ 4. Bend your knees and hips.

If the client is alert and able:

_____ 5. Instruct the client to bend his knees and place his feet flat against the bed surface.

If the client is unable to move his legs but can move his arms:

_____ 6. Instruct the client to hold onto the siderail so that he can push himself against it, on the rail opposite you.

_____ 7. Place your hand and arm under the client's near shoulder, just at the level of the scapula. Place your other hand below the client's hip, under his thigh.

_____ 8. Instruct client to breathe out as he moves.

_____ 9. Rock back toward the foot of the bed and simultaneously tell the client to "push off" with his legs or arm. Rock forward toward the head of the bed, pushing the client's body toward the head of the bed, as far as possible.

_____ 10. If the client has a trapeze, instruct him to pull himself up from the bed, while you propel his body toward the head of the bed.

_____ 11. Repeat steps 7–9 until the client's head reaches the head of the bed.

_____ 12. Position the client comfortably and attach his call signal within his reach.

_____ 13. Raise the siderails.

_____ 14. Wash hands.

To move the client up in bed using a turning sheet, *two* nurses will:

_____ 1. Prepare for the move.

_____ 2. Fold a sheet in half and turn the client to one side; tuck the sheet under the client and roll back; pull sheet under body.

_____ 3. Position the client's arms on his chest, one arm folded on the other.

_____ 4. If the client is able to use the trapeze, instruct him to grasp the bar of the trapeze.

_____ 5. Turn to face the head of the bed and position your feet about 2 feet apart, one foot in front of the other.

_____ 6. Bend your knees and hips.

_____ 7. Gather or roll the turning sheet close to the client's body on both sides.

_____ 8. Grasp the turning sheet roll near the shoulder and the hip.

_____ 9. Instruct the client to bend his knees and place his feet flat on the bed, if possible.

_____ 10. Rock back toward the foot of the bed and simultaneously tell the client to "push off" with his legs or arms. Rock forward toward the head of the bed, lifting and pulling the turning sheet with the client's body in the same direction.

_____ 11. Repeat steps 8–10 until the client's head is at the head of the bed.

_____ 12. Position the client comfortably and attach his call signal within his reach.

_____ 13. Raise the siderails.

_____ 14. Wash hands.

C. Moving the supine client from the center to the side of the bed:

_____ 1. Prepare for the move.

_____ 2. Place the client's arms on his chest, one arm folded on top of the other arm.

_____ 3. Stand near the head of the bed, and bend your knees and hips. Position your feet about 2 feet apart, with one foot in front of the other. Bend the upper body toward the bed.

_____ 4. Place the arm nearest the head of the bed under the client's head and shoulders, so that his head rests in the antecubital fossa.

_____ 5. Place your other arm under the client's waist in the lumbar region.

_____ 6. Pull the client's upper body toward you by rocking backward.

_____ 7. Place the arm nearest the head of the bed under the client's waist, the lumbar region, and place the other arm under the thighs.

_____ 8. Repeat step 6.

_____ 9. Place the arm nearest the head of the bed under the client's knees and the other arm under his ankles.

Name ______________________________ Date ______________

Observed by ____________

____ 10. Repeat step 6.

____ 11. Raise the siderails before leaving the client in this position.

____ 12. Wash hands.

D. Moving the supine client from the center to the side of the bed using a turning sheet:

____ 1. Prepare for the move.

____ 2. Place the client's arms on his chest, one arm folded on top of the other arm.

____ 3. Stand near the head of the bed, with bent knees and hips and with feet about 2 feet apart, one foot in front of the other. Tilt your upper body toward the bed.

____ 4. Gather or roll the turning sheet close to the client's body.

____ 5. Pull the turning sheet under the client's shoulders toward you, rocking backward.

____ 6. Pull the turning sheet under the client's hips by rocking backward.

____ 7. Pull the turning sheet under the client's knees by rocking backward.

____ 8. Position the client's feet near the side of the bed.

____ 9. Raise the siderails before leaving the client in this position.

____ 10. Wash hands.

E. Moving the client from supine to lateral:

____ 1. Prepare for the move.

____ 2. Move the client to the side of the bed nearest the nurse.

____ 3. Raise the siderail.

____ 4. Move to the opposite side of the bed and lower the siderail.

____ 5. Place the client's far leg over the near leg. Flex the far arm and place it on the abdomen. Draw the other arm toward you.

____ 6. Flex your knees and position your feet in a broad stance, with one foot ahead of the other.

____ 7. Reach across the bed and grasp the client's body at the shoulder and hip. Roll the client by gently pulling him toward the center of the bed, shifting your weight from the forward to the back foot.

____ 8. Position the client in correct alignment for the lateral position when his body rests on its side. Use supportive aids as necessary.

____ 9. Raise the siderails and attach the call signal within the client's reach.

____ 10. Wash hands.

F. **Moving the client from lateral to prone:**

_____ 1. Prepare for the move.

_____ 2. Place the client's upper leg in front of the lower leg. Straighten the lower arm and place it next to the client's side.

_____ 3. Flex your knees and position your feet in a broad stance, with one foot ahead of the other.

_____ 4. Reach across the bed and grasp the client's body at the shoulder and hip. Roll the client by gently pulling him toward the center of the bed, shifting your weight from the forward to back foot.

_____ 5. Roll the client until he has rolled completely over the arm that is under him. His body is now resting on the chest and abdomen.

_____ 6. Adjust the client's limbs and head to the correct alignment for the prone position.

_____ 7. Raise the siderails and attach the call signal within the client's reach.

_____ 8. Wash hands.

G. **Moving the client from prone to supine:**

_____ 1. Prepare for the move.

_____ 2. Place the client's near arm directly parallel to his side.

_____ 3. Flex your knees and position your feet in a broad stance, with one foot ahead of the other.

_____ 4. Reach across the bed and grasp the client's body at the shoulder and hip. Roll the client by gently pulling him toward the center of the bed, shifting your weight from the forward to the back foot.

_____ 5. Position the client in correct alignment for the supine position, using supportive aids as necessary.

_____ 6. Raise the siderails.

_____ 7. Attach the call signal within the client's reach.

_____ 8. Wash hands.

H. **Moving the client by logrolling (two workers):**

_____ 1. Prepare for the move.

_____ 2. Cross the client's arms on his chest.

_____ 3. One nurse places her arms under the client's neck and thoracic spine and the second nurse places her arms under the client's lumbar spine and knees.

_____ 4. Both nurses assume the bent-knee, broad-based stance.

_____ 5. Together they pull the client's body toward the near side of the bed as a unit.

_____ 6. Raise the siderail, and move to the opposite side of the bed.

_____ 7. Lower the siderail, and assume the same flexed-knee, broad-based stance.

_____ 8. Place a pillow lengthwise between the client's knees and thighs.

_____ 9. Roll the client's body from his back to his abdomen, toward the nurses simultaneously so that all parts of the body move as a unit.

Name ______________________ Date ______________________

Observed by ____________

_____ 10. Place the client's body in correct alignment for the prone position.

_____ 11. Attach the call signal within the client's reach and raise siderails.

_____ 12. Wash hands.

I. Moving the client from back to a sitting position:

_____ 1. Explain to the client that he will be moved and why. Tell the client how he can help.

_____ 2. Wash hands.

_____ 3. Assist the client to a lateral position facing you.

_____ 4. Raise the head of the bed to its highest position.

_____ 5. Place the client's feet and lower legs over the edge of the bed.

_____ 6. Place one arm and hand behind the client's shoulder next to the bed, and place your other hand and arm under the client's thigh and knees.

_____ 7. Bend your knees and hips, and assume a broad stance with one foot ahead of the other.

_____ 8. Pull the client's shoulder up and away from the bed and simultaneously pull the client's thighs and knees toward the edge of the bed. Rotate his body to do this until the client is sitting upright with his feet dangling over the edge of the bed.

_____ 9. Continue to hold the client's shoulder for balance and contact, and assess his response to the movement.

To return the client to supine position after sitting:

_____ 10. Lower the client's shoulder to the elevated head of the bed. Place a pillow behind the client's head for comfort.

_____ 11. Raise and place his feet and legs on the surface of the bed.

_____ 12. Lower the head of the bed and assist the client to assume a supine position.

_____ 13. Raise the siderails and attach the call signal within the client's reach.

_____ 14. Wash hands.

Name ____________________ Date ____________________

Observed by ____________

SKILL 16.4 Transferring the Client

A. Transfer from bed to chair or wheelchair:

____ 1. Assess the client to determine the nursing diagnosis.

____ 2. Plan the nursing objectives and expected outcomes.

____ 3. Gather the necessary equipment.

____ 4. Explain to the client that he will be moved to a chair (or wheelchair).

____ 5. Wash hands.

____ 6. Lower the siderails on the side of the bed where the client will exit.

____ 7. Move the client so that he is lying near the side of the bed where he will exit. Raise the siderails.

____ 8. Place the client in a high Fowler's position.

____ 9. Draw the curtains around the bed. Remove top bed linens.

____ 10. Place the client's slippers or shoes on his feet.

____ 11. Lower the entire bed to its lowest position. Lock the wheels on the bed.

____ 12. Place the chair with its side next to the side of the bed, facing toward the head of the bed. (If the client has one weight-supporting leg, place the chair on the side of the bed next to that leg.) Lock the wheels on the wheelchair and move the leg and foot rests out of position.

____ 13. Lower the siderails between the client and the chair.

____ 14. Assist the client into a dangling position. Wait several moments to determine if the client is lightheaded. When he is comfortable and without lightheadedness, proceed. Support him by holding his shoulders.

____ 15. Bend your knees and hips so that your upper body is at the same level as the client's upper body. Place your feet in a wide stance with one foot forward.

____ 16. Instruct the client to place his arms and hands on your shoulders. Place your hands on the client's ribs, just above waist level.

____ 17. Help the client move his buttocks to the edge of the bed, so that his feet touch the floor or are close to the floor.

____ 18. Instruct the client to rise slowly to a standing position. Continue supporting him by holding his waist and raising your body as the client rises. Place your front knee against the client's opposite knee. Move both bodies with a backward rocking motion.

____ 19. Steady the client when you both are standing. Help him pivot his body by turning on the ball of his foot until his back is next to the chair seat.

____ 20. Instruct the client to sit down when he feels the edge of the chair seat against the back of his legs.

_____ 21. Bend your knees and hips to lower your body while the client lowers his body, holding the client under the axilla until he is seated.

_____ 22. Assess the client's body posture to determine if he is in correct alignment for sitting. Make necessary adjustments.

_____ 23. Help the client raise his legs and reposition the leg and foot rests on the wheelchair, and help him securely place his feet and legs on the rests.

_____ 24. Place a safety belt around the client's body trunk.

_____ 25. Unlock the wheels of a wheelchair before moving it.

To transfer the client from the wheelchair back to bed:

_____ 26. Place the chair next to the bed so that it faces the head of the bed. Lock the wheels on a wheelchair.

_____ 27. Help the client raise his legs and move the leg and foot rests out of position.

_____ 28. Bend your hips and knees so your body is at the same level as the client's body, and place your feet in a wide stance, with one foot forward.

_____ 29. Instruct the client to place his arms and hands on your shoulders. Place your hands on his ribs, just above the waist.

_____ 30. Brace your forward knee against the client's opposite knee.

_____ 31. Instruct the client to rise. Rise at the same time, straightening your hips and knees until both of you are standing upright.

_____ 32. Instruct the client to pivot so that his back is next to the bed.

_____ 33. Instruct the client to sit on the bed when he feels the edge of the bed against his legs. Move downward with him, flexing your knees and hips and keeping your back straight.

_____ 34. Instruct the client to lower his arm and shoulder against the bed. Simultaneously, lift his knees and lower legs onto the bed. (He will be laterally semisitting.)

_____ 35. Assist the client to his back. (He will be in Fowler's position near the edge of the bed.)

_____ 36. Remove the client's shoes and socks.

_____ 37. Move the client toward the center of the bed. Help him assume a position of comfort.

_____ 38. Replace the client's bedcovers. Attach his call signal within reach.

_____ 39. Open the bed curtains, if necessary.

_____ 40. Wash hands.

B. Preparing for transfer from a bed to a stretcher:

_____ 1. Assess the client to determine the nursing diagnosis.

_____ 2. Plan the nursing objectives and expected outcomes.

_____ 3. Determine and prepare the necessary equipment.

_____ 4. Explain to the client that he will be moved to a stretcher.

_____ 5. Wash hands.

Name ______________________ Date ______________

Observed by ________

_____ 6. Close the doors to the client's room. Draw the curtains between the bed units if other clients are in the room.

_____ 7. Raise the siderails on both sides of the bed.

_____ 8. Raise the bed level to its maximum height. Lock the wheels in place.

_____ 9. Lower the siderail on the side of the bed where the stretcher will be placed.

_____ 10. Place the client in a supine position. Remove pillows if the client is able to tolerate it. Untuck the top bedcovers or remove them and place a bath blanket over the client.

_____ 11. Lower the siderail of the stretcher on the side nearest the bed and roll it directly next to the bed.

C. Transferring from bed to stretcher with the client assisting:

_____ 1. Prepare for transfer.

_____ 2. Stand next to the stretcher and instruct the client to raise his hips and move his body toward the stretcher. Encourage him to use the siderails to provide leverage. Help him remain covered with the bath blanket or top covers.

_____ 3. Place a pillow under the client's head and cover the client with a bath blanket when he is resting completely on the stretcher. Secure safety belts if present. Raise the remaining siderail.

_____ 4. Unlock the stretcher wheels and move it away from the bed.

_____ 5. Reverse these steps to return the client to bed.

D. Transferring from bed to stretcher when the client is unable to move:

_____ 1. Prepare for transfer.

_____ 2. Place a turning sheet under the client.
OR
Place a roller pad or apparatus under the client.

_____ 3. Lower the siderail of the stretcher on the side nearest to the bed and roll it directly next to the bed. Lock the wheels in place.

_____ 4. Position two workers on side of stretcher; position another one or two workers on the other side of the client in bed.

Using turning sheet:

_____ 5. (All workers) Grasp edges of turning sheet close to the client's body.

_____ 6. Lift sheet and client in unison; move to stretcher.

Using roller pad or apparatus:

_____ 5. Pull pad toward the stretcher; the client will roll over it onto the stretcher.

_____ 6. Monitor client's extremities and assist with their movement as necessary.

_____ 7. Place a pillow under the client's head and cover him with a bath blanket.

_____ 8. Secure safety belts, if present, and raise siderails on the stretcher.

_____ 9. Unlock the stretcher wheels before moving it.

_____ 10. Reverse these steps to return the client to bed.

E. Using a mechanical lift:

_____ 1. Assess the client to determine the nursing diagnosis.

_____ 2. Plan the nursing objectives and expected outcomes.

_____ 3. Determine and prepare the necessary equipment.

_____ 4. Explain to the client that he will be moved and explain how the machine works. Assure him that he will be safe at all times.

_____ 5. Inspect the machine to determine that it is in good, safe working order. Be very familiar with the working mechanism and all safety features.

_____ 6. Position the chair near the client's bed.

_____ 7. Remove furniture near the client's bedside and position the lift near the client's bed.

_____ 8. Raise the client's bed to a good working level for the nurse. Lower the siderails.

_____ 9. Place the canvas chair straps under the client's body by rolling the client from side to side. Be sure they are positioned exactly.

_____ 10. Lower the bed to its lowest level. Lock the bed wheels.

_____ 11. Roll the lift so that its footbars are directly under the bed and the lift arm is above the client. Lock it into position, if possible.

_____ 12. Instruct the client to cross his arms on his chest, or position his arms for him.

_____ 13. Attach the hooks from the canvas straps to the chain or bar attached to the lift arm. Be sure that both sides are attached at equal distances.

_____ 14. Tightly close the pressure valve on the hydraulic mechanism. Pump the lift so that the client's buttocks are completely off the bed surface.

_____ 15. Unlock the lift and slowly roll it until the client is directly over the chair. (A second worker guides the client on the canvas chair.) Lock lift in place.

_____ 16. Release the pressure valve and lower the client into the chair. (A second worker guides the client into the chair.)

_____ 17. Carefully unhook the canvas chair straps from the chair or bar, preventing the bar from swinging against the client or workers.

_____ 18. Unlock the lift and roll it away from the chair. Secure the bar and chain so that it doesn't swing against the client and workers.

_____ 19. Leave the client sitting on the canvas straps. Adjust him for correct alignment as necessary.

_____ 20. Reverse the above steps to return the client to bed.

Name ______________________________ Date ______________

Observed by ____________

CHAPTER 17 BEDMAKING

SKILL 17.1 Bedmaking

A. Unoccupied bed:

____ 1. Assess the client and determine the nursing diagnosis.

____ 2. Plan the expected outcomes.

____ 3. Explain the procedure to the client.

____ 4. Wash hands and put on clean gloves.

____ 5. Raise bed to a working level that prevents back strain for the nurse.

____ 6. Assess used linens to determine which linens will be changed.

____ 7. Bring clean linens to the bedside and place on an adjacent overbed table or chair. Stack in the reverse order of use.

____ 8. If a laundry bag or cart is not present at the bedside, remove pillowcase, fold the cuff outward, and place the cuff over the back of the chair so that the pillow hangs open as a bag.

If the top linens are to be saved and reused:

____ 9. Loosen all soiled linens by pulling them out from under the mattress. Start at the head of the bed and work around the foot of the bed and then move up toward the head of the bed on the opposite side. Return to the side of the bed near the overbed table.

____ 10. Grasp top edge of the spread with both hands and pull it toward the bottom edge, folding it in half. Pick up the spread in the center and fold it in half a second time. Place the folded spread over the nearby chair.

____ 11. Repeat steps 9 and 10 for the top sheet.

____ 12. Roll loosened bottom sheets toward the bottom of the bed and place the ball of linens in the laundry cart or pillowcase. If the mattress pad is soiled, remove it too.

If all linens are to be removed:

____ 9. Loosen all the soiled linens by pulling them out from under the mattress. Roll them toward the center of the bed. Start at the head of the bed and work around the foot of the bed and then move up toward the head of the bed on the opposite side.

____ 10. Return to the side of the bed near the overbed table.

____ 11. Roll loosened linens into a ball toward the foot of the bed. If the mattress pad is soiled, remove it also.

____ 12. Place ball of linens in the laundry cart or pillowcase.

After all linens are removed from the bed:

_____ 13. Reposition and smooth the mattress pad or place a clean pad on the bed, and unfold it into place.

_____ 14. Place clean bottom sheet on the lower end of the bed so that the center fold of the sheet is placed on the center of the bed.

_____ 15. Unfold sheet lengthwise so that the bottom hem extends about 1 inch over the foot end of the mattress.

_____ 16. Unfold sheet crosswise toward the working side of the bed until that half of the sheet is open. Smoothly push the unopened half of the sheet toward the opposite side of the bed.

_____ 17. Tuck top of the opened half of the sheet under the head of the mattress.

To miter the corner of the bedsheet:

_____ 18. Lift untucked sheet about 10–12 inches from the head of the bed. Place this portion of the sheet on the top of the bed so that it forms a triangle. The side hem of the sheet will be parallel to the head of the bed.

_____ 19. Tuck portion of sheet that hangs below the lower mattress edge under the mattress while holding the triangle portion snugly against the top of the mattress.

_____ 20. Fold sheet so that it hangs down over the edge of the bed.

_____ 21. Tuck remainder of the side of the sheet under the mattress, working from the head to the foot of the bed.

_____ 22. Place protective drawsheet on the center of the bed, and unfold it so that it lies centered on the bed.

_____ 23. Place drawsheet on top of the protective drawsheet and unfold it so that it completely covers the protective drawsheet. Tuck the sheet under the mattress. If no protective sheet is used, place the drawsheet in this fashion. If neither is used, omit these steps.

_____ 24. Place top sheet on the drawsheet so that the center fold is in the middle of the mattress.

_____ 25. Unfold top sheet toward the head and foot of the mattress. Unfold half of the sheet toward the working side of the mattress and smooth over the side.

_____ 26. Place a blanket or a bedspread in the same manner as the top sheet.

_____ 27. Smooth top linens (sheet, blanket, and spread) together over the foot of the bed, and lifting the foot end of the mattress, tuck the linens together under the mattress.

_____ 28. Miter corner of the top linens using steps 18–20.

_____ 29. Move to unmade side of the bed.

_____ 30. Smooth the mattress pad and unfold the bottom sheet in place.

_____ 31. Miter the bottom sheet at the head of the bed using steps 18–20.

_____ 32. Tug gently on the bottom sheet and smooth and tighten it toward the edge of the mattress, tucking it under the mattress.

_____ 33. Unfold and smooth into place the protective pad and drawsheet.

Name ______________________ Date ______________________

Observed by ____________

_____ 34. Tug gently on the drawsheets and tuck under the mattress in the center of the drawsheets.

_____ 35. Pull edge of the drawsheet toward the head of the bed and over the edge of the mattress and tuck in place.

_____ 36. Repeat pulling and tucking motion on the drawsheet edge toward the foot of the bed.

_____ 37. Unfold sheet, blanket, and top spread and smooth in place.

_____ 38. Smooth top linens (sheet, blanket, and spread) together over the foot end of the bed and lifting the lower end of the mattress, tuck the linens together under the mattress.

_____ 39. Miter corner of the top linens using steps 16–19.

_____ 40. Unfold clean pillowcase and reach inside to the seam opposite the case opening with nondominant hand. Fanfold the case with hand so that the seam is just inside the opening.

_____ 41. Lay pillow on the bed. Grasp an end of the pillow with the dominant hand. Gently ease the pillowcase over the end of the pillow, and roll the case toward the opposite end so that the case completely covers the pillow.

To make an open bed:

_____ 42. Fold back the top linens to make a 6–8-inch cuff at the head end.

_____ 43. Fanfold top sheets in two or three folds at the foot end of the bed.

For both closed and open bed:

_____ 44. Place pillow at the head of the bed.

_____ 45. Wash hands.

B. Anesthesia bed:

Before tucking in the top linens:

_____ 1. Fold the bottom hems of the top linens back toward the head of the bed, so that the edge of the fold is about 2 inches from the foot of the mattress.

_____ 2. Fold the top hems of the top linens back toward the foot end of the bed, so that the edge of the fold is about 10–20 inches from the head of the mattress.

_____ 3. Grasp the folded edge of the top sheets at the foot of the bed on the side of the bed facing the door of the client's room. Place this edge on top of the bed on the far side so that the folded top linens make a triangle.

_____ 4. Repeat step 38 with the remaining half of the top linens that are on the head of the bed. The linens form a triangle on the bed, with an angle pointing toward the floor on the side of the bed facing the door.

_____ 5. Pick up the lowest corner of the linen triangle and fanfold the top linens on the side of the bed farther from the door.

_____ 6. Place the pillow upright at the head of the bed.

_____ 7. Remove gloves and wash hands.

C. Occupied bed:

_____ 1. Assess client and determine the nursing diagnosis.

_____ 2. Plan expected outcomes.

_____ 3. Explain procedure to the client.

_____ 4. Wash hands and put on clean gloves.

_____ 5. Raise the siderails.

_____ 6. Raise bed to a level so that you can remain standing upright while working.

_____ 7. Assess used linens to determine which linens will be changed.

_____ 8. Bring clean linens to the bedside and place on an adjacent overbed table or chair.

_____ 9. Remove pillowcase and fold the cuff over the back of the chair so that the pillowcase hangs open like a bag. Set pillow aside.

_____ 10. Place a fresh pillowcase on the pillow and position it under the client's head.

_____ 11. Lower siderails, and loosen all linens by pulling them out from under the mattress. Start at the head of the bed. Raise the siderails when one side of the bed is completed. Lower siderails on opposite side, loosen linens, and raise the siderails again.

If a bath blanket is used:

_____ 12. Place a bath blanket over the top linens.

_____ 13. Instruct client to hold the top edge of the bath blanket, if he is able to do so.

_____ 14. Reach under bath blanket, and grasp the top edge of the spread with both hands and pull it toward the bottom edge, folding it in half. Pick up the spread in the center and fold it in half a second time. Place the folded spread over the nearby chair.

_____ 15. Repeat step 12 for the top sheet. If all linens are discarded, remove all at once and place in the laundry receptacle.

If no bath blanket is used, remove only the spread and use the top sheet as a cover during the bath.

_____ 16. Move client to the opposite side of the bed, or have the client grasp the siderails and roll himself to that side.

_____ 17. Raise near the edge of the bottom linens and tuck and fanfold them under the client.

_____ 18. Reposition and smooth mattress pad or place a clean pad on the bed, unfolding half of the pad and fanfolding and tucking *under* the fanfolded soiled linen that is now under the client.

Name ______________________ Date ______________________

Observed by ______________

_____ 19. Place clean bottom sheet on the lower end of the bed so that the center fold of the sheet is at the center of the bed, next to the client.

_____ 20. Unfold sheet lengthwise so that the bottom hem extends about 1 inch over the end of the mattress.

_____ 21. Unfold half of the sheet toward you so that it hangs below the mattress.

_____ 22. Fanfold and tuck the opposite half of the sheet under the client.

_____ 23. Tuck hanging edge of the sheet under the mattress. Miter the corner at the head.

_____ 24. Place protective pad and drawsheet on the bed crosswise, open toward the head and foot of the bed and smooth. Tuck the sheets under the mattress.

_____ 25. Fanfold and tuck drawsheet under the client.

_____ 26. Place top sheet on the client and unfold it so that the client and the bath blanket are covered.

_____ 27. Place a blanket (if necessary) and the bedspread on top of the sheet.

_____ 28. Tuck top linens at the foot of the bed, mitering the corner.

_____ 29. Raise siderail on the working side and roll or instruct the client to roll toward you. Hold the covers in place during this movement. Instruct the client, "You will roll over a lump—that is the linen folded under you."

_____ 30. Move to the other side of the bed, and lower the siderails.

_____ 31. Pull remaining lower sheets out from under the client, gathering them in a bundle. Dispose in the laundry receptable.

_____ 32. Locate edges of the clean linen and pull them toward the nurse. Smooth and straighten as the linens are pulled.

_____ 33. Tighten lower bed linens at the head of the bed, and tuck smoothly into place.

_____ 34. Miter bottom linens at the head of the bed.

_____ 35. Pull, tighten, and smooth the remaining bottom sheet and tuck under the mattress, working from head to foot of the bed.

_____ 36. Pull, tighten, and smooth protective pad and drawsheet. Tuck under the mattress, beginning at the middle of the drawsheets and working toward the outer edges.

_____ 37. Unfold and smooth the top covers over the client.

_____ 38. Fold back the covers at the head of the bed to make a cuff about 8 inches at the head.

_____ 39. Smooth and tuck the covers at the foot of the bed under the mattress. Miter the corner.

_____ 40. Pull bath blanket from under the top covers and discard in the laundry receptacle.

_____ 41. Assist client to a position of comfort. Reposition the pillow if necessary.

_____ 42. Attach call light in a place where the client can readily reach it.

_____ 43. Wash hands.

D. Suggestions for bedmaking in home care:

_____ a. Advise the caregivers that hospital beds can be rented from hospital supply outlets or borrowed from charitable agencies.

_____ b. If a hospital bed is not available and the client is on total bed rest, raise the height of a bed by placing each leg of the bed in a small bucket (or used coffee can) filled with 5–6 inches of sand. Add moisture to the sand for stability.

_____ c. Raise height of the bed by placing legs on 6 inch by 6 inch blocks, taking care to ensure that legs cannot be dislodged from the block.

_____ d. Rented siderails can be attached to the home bed if client remains on total bed rest.

_____ e. Suggest that caregivers move one edge of the bed next to a wall if client remains on bed rest and siderails are not available.

_____ f. Place back of a chair next to the bed with weighted objects on the seat to create a makeshift siderail.

_____ g. Use a large piece of plastic such as a trash bag cut open or an old shower curtain as a protective bed pad if the client is incontinent.

_____ h. Make drawsheets by folding a regular size flat sheet in half.

_____ i. Teach caregivers how to change the bed using correct body mechanics.

_____ j. Advise the caregivers to launder linens in the hottest water available and dry in a hot air dryer if possible.

Name ______________________________ Date ______________

Observed by __________

CHAPTER 18 EXERCISING AND AMBULATING

SKILL 18.1 Performing Joint Range of Motion Examples

____ 1. Assess the client to determine the nursing diagnosis.

____ 2. Plan the expected outcomes.

____ 3. Explain to the client that the nurse will bend, straighten, or rotate each of his joints in a smooth and rhythmic fashion at least three times. Explain that these exercises prevent joint stiffness and muscle wasting. Encourage the client to relax.

____ 4. Wash hands.

____ 5. Draw·the curtains around the client's bed or close the door to his room.

____ 6. Raise the bed to a comfortable working height and place the bed in a flat, horizontal position.

____ 7. Remove any restrictive clothing from the client. Remove top bed linens and drape him as necessary to provide privacy.

____ 8. Lower the siderails on the side of the bed where the nurse is standing.

____ 9. Move the client's body toward the side of the bed where the nurse stands.

____ 10. Place your hands under the client's neck and back of the head, and gently raise the head, moving the face toward the chin, flexing the neck. Lower the head so that the neck is in its functional position. Extend the neck by lowering the head toward the bed, and return to the functional position. Repeat this maneuver three times.

____ 11. Explain how to do each step to the client and caregiver and explain the reasons for the exercise as the joints are moved.

____ 12. Flex the client's neck laterally by tilting the head toward one shoulder and then tilting the head toward the other shoulder. Repeat three times.

____ 13. Rotate the head three times, placing the head in its resting position when this is completed.

____ 14. Grasp the client's arm by the elbow and hand, and flex the shoulder by raising the arm in an arc from the bed to above the client's head. Extend the shoulder by lowering the arm to the client's side on the bed. Repeat three times.

____ 15. Abduct the shoulder by moving the arm away from the client's side by holding at the wrist and elbow; adduct the shoulder by returning the arm over the client's abdomen toward the opposite arm. Repeat three times.

____ 16. Place the upper arm out from the body at shoulder level, flex the elbow at 90° by holding the elbow and grasping the palm, raising the hand above the head level. Internally rotate the shoulder by turning the lower arm down so that the palm faces the bed. Externally rotate by returning the hand above the head. Repeat three times.

_____ 17. Flex the elbow by grasping the palm, and holding the arm under the elbow, moving the forearm toward upper arm. Extend the elbow by straightening the arm. Repeat three times.

_____ 18. Supinate the forearm by holding the elbow and palm, rotating the forearm so that the palm faces upward. Pronate by turning the palm downward. Repeat three times.

_____ 19. Flex the wrist by turning the hand toward the inner forearm. Extend by straightening the wrist. Hyperextend by moving the hand toward the back of the arm. Repeat three times.

_____ 20. Deviate the wrist by rotating the thumb toward the radial surface of the arm, and then rotate the ulnar edge of the palm toward the outer surface of the arm. Repeat three times.

_____ 21. Flex the finger joints by closing your hands and fingers around the client's fingers while holding his hand at the wrist. Extend the joints by opening the hand. Repeat three times.

_____ 22. Abduct and adduct the fingers one by one by separating and then closing them. Repeat three times.

_____ 23. Move the thumb toward the little finger and back again. Repeat three times.

_____ 24. Repeat steps 11–20 for the near arm.

_____ 25. Place one of your hands under the client's knee and the other hand under the heel of the far leg from the nurse.

_____ 26. Raise the client's lower leg so that both hip and knee are flexed. Lower the leg so that hip and knee are extended. Repeat three times.

_____ 27. Abduct the hip by moving the entire leg away from the midline of the body by holding the leg at the knee and ankle; adduct the hip by moving the leg toward the midline and over the opposite leg. Repeat three times.

_____ 28. Grasp the client's heel; rotate the entire leg externally and internally; repeat slowly two times.

_____ 29. Place the nurse's hand under the heel so that the nurse's forearm rests against the bottom of the foot. Dorsiflex the heel by pushing the foot toward the client's lower leg with nurse's hand and arm. Plantar flex by pushing the foot down and away from the client's lower leg. Repeat three times.

_____ 30. Hold the client's heel with one hand and invert or turn the foot inward and then evert or turn outward with the other hand. Repeat three times.

_____ 31. Hold the client's foot at the arch, and use your fingers and hand to bend or flex the toes forward and straighten or extend the toes. Repeat three times. Abduct and adduct toe by toe by separating and placing them together.

_____ 32. Repeat steps 21–27 for the near leg.

_____ 33. Remove drapes and replace client's clothing and top covers.

Name ______________________________ Date ______________

Observed by ____________

_____ 34. Place client in a comfortable position and attach call signal within client's reach.

_____ 35. Lower bed to a safe level for the client and raise the siderails. Open the curtains or door as necessary.

_____ 36. Wash hands.

Name ________________________________ Date ________________

Observed by ____________

SKILL 18.2 Assisting with Ambulation

To prepare the client for ambulation, the nurse will:

_____ 1. Assess the client to determine his readiness for walking and identify the nursing diagnosis.

_____ 2. Plan the expected outcomes of preparing the client to walk.

_____ 3. Explain to the client that he will soon be walking and he is now going to exercise to prepare for that.

_____ 4. Position the client in a high Fowler's position in bed.

_____ 5. Teach the client to do the following isometric exercises: (Explain that he should contract his muscles, slowly count to five, relax the muscles, slowly count to five, and then repeat.)

a. Push his knee toward the mattress.

b. Pinch the buttocks together.

c. Push down against the mattress with his hands, and slowly lift his buttocks.

_____ 6. Encourage the client to start these exercises by doing them five or six times every other hour, and then increase the number of contractions and relaxations as well as the frequency of the exercise.

_____ 7. Provide positive reinforcement for the client.

To assist the client to walk, the nurse will:

_____ 1. Assess the client to determine his readiness for walking and identify the nursing diagnosis.

_____ 2. Plan the expected outcomes of assisting the client to walk.

_____ 3. Explain to the client that he will be walking and the nurse will walk with him for support and strength. Explain the necessity for exercise if the client seems unsure or reluctant. Set a specific goal of how far the walk will be.

_____ 4. Be sure the pathway of the walk is cleared of obstacles.

_____ 5. Wash hands.

_____ 6. Assist the client from his bed to a standing position.

To walk arm in arm:

_____ 7. Stand next to the client, and place your lower arm under the client's lower arm, grasping his hand with your hand.

To walk with the nurse's arm around the client's waist:

_____ 7. Stand next to the client, and place your arm around his waist. Hold the near hand with your opposite hand.

To walk using a walking belt:

_____ 7. Stand to the side and slightly behind the client, grasping the hand grip on the bed.

To walk assisted by two nurses:

_____ 7. Position a nurse on each side, each placing her lower arm under the client's lower arm, grasping his hand with her hand. (One nurse may prepare to hold an arm around the client's waist.)

For each type of assistance:

_____ 8. Step forward as the client steps forward. Ask the client how he feels.

_____ 9. Continue walking until the predetermined goal is achieved or until the client expresses a desire to stop or demonstrates increased fatigue or weakness.

_____ 10. Positively reinforce the client's efforts, no matter how limited those efforts may be. Encourage the client to do as much as he can.

_____ 11. Assess continually the client's response to exercise: posture, gait, pulse, and respirations.

_____ 12. Walk with the client to his bedside to sit in a chair, or if he desires, to his bed. Provide whatever comfort measures are necessary (a drink of water, for example).

_____ 13. Discuss with the client and plan a goal greater than the one just achieved for the next walk.

_____ 14. Attach the client's call signal within his reach.

_____ 15. Wash hands.

Name ______________________ Date ______________________

Observed by ______________

SKILL 18.3 Teaching the Client to Use an Assistive Device with Ambulation

A. Teaching the client to walk with a cane:

_____ 1. Assess the client to determine if he meets the criteria for using a cane.

_____ 2. Identify the client's nursing diagnosis and plan the expected outcomes of teaching cane walking.

_____ 3. Explain to the client that he will learn how to use a cane to help him stabilize himself when walking.

_____ 4. Provide the cane for the client to inspect and examine.

_____ 5. Demonstrate the use of the cane, explaining the reason for each action:

a. Hold the cane so that it touches the floor approximately 6 inches to the client's side and about 12–18 inches in front of the client. Maintain body balance.

b. Lift and move the cane forward about 12 inches.

c. Move the affected leg toward the cane.

d. Move the unaffected leg toward the cane.

e. Lift and move the cane forward again, and repeat the process.

_____ 6. Help the client to a standing position and give him the cane.

_____ 7. Instruct the client to walk, using the cane as demonstrated. Set a goal of how far the client will walk. Walk beside the client on his affected side.

_____ 8. Observe the client's walking, and provide encouragement and make suggestions as necessary to help him improve his use of the cane and enhance his stability and safety.

_____ 9. Ask the client about how he feels his walk has been. Answer any questions. Arrange another time for the client to practice walking with a cane again.

B. Teaching the client to walk with a walker:

_____ 1. Assess the client to determine if he meets the criteria for using a walker.

_____ 2. Identify the client's nursing diagnosis and plan the expected outcomes of teaching use of a walker.

_____ 3. Explain to the client that he will learn how to use a walker to help him support and stabilize himself when walking.

_____ 4. Provide the walker for the client to inspect and examine.

_____ 5. Demonstrate the use of the walker.

a. Place the walker in front of the nurse so that the open side of the frame faces the nurse. Place hands on the hand grips.

b. Lift and move the walker forward about 12 inches.

c. Step toward the walker one foot at a time, keeping the hands placed on the hand grips and leaning toward the walker. Balance weight on the walker.

If the client has one affected leg:

c. Step toward the walker with the affected leg first.

d. Repeat steps b and c.

_____ 6. Help the client to a standing position and place the walker in front of him. Instruct him to hold the hand grips and lean into the walker.

_____ 7. Instruct the client to walk using the walker as demonstrated. Set a goal of how far the client will walk. Walk beside the client.

_____ 8. Observe the client's walking, and provide encouragement and make suggestions as necessary to help him improve his use of the walker and enhance his stability and safety.

_____ 9. Ask the client how he feels his walk has been. Answer any questions.

_____ 10. Arrange a time for the client to practice walking with the walker again.

C. Preparing the client to walk with crutches:

_____ 1. Assess the client to determine if he meets the criteria for using crutches.

_____ 2. Identify the client's nursing diagnosis and plan the expected outcomes of teaching crutch walking.

_____ 3. Measure the client to determine the correct fit for the crutches.

a. Place the client in a supine position with his shoes on.

b. Place one end of a tapemeasure under the axillary fold.

c. Measure the distance from the axilla to the heel and add 2 inches. This is the correct length for the crutches, including the axillary pads and rubber tips.

OR

a. Have the client stand and hold a crutch under each arm, grasping the handgrip.

b. Instruct the client to place each crutch tip 4–6 inches to the front and side of each foot while supporting his weight on the handgrips. Instruct him to place the tips on only dry and hard surfaces.

c. Measure the gap between the axillary pad and the client's axilla to determine if it is two fingers wide. If it is not, adjust the crutch height so that the gap is two fingers wide.

d. Slide the central strut at the bottom of the crutch upward or outward by removing the bolt and wing nut. Adjust the height, and tightly secure the bolt and wing nut.

_____ 4. Adjust the handgrip on the crutches to the correct fit.

a. Instruct the client to grasp the handgrips to determine if his elbows are flexed 30° when he is standing and holding the crutch.

b. If the elbow angle is not 30°, remove the bolt and wing nut and slide the handgrip level to the desired level. Tightly secure the bolt and wing nut on the handgrip.

Name ______________________________ Date ______________________________

Observed by ______________

_____ 5. Build the client's muscular strength by instructing him to do these exercises:

a. Sitting in high Fowler's position in bed, push down against the bed with his hands and arms until he raises his entire body from the surface of the bed.

b. Grasp a rubber ball in the hand and squeeze.

c. Lying in a supine position, extend the arms forward and stretch, raising the body to a sitting position.

D. Instructing the client to use crutches:

_____ 1. Explain to the client that he will learn to use crutches because this will enable him to walk even though he cannot put weight on one or both legs. Provide support as needed.

_____ 2. Place the client in a dangling position with the bed level slightly elevated from the floor.

_____ 3. Hand the crutches to the client, instructing him to hold the handgrips and raise and lower the crutches.

_____ 4. Help the client push himself to the edge of the bed, so that his legs are extended and his feet rest lightly on the floor but his body weight is still resting on the bed.

_____ 5. Instruct the client to place the crutches in position under his axilla without supporting his body weight on the axillary rest.

_____ 6. Instruct the client to place the tips of the crutches forward and to the side of his feet about 4–6 inches.

_____ 7. Instruct the client to push himself off the bed and stand upright with the crutches properly positioned and supporting his body weight on his unaffected leg and hand.

_____ 8. Assess the client to determine that:

a. The crutch tips are 4–6 inches to the front and side of each foot.

b. The client's axilla is two fingers above the axillary rest.

c. The client's hands grasp the handgrips and his arms support his body weight.

d. The client's body is upright with his head looking forward.

Using a three-point or swing-through gait:

_____ 9. Give these instructions:

a. "Move the crutch tips directly forward about 12 to 15 inches on the side of your feet and simultaneously move your *affected* foot forward about 12 to 15 inches."

b. "Move the *unaffected* foot forward to the same area as the crutch tips and your affected foot."

c. "Repeat these steps to continue walking with the crutches."

_____ 10. Encourage the client to place the *unaffected* foot about 12–15 inches in front of the crutch tips and *affected* foot to change his gait to a swing-through gait, when he is using the three-point gait safely and effectively.

Using a two-point gait:

_____ 9. Give these instructions:

a. "Move your *right* foot and *left* crutch tip forward about 12–15 inches.

b. "Move your *left* foot and *right* crutch tip forward about 12–15 inches in front of the other foot and crutch."

_____ 10. Encourage the client to continue this gait by repeating steps a and b.

Using a four-point gait:

_____ 9. Give these instructions:

a. "Move your *right* crutch tip forward about 12–15 inches, and then move your *left* foot to the same level as the *right* crutch tip."

b. "Move your *left* crutch tip forward about 12–15 inches and then move your *right foot* to the same level as the *left* crutch.

_____ 10. Instruct the client to repeat steps a and b to continue using the gait.

Using each type of crutch gait:

_____ 11. Assess the client's posture and balance. Help him correct any problems with the technique. Encourage him frequently and praise his efforts. Arrange to practice crutch-walking again.

E. Teaching the client to sit down in and get up from a chair while using crutches:

_____ 1. Explain to the client that he will learn how to sit and get up from a chair while maintaining his balance using crutches.

_____ 2. Select a chair with arms and place it against the wall.

_____ 3. Instruct the client to do these steps to sit in the chair:

a. "Stand facing the front of the chair with your toes about 12–15 inches away."

b. "Hold both crutches in your affected hand under your affected arm. Place your unaffected hand on the chair arm nearest the hand."

c. "Lean both crutches over the back of the chair near the affected side of your body. Balance your body weight on your unaffected leg and keep your affected leg elevated from the floor."

d. "Holding the chair arm with your unaffected hand, pivot on your unaffected foot and swing your body 180°, lowering it as you move, so that your body moves into the seat of the chair. Grasp the chair arm with your affected arm as you turn to propel your body."

_____ 4. Encourage and praise the client's efforts.

Name ______________________________ Date ______________________________

Observed by ______________

_____ 5. Allow the client a short time of rest before proceeding.

_____ 6. Instruct the client to do these steps to rise from the chair:

a. "Hold the crutches with your affected hand and place both crutch tips about 4–6 inches to the front and side of the affected foot."

b. "Place your unaffected arm on the chair arm near it."

c. "Rise with a simple movement, bearing weight on the unaffected foot and hand."

_____ 7. Encourage and praise the client's efforts.

_____ 8. Instruct the client to repeat the steps sitting in and rising from the chair.

_____ 9. Arrange a time when the client can practice again.

F. Teaching the client to walk up and down stairs with crutches:

_____ 1. Explain to the client that he will learn how to walk up and down stairs with crutches.

_____ 2. Walk with the client to the bottom of a flight of stairs.

_____ 3. Stand behind the client and toward his affected side.

_____ 4. Instruct the client to do these steps to go up the stairs:

a. "Place the crutches and your unaffected leg in the three-legged position."

b. "Transfer your weight to the crutches and lift your unaffected leg to the first step."

c. "Transfer your weight to the unaffected leg on the first step."

d. "Move the crutches and affected leg to the first step."

e. "Repeat these steps until you reach the top of the stairs."

_____ 5. Instruct the client to do these steps to go down the stairs:

a. "Place the crutches and your unaffected leg in the three-legged position."

b. "Balance your weight on your unaffected leg and place crutches and affected leg on the first lower step."

c. "Transfer your weight to the crutches and affected leg and move your unaffected leg to the lower step."

d. "Repeat these steps until you reach the bottom of the stairs."

_____ 6. Observe the client as he practices. Offer assistance as needed.

_____ 7. Encourage and praise the client's efforts.

_____ 8. Instruct the client to repeat his performance.

_____ 9. Arrange a time when the client can practice again.

Name ________________________ Date ____________

Observed by ____________

CHAPTER 19 PROTECTING THE IMMOBILE CLIENT

SKILL 19.1 Placing the Client on a Protective Mattress or Pad

_____ 1. Assess the client to determine the nursing diagnosis.

_____ 2. Plan the nursing objective and expected outcomes; gather the necessary equipment.

_____ 3. Explain to the client what will be done.

_____ 4. Close the door to the client's room or close the curtains around his bed.

_____ 5. Wash hands.

If the bed is unoccupied:

_____ 6. Change the bottom sheet and place the supportive pad on the bed.

If the client is in bed:

_____ 6. Move the client to one side of the bed and raise the siderails.

_____ 7. Replace the bottom sheet with a clean one.

If placing a foam mattress, sheepskin, or deflated air mattress:

_____ 8. Fold the supportive pad lengthwise and place on the bottom sheet next to the client.

_____ 9. Place a sheet over an air mattress or foam mattress.

If placing a flotation pad:

_____ 8. Place pad in a pillowcase and fold the edges neatly around the pad.

_____ 9. Tuck the far edge of the supportive pad under the client's body.

_____ 10. Raise the siderail and move to the side of the bed where the client lays.

_____ 11. Lower the siderail and move the client over the folded supportive pad.

_____ 12. Pull the tucked pad from under the client and smooth in place.

_____ 13. Inflate the air mattress or attach the mattress to the pressure pump. Check to determine that the mattress inflates and deflates alternatively.

_____ 14. Place a waterproof pad under the client's hips over a foam pad or air mattress if client is incontinent.

_____ 15. Reposition the client comfortably and attach the call signal.

_____ 16. Wash hands.

_____ 17. Open curtains or door of the room.

Name ______________________________ Date ______________

Observed by ____________

SKILL 19.2 Turning the Client on a Special Frame

A. Turning the client from supine to prone on a wedge frame:

_____ 1. Assess the client to identify the nursing diagnostic category.

_____ 2. Plan the nursing objective and the expected outcomes and prepare the necessary supplies and equipment.

_____ 3. Explain to the client exactly what will be done: safety features, direction of turn, change of linens. Answer his questions.

_____ 4. Wash hands.

_____ 5. Close the door to the client's room or draw the curtains around his bed.

_____ 6. Prepare the anterior frame for use by covering with a sheet.

_____ 7. Offer a bedpan to the female client.

_____ 8. Check the locking feature on the bed to ensure that it is in place.

_____ 9. Open the turning ring.

_____ 10. Place protective pads (sheepskin) on the client's chest, abdomen, or legs, as needed.

_____ 11. Place the head end of the anterior frame over the client's face and into the securing bolt on the bed frame. Tighten the nut.

_____ 12. Secure the foot end of the frame by tightening the nut.

_____ 13. Instruct the client to clasp his arms and hands around the posterior frame.

If the client cannot grasp the frame:

_____ 13. Secure a safety strap around both frames at the client's waist level, ensuring that the client's arms and hands are between the frames.

_____ 14. Close and lock the turning circle.

_____ 15. Check the security of the nuts and the safety straps again.

_____ 16. Remove the lock pin at the head of the frame and pull out the bed-turning lock.

_____ 17. Grasp the handles of the turning circle, inform the client that he will now be turned.

_____ 18. Rotate the turning circle to the client's right, the narrower side of the wedge, slowly and smoothly, until the client is prone and the frame automatically locks.

_____ 19. Replace the lock pin.

_____ 20. Open the turning circle.

_____ 21. Unscrew the nuts, remove the safety straps, and remove the posterior frame.

_____ 22. Adjust the client's position as necessary. Cover him with linens.

_____ 23. Attach arm supports or other aids as desired by the client.

_____ 24. Attach the call signal within the client's reach; open curtains or door to the room.

_____ 25. Wash hands.

B. Turning the client from prone to supine on a wedge frame:

_____ 1. Assess the client to identify the nursing diagostic category.

_____ 2. Plan the nursing objective and the expected outcomes and prepare the necessary supplies and equipment.

_____ 3. Explain to the client exactly what will be done: safety features, direction of turn, change of linens, etc. Answer his questions.

_____ 4. Wash hands.

_____ 5. Close the door to the client's room or draw the curtains around his bed.

_____ 6. Prepare the posterior frame for use by covering with a sheet.

_____ 7. Offer a urinal to the male client.

_____ 8. Check the locking feature on the bed to ensure that it is in place.

_____ 9. Open the turning ring.

_____ 10. Place protective pads (sheepskin) on the client's back, buttocks, or legs as desired.

_____ 11. Place the head end of the posterior frame over the client's face and into the securing bolt on the bed frame. Tighten the nut.

_____ 12. Secure the foot end of the frame by tightening the nut.

_____ 13. Instruct the client to clasp his arms and hands around the posterior frame.

If the client cannot grasp the frame:

_____ 13. Secure a safety strap around both frames at the client's waist level, ensuring that the client's arms and hands are between the frames.

_____ 14. Close and lock the turning circle.

_____ 15. Check the security of the nuts and the safety straps again.

_____ 16. Remove the lock pin at the head of the frame and pull out the bed-turning lock.

_____ 17. Grasp the handles of the turning circle, and inform the client that he will now be turned.

_____ 18. Rotate the turning circle to the client's right, the narrower side of the wedge, slowly and smoothly, until the client is prone and the frame automatically locks.

_____ 19. Replace the lock pin.

_____ 20. Open the turning circle.

_____ 21. Unscrew the nuts, remove the safety straps, and remove the posterior frame.

_____ 22. Adjust the client's position as necessary. Cover him with linens.

_____ 23. Attach arm supports or other aids as desired by the client.

Name ______________________________ Date ______________

Observed by ______________

_____ 24. Attach the call signal within the client's reach; open curtains or door to the room.

_____ 25. Wash hands.

C. Placing the client on a Rotokinetic bed:

_____ 1. Close the door to the room or draw curtains around the bed.

_____ 2. Wash hands.

_____ 3. Place the bed in a horizontal position and remove supportive devices.

_____ 4. Lock gatch; unplug electric cord.

_____ 5. Transfer the client from hospital bed to Rotokinetic bed.

_____ 6. Secure safety devices as described in the manufacturer's instructions.

_____ 7. Cover the client with a sheet.

_____ 8. Plug in electricity.

_____ 9. Adjust degree of rotation as instructions indicate.

_____ 10. Monitor the client's responses for feelings of lightheadedness, disorientation, or nausea.

_____ 11. Stop the bed by releasing the gatch and manually rotating the bed to desired position.

D. Turning the client from prone to supine on a CircOlectric bed:

_____ 1. Assess the client to identify the nursing diagnostic category.

_____ 2. Plan the nursing objective and expected outcomes and prepare the necessary supplies and equipment.

_____ 3. Explain to the client exactly what will be done: safety features, direction of turn, change of linens. Answer his questions.

_____ 4. Wash hands.

_____ 5. Close the door to the client's room or draw the curtains around his bed.

_____ 6. Prepare the anterior frame for use by covering with a sheet.

_____ 7. Offer a bedpan to the female client.

_____ 8. Place a small pillow or support over the client's ankles.

_____ 9. Place footboard securely against the client's feet.

_____ 10. Bring the anterior frame through the sides of the circular frame with the help of a second worker.

_____ 11. Position frame on top of the client, with his face centered in the opening.

_____ 12. Secure the ends of anterior frame to the circular frame by fastening the bolts.

_____ 13. Instruct the client to hold the sides of the frame.

If the client cannot hold the frame:

_____ 13. Place the client's arms at his sides and secure with a safety belt around both frames at waist level. Or place his arms in the safety slings.

_____ 14. Check the security of the bolts and the safety straps again.

_____ 15. Plug in the bed's electric cord. Ensure that the bed will move without obstruction.

_____ 16. Inform the client that the turn will begin. Tell him to inform you if he is feeling weak or lightheaded or has other discomfort.

_____ 17. Rotate bed by turning the control marked "Face." Release if the client states he is experiencing untoward difficulty.

_____ 18. Release control when the client is prone.

_____ 19. Remove safety belts; remove locking bolt on the posterior frame.

_____ 20. Pull support bar in the bed frame forward and raise the posterior frame until it locks in place.

_____ 21. Check to ensure that the client's feet are positioned properly and not compressed by the footboard of the posterior frame. Ensure that the client's face is unobstructed.

_____ 22. Check the client's body alignment for correctness.

_____ 23. Attach side arms to the anterior frame. Secure safety belts as necessary.

_____ 24. Cover the client with sheets or blankets as desired.

_____ 25. Attach the call signal within the client's reach.

_____ 26. Unplug the electric cord.

_____ 27. Open curtains or door to the room.

_____ 28. Wash hands.

E. Turning the client from prone to supine on a CircOlectric bed:

_____ 1. Assess the client to identify the nursing diagnostic category.

_____ 2. Plan the nursing objective and the expected outcomes and prepare the necessary supplies and equipment.

_____ 3. Explain to the client exactly what will be done: safety features, direction of turn, change of linens, etc. Answer his questions.

_____ 4. Wash hands.

_____ 5. Close the door to the client's room or draw the curtains around his bed.

_____ 6. Prepare the posterior frame for use by covering with a sheet.

_____ 7. Offer a urinal to the male client.

_____ 8. Bring the posterior frame through the sides of the circular frame with the help of a second worker.

_____ 9. Position frame on back of the client.

_____ 10. Secure ends of posterior frame to the circular frame by fastening the bolts.

Complete steps 11–16 as above.

_____ 17. Release control when the client is supine.

Name ________________________________ Date ________________

Observed by ____________

_____ 18. Remove safety belts; remove locking bolt on the anterior frame.

_____ 19. Remove the anterior frame from the circular frame with the help of a second worker.

_____ 20. Check the client's body alignment for correctness.

_____ 21. Attach side arms to the anterior frame. Secure safety belts as necessary.

_____ 22. Cover the client with sheets or blankets as desired.

_____ 23. Attach call signal within the client's reach.

_____ 24. Unplug the electric cord.

_____ 25. Open curtains or door to the room.

_____ 26. Wash hands.

Name ____________________ Date ____________________

Observed by ____________

SKILL 19.3 Managing the Client on an Air-Fluidized Bed

_____ 1. Assess the client to determine his nursing diagnostic categories.

_____ 2. Plan the expected outcomes of Clinitron therapy and prepare the required equipment and supplies.

_____ 3. Ask the client if he has questions or concerns regarding his Clinitron therapy.

_____ 4. Maintain fluidization by depressing the continuous mode switch.

_____ 5. Regulate the air temperature to a level recommended by the physician or to provide comfort for the client.

_____ 6. Smooth the filter sheet under the client and keep a clean bottom sheet spread smoothly under the client.

_____ 7. Change the bottom sheet when it becomes soiled or damp from perspiration.

_____ 8. Place a layer of top covers over the client if he desires.

_____ 9. Ask the client if he feels the effects of floating. Ask him to describe his feelings.

_____ 10. Assess the client's level of awareness.

_____ 11. Encourage the client to drink liquids frequently, if fluid intake is unlimited.

_____ 12. Apply moisturizing lotion liberally and frequently to the client's skin.

To place a bedpan under the client:

_____ 13. Set intermittent fluidization mode.

_____ 14. Place and remove bedpan.

_____ 15. Reset continuous fluidization mode.

To turn the client:

_____ 16. Set intermittent fluidization mode.

_____ 17. Turn and position the client.

_____ 18. Reset continuous fluidization mode.

To prepare the client for meals:

_____ 19. Set intermittent fluidization mode.

_____ 20. Assist the client to a low Fowler's position and place wedge pillow behind his upper back and shoulders.

_____ 21. Adjust position with additional pillows as desired.

_____ 22. Reset continuous fluidization mode.

Name ______________________ Date ______________

Observed by ____________

CHAPTER 20 MAINTAINING THERAPEUTIC IMMOBILITY

SKILL 20.1 Applying and Managing a Splint or Brace

A. Preparation:

____ 1. Assess the client to determine the nursing diagnosis.

____ 2. Plan the expected outcomes of the procedure and gather the necessary equipment.

____ 3. Tell the client that he is to have a splint or brace applied to the body part and explain the reason for it.

____ 4. Close the door to the client's room or draw the privacy curtains around his bed.

B. Applying a soft or hard cervical collar:

____ 5. Position the client in a sitting position with his head erect, chin pointing slightly forward.

____ 6. Place the collar around the neck and fasten securely with the straps or Velcro.

____ 7. Assess the position of the collar to ensure that it is snug, effectively immobilizes the neck, but does not obstruct the airway or impair the client's ability to swallow.

____ 8. Assess the underlying soft tissues; readjust collar if tissues are compressed because of poor fit. Pad with soft fabrics or cotton if fit is correct but client reports skin discomfort.

C. Applying a clavicle splint:

____ 5. Position the client sitting upright with his arms abducted and elevated away from his body.

____ 6. Place the neck portion of the strap on the posterior neck and position the axillary straps under the axillae. Draw the ends of the straps through the posterior buckle and secure.

____ 7. Assess the position of the straps to ensure that they do not place excessive pressure on the axilla.

____ 8. Assess the underlying soft tissues; readjust splint if tissues are compressed because of poor fit. Pad with soft fabrics or cotton if fit is correct but client reports skin discomfort.

D. Applying a wrist, ankle, or knee splint:

____ 5. Place the client's affected joint in the prescribed joint position, usually extension.

____ 6. Place the parts of the splint in position around the joint and fasten the straps, hooks, or Velcro.

_____ 7. Assess the client's limb to determine if the correct degree of immobilization is achieved.

_____ 8. Assess the underlying soft tissues; readjust splint if tissues are compressed because of poor fit. Pad with soft fabrics or cotton if the fit is correct but client reports skin discomfort.

For each type of splint:

_____ 9. Assess the color, movement, and sensation of the affected limbs immediately after application of the splint and again at regular intervals.

_____ 10. Teach the client how to apply and remove splint at intervals recommended by the physician; encourage questions; have client demonstrate the application.

_____ 11. Explain to the client how to assess neurovascular status; have the client demonstrate the assessment.

_____ 12. Instruct and encourage the client to actively exercise body parts that are not immobilized.

_____ 13. Remove the splint at regular intervals and stimulate the underlying skin surfaces through washing and gentle massage.

E. Applying a brace:

_____ 5. Assist the client to dress the body part (shirt for a back brace, stockings for a leg brace).

_____ 6. Assist the client to a position that permits application of the brace.

_____ 7. Check hinges of splint and apply lubrication as needed.

_____ 8. Fit the brace against body part and check for proper alignment and comfort.

_____ 9. Secure the brace with straps and buckles so that it is snug but not tight.

_____ 10. Assess the underlying tissues for evidence of compression; adjust the brace if necessary or pad the tissues with soft fabric or cotton padding.

_____ 11. Assess the color, movement, and sensation of the affected limbs immediately after application of the brace and again every two hours.

_____ 12. Teach the client how to apply and remove the brace; encourage questions; have client demonstrate the application.

_____ 13. Explain to the client how to assess neurovascular status; have the client demonstrate the assessment.

_____ 14. Instruct and encourage the client to actively exercise body parts that are not immobilized.

Name ______________________________ Date ______________

Observed by ____________

SKILL 20.2 Managing the Client with a Cast

A. Assisting with the application of a cast:

_____ 1. Assess the client to determine his nursing diagnosis.

_____ 2. Plan the expected outcomes of the cast application and gather the necessary supplies.

_____ 3. Explain the procedure to the client, answering his questions and addressing his concerns. Instruct him to report pain or discomfort to the physician during the procedure.

_____ 4. Place waterproof padding under the affected body part or over the entire bed and other nearby furniture.

_____ 5. Measure and cut the stockinette so that it will be slightly longer than the affected body part.

_____ 6. Roll the stockinette.

_____ 7. Hold the affected limb in a neutral position, grasping the joints or uninjured portion, while the physician applies the stockinette.

_____ 8. Hold the affected limb while the physician applies one to three layers of padding.

_____ 9. Don disposable gloves.

_____ 10. Immerse the cast roll in the water for the required period of time. Squeeze to remove excess water.

_____ 11. Support the body part by grasping and holding the distal portion or the unaffected areas of the part above the bed while the physician unrolls the cast material and forms the cast dressing.

_____ 12. Apply lubricant to the physician's gloves, if he or she desires, to assist with molding the shape of the cast.

_____ 13. Assist the physician to fold the ends of the stockinette back over the distal and proximal edges of the cast. Trim with scissors, as necessary.

_____ 14. Remove excess materials and clean the area as needed.

_____ 15. Assess the client's response to the cast: discomfort, pain, chilling, color, movement, and sensation of distal parts of casted extremities.

_____ 16. Support the cast on a pillow until it has dried.

B. Maintaining the integrity of the cast:

_____ 1. Handle the cast with the palms of the hands while the cast is drying.

_____ 2. Elevate the casted limb above the level of the client's heart by using pillows, blankets, or the bed knee gatch.

_____ 3. Reassess the neuromuscular and circulatory status of the distal part at regular intervals.

_____ 4. Apply ice bags to the cast, if directed by the physician.

_____ 5. Examine the cast for drainage stains, if the client has had surgery or an open wound injury. Measure the size of the stain and note the size and time. Or draw a line around the stain and note the time directly on the cast.

To petal the cast edges, the nurse will:

_____ 1. Examine the cast for rough edges.

_____ 2. Cut several 2–3-inch-long strips of 1-inch-wide adhesive tape.

OR

Cut several strips of moleskin of this size and shape.

_____ 3. Cut curved edges on one end of each adhesive tape strip.

_____ 4. Slip the adhesive side of the square end of the tape about 1 inch into the inside of the cast edge and press into place.

_____ 5. Smooth the remainder of the tape over the outside of the cast.

_____ 6. Repeat steps 4 and 5 until the entire edge of both distal and proximal ends of the cast is covered.

Name ______________________________ Date ______________

Observed by ____________

SKILL 20.3 Managing the Client in Traction

A. Placing the client in skin traction:

_____ 1. Assess the client's affected body part and determine the nursing diagnosis.

_____ 2. Prepare the plan of expected outcomes and gather the equipment necessary.

_____ 3. Explain the procedure and the reason for it to the client.

_____ 4. Inspect the traction frame attached to the bed to ensure that it will provide the correct amount and direction of force.

_____ 5. Wash and dry carefully the body part that will be placed in the traction garment.

B. For Buck's extension:

_____ 6. Place the client in a supine position in alignment with the traction apparatus at the foot of the bed.

_____ 7. Position the client's leg in the traction half-boot.

_____ 8. Fasten the straps or Velcro strips securely around the boot and leg.

_____ 9. Place two fingers between the boot straps and the leg to ensure adequate space.

_____ 10. Attach the foot of the boot to the traction rope and weight carrier.

_____ 11. Apply the prescribed weight to the weight carrier slowly and deliberately. Ensure that the weights hang freely.

C. For cervical traction:

_____ 6. Place the client in a supine position with the head directly aligned with the traction apparatus at the head of the bed.

_____ 7. Place the client's head and neck into the cervical collar or halter.

_____ 8. Inspect for centering, proper fit, and pressure points.

_____ 9. Attach ends of the spreader bar to the collar or halter attachments.

_____ 10. Attach the weight carrier to the rope on the spreader bar.

_____ 11. Apply the prescribed weights to the weight carrier slowly and deliberately. Ensure that the weights hang freely.

D. For pelvic traction:

_____ 6. Assist the client to a side-lying position.

_____ 7. Fold the belt or girdle and tuck it just beneath the client's waist.

_____ 8. Assist the client to turn to the other side. Smooth the belt or girdle under the waist as he moves.

_____ 9. Attach the belt or girdle securely into position around the waist and upper hips.

_____ 10. Place two fingers between the belt or girdle and the hips to ensure adequate space.

_____ 11. Place the client to a supine position and align body with the traction apparatus at the foot of the bed.

_____ 12. Adjust the straps from the belt or girdle to lay along the client's legs.

_____ 13. Attach the spreader bar to the straps.

_____ 14. Attach the weight carrier to the rope on the spreader bar.

_____ 15. Apply the prescribed weights to the weight carrier slowly and deliberately. Ensure that the weights hang freely.

E. To maintain the client in skin traction, the nurse will:

_____ 1. Reassess the client's neuromuscular and circulatory status after applying traction and at periodic intervals.

_____ 2. Inspect the ropes, knots, pulleys, and traction bars to ensure their intactness at regular intervals.

_____ 3. Ensure that the weights hang freely at all times.

_____ 4. Check the client's body alignment in relationship to the traction apparatus at regular intervals.

_____ 5. Remove the traction garment at intervals and inspect the skin for pressure, redness, abrasions and edema.

_____ 6. Provide skin cleansing and gentle massage when the traction garment is removed.

_____ 7. Encourage the client to perform active joint range of motion exercises on all his nonaffected joints. Perform passive exercises if he is unable to do so.

F. To maintain the client in skeletal traction, the nurse will:

_____ 1. Inspect the client's alignment with the traction apparatus at regular intervals.

_____ 2. Inspect the ropes, knots, pulleys, and traction bars to ensure their intactness at regular intervals.

_____ 3. Ensure that the weights hang freely at all times.

_____ 4. Reassess the client's neuromuscular and circulatory status at regular intervals.

_____ 5. Inspect the pin or wire insertion into the body at regular intervals to look for change of position, signs of inflammation, or any unusual drainage.

_____ 6. Cleanse the pin site with an antiseptic solution or ointment at regular intervals.

_____ 7. Encourage the client to perform active joint range of motion exercises on all his nonaffected joints. Perform passive exercises if he is unable to do so.

Name ____________________ Date ____________________

Observed by ____________

CHAPTER 21 MANAGING ANXIETY

SKILL 21.1 Managing Anxiety

_____ 1. Assess the client to identify actual and potential nursing diagnoses of anxiety.

_____ 2. Plan the expected outcomes.

_____ 3. Promote a therapeutic environment.

- Move the client from a large, open, and noisy space to a smaller, quiet enclosure.
- Stay with the client and remain calm.
- Ensure that the lighting is not too bright or too dim.

_____ 4. Demonstrate acceptance of the client and respect for the individual.

- Remain present and demonstrate interest and concern.
- Use active listening skills.

_____ 5. Facilitate the client's expression of feelings.

- Use therapeutic skills of communication to facilitate the expression of feelings the client is experiencing.
- Communicate in short, simple sentences; give only one direction at a time.
- Use a quiet, firm tone of voice to communicate assurance to the client that you are in control of the situation and will not allow harm to come to the client.
- Avoid the use of the false reassurance, "Everything is going to be o.k."
- Accept the expression of negative feelings.
- Demonstrate sensitivity to the client's feelings and needs.
- Avoid negating, belittling, or discounting the client's feelings or experiences.
- Express an empathetic, sensitive understanding of the client's feelings.
- Use touch if rapport has been established; if not, avoid touch.

_____ 6. Promote a sense of security.

- Maintain an awareness of anxious feelings in yourself and develop control over your responses.
- Convey confidence that a constructive resolution to the client's conflicts will be found.
- Describe briefly and clearly any procedures the client is to undergo.
- Avoid threatening the client through indiscriminate use of medical or psychiatric terminology, insincerity, judgmental attitudes, etc.
- Counteract feelings of guilt in the client.
- Use nonverbal communication such as touch and a close, quiet presence.
- Accept or encourage crying.
- Administer an antianxiety agent as ordered by the physician.

- Assure client that some anxiety must be endured in order for new coping mechanism to develop.

_____ 7. Promote problem solving.

- Explore possible sources of anxiety: "What were you doing when this feeling came upon you?" "When did you start to feel anxious?" "What was happening?"
- Determine the client's usual coping patterns: "What do you usually do when you feel this way?" "Is that helpful?"
- If past coping mechanisms are not helpful in the present situation, encourage the client to explore options: "What else might you do to prevent or alleviate the anxiety?"
- Provide opportunities for the client to role play or try out new behaviors.
- Positively reinforce new, more adaptive coping mechanisms.
- Emphasize that some anxiety is inherent in living and that a mild amount motivates productivity and assists one toward self-actualization.

Name ______________________ Date ______________

Observed by __________

CHAPTER 22 MANAGING PAIN

SKILL 22.1 Managing Pain

A. Removing painful stimuli:

_____ 1. Explain to the client what will be done to alleviate his discomfort or pain.

_____ 2. Wash hands.

_____ 3. Alter environmental factors.

- Change the intensity or direction of the lighting.
- Reduce sound intensity from radio or television.
- Close the door to client's room.
- Regulate temperature controls to more comfortable level.

_____ 4. Remove possible sources of discomfort from bed or bedside.

- Smooth wrinkles in bed sheets.
- Change position of tubing or equipment.
- Loosen bedclothes.
- Alter dressing if necessary.

_____ 5. Help the client move to a more comfortable position with proper alignment. Use pillows or blankets as necessary.

_____ 6. Check with client to determine if he is more comfortable. If not, reassess and use the measures you deem necessary.

_____ 7. Wash hands.

B. Using relaxation techniques:

_____ 1. Ask client if he has a way of relaxing.

_____ 2. Encourage him to use his own method.

If time is brief for teaching:

_____ 3. Identify simple methods of relaxation: stretching, sighing, yawning, deep breathing. Suggest client use a combination of these methods.

For long-term use of relaxation:

_____ 4. Close the door to room or draw curtains.

_____ 5. Instruct the client to assume a position of comfort and close his eyes.

_____ 6. Instruct him to breathe in and out slowly, using the abdomen to exhale.

_____ 7. Instruct the client to follow your cues while maintaining steady breathing pattern with the eyes closed.

_____ 8. Use a calm, steady voice to give instructions.

_____ 9. Instruct the client to tighten and then relax muscles one by one, moving from head to toes or toes to head. Use sequence of instructions:

a. "Raise both arms above head and stretch as far as you can reach; breathe in and out one time. Relax arms at side and breathe in and out two times."

b. "Grimace and tighten your eyes and breathe in and out one time; relax your facial muscles and breathe in and out two times."

c. "Press your chin toward your chest and breathe in and out one time; relax the chin and breathe in and out two times."

d. "Raise your shoulders toward your ears and breathe in and out one time. Relax your shoulders and breathe in and out two times."

e. "Tighten the abdominal muscles; breathe in and out one time. Relax the muscles and breathe in and out two times."

f. "Tighten your hips and buttocks; breathe in and out one time. Relax muscles and breathe in and out two times."

g. "Stretch your legs as far as you can; breathe in and out one time. Relax your legs and breathe in and out two times."

h. "Bend your knee slightly; breathe in and out one time; stretch your knee and breathe in and out two times."

i. "Tighten the muscles of your calf; breathe in and out one time. Relax the muscles and breathe in and out two times."

j. "Bend your ankle and point the toes toward the skin; breathe in and out one time; relax the ankle and breathe in and out two times."

k. "Curl and point your toes downward; breathe in and out one time; relax your toes and breathe in and out two times."

_____ 10. Remind the client that he is now relaxed and warm and may feel he is floating.

_____ 11. Ask the client to say, "I am awake and I feel relaxed."

_____ 12. Encourage the client to repeat the sequence on his own when he has learned it.

C. Using distraction:

_____ 1. Ask the client to think of an activity or hobby that is very enjoyable for him. Good choices to use as distraction include music, sports, watching television, participating in relationships with others, video or board games, needlework.

_____ 2. Position the client so that he can look out a window or sit in the doorway to his room to watch activities of other people.

Use a favorite activity for distraction:

_____ 3. Encourage the client to listen to his favorite music on a radio or tape recorder while using relaxation techniques.

a. Instruct the client to tap his hands or feet in rhythm with the music or to sing along (silently or out loud).

b. Encourage the client to adjust volume of music with the intensity of pain.

Name ______________________ Date ______________

Observed by ____________

_____ 4. Encourage the client to interact with family or friends.

_____ 5. Encourage the client to watch sports events or other programs of great interest on television.

_____ 6. Suggest the client use deep breathing exercises and massage the painful body area simultaneously.

_____ 7. Employ any other available means of distraction identified by the client.

D. Using guided imagery:

_____ 1. Explain to the client that he will call on his memories, experiences, or imagination to help manage his pain.

_____ 2. Ask the client to remember a favorite, enjoyable place that he has visited.

_____ 3. Dirêct client to close his eyes and visualize that place; tell him to savor the sights, sounds, and smells while breathing rhythmically.

_____ 4. Pause for several minutes; ask the client to describe what he feels.

_____ 5. Suggest the client repeat the experience at other times if he describes the visualization rather than the pain.

E. Using therapeutic touch:

_____ 1. Explain to the client that you will massage the painful area to help relieve pain. Ask him to signal what feels good and what feels bad as he is massaged.

_____ 2. Close the door to the room or draw the curtains around the bed.

_____ 3. Wash your hands; rub them together to ensure warmth.

_____ 4. Warm a bottle of lotion in a basin of warm water.

_____ 5. Place the client in a comfortable position and expose the body area that is painful to him.

_____ 6. Apply warmed lotion to your hands.

_____ 7. Direct the client to close his eyes and breathe deeply and rhythmically.

_____ 8. Massage the painful body area very slowly and steadily; use the amount of pressure that is most soothing to client.

_____ 9. Massage near the painful area if that is more comfortable to client.

_____ 10. Continue massage until client seems relaxed.

_____ 11. Wash hands.

_____ 12. Teach client's caregiver to use the same technique if it is effective.

F. Applying a TENS unit:

_____ 1. Explain to the client how the TENS unit works: "When placed on your skin, this unit will produce a buzzing or vibrating sensation. Soon you will notice your pain is less or absent."

_____ 2. Close the door to the client's room or draw the bedside curtains.

_____ 3. Wash your hands.

_____ 4. Check the instructions on the TENS unit for proper placement of electrodes.

_____ 5. Demonstrate to the client how to adjust the intensity of the skin stimulation.

_____ 6. Assist the client to expose the body area for application.

_____ 7. Apply conductive gel or water against application points.

_____ 8. Attach electrodes.

_____ 9. Instruct the client to adjust the stimulators until he feels a pleasant sensation.

_____ 10. Remain with the client until he has made adjustments and is comfortable using the unit.

_____ 11. Monitor the client at regular intervals for response to the unit.

G. Administering analgesics:

Before the client has pain, prepare for analgesic administration:

_____ 1. Check the physician's orders to determine what medication, dose, route, and interval of administration is ordered.

_____ 2. Look up the drug, action, effects, and side effects if you are unsure of this information.

_____ 3. Check the medication administration record to determine when the drug was last given.

To determine when to administer the analgesic:

_____ 4. Monitor the client for pain behaviors.

_____ 5. Administer medication when client's behavior reflects

- the onset or return of pain
- moderate to severe pain

After the analgesic is given:

_____ 6. Monitor for the medication's effects at frequent intervals.

Name ______________________________ Date ______________

Observed by ____________

CHAPTER 23 ASSESSING FLUID BALANCE AND NUTRITION

SKILL 23.1 Measuring Intake and Output

A. Measuring and recording intake and output:

_____ 1. Assess the client to determine the nursing diagnostic category.

_____ 2. Plan the nursing objectives and expected outcomes.

_____ 3. Indicate that I & O is monitored on the nursing care plan.

_____ 4. Place I & O record where all staff members have access to it.

_____ 5. Post a sign near the client's bedside stating "Intake and Output."

_____ 6. Monitor, measure, and record the client's intake.

_____ 7. Monitor, measure, and record the client's output.

B. Teaching the client and caregivers to measure and record intake and output:

_____ 1. Assess the client to determine the nursing diagnostic category.

_____ 2. Plan the nursing objectives and expected outcomes.

_____ 3. Indicate that I & O is monitored on the nursing care plan.

_____ 4. Place I & O record where all staff members have access to it.

_____ 5. Post a sign near the client's bedside stating "Intake and Output."

_____ 6. Explain to the client that all of his fluid intake and output is being measured and recorded. Explain why.

_____ 7. Explain what fluids are to be included on intake.

_____ 8. Demonstrate how to measure liquids with a marked medication measuring cup. Or show the client a prepared sheet listing amounts of liquids held in commonly used cups or glasses.

_____ 9. Provide the client with a pad and pencil and ask him to write down the time and amount of all liquids he drinks.

OR

_____ 10. Show the client the Intake and Output record and how to record his intake.

_____ 11. Explain that the client's urine is measured as output.

_____ 12. Provide the client with urinary collection hat and measuring cup.

_____ 13. Demonstrate the method for recording output on Intake and Output flow sheet.

_____ 14. Ask client to demonstrate how to measure and record fluids.

_____ 15. Explain to the client's family, if present, that all liquid intake and output is to be recorded; explain why. Ask them to monitor intake and report to staff.

_____ 16. Check on the client's progress from time to time.

C. Monitoring and recording fluids in the client's home:

_____ 1. Explain to client and caregivers why fluid balance is being monitored.

_____ 2. Explain how to measure fluid intake using these suggestions:

- A household measuring cup can be used to determine volume of commonly used cups or glasses.
- Encourage the client to make a chart listing volume of commonly used cups or glasses.
- If no measuring cup is available, suggest using a jelly jar that has volume labeled on the bottom or side.

_____ 3. Explain how to collect and measure fluid output using these suggestions:

- Always use a different container for output than that used for intake.
- Collect urine in an empty, washed fruit juice bottle or metal can that has volume printed on it.

_____ 4. Explain how to record measurements using these suggestions:

- A notebook or paper may be prepared with separate sections for intake and output, for documenting their amounts.
- Each item entered on the record must be appropriately documented.
- Have the client who is unable to comprehend how to measure or has difficulty measuring because of visual losses simply record that "one juice glass" or "one bowl of soup" was consumed. Later the nurse can measure and record the exact volume.
- Instruct the client to keep the intake and output record in a convenient location (in the kitchen or in the bathroom).

_____ 5. Ask the client to demonstrate both how to measure and how to record. Check the records on subsequent visits.

Name ____________________ Date ____________

Observed by ________

SKILL 23.2 Assessing Nutritional Status

____ 1. Interview the client to obtain a diet history.

____ 2. Explain to the client that basic body measures will be taken to help evaluate his nutritional status.

____ 3. Measure the client's height.

____ 4. Weigh the client.

____ 5. Compare the height and weight to standards for the client's age and sex. If he is not within normal limits, determine what percentage his weight is over or under the norm for his age and sex.

____ 6. Instruct the client to flex the elbow of his nondominant arm.

____ 7. Locate the olecranon of the ulna and the acromial process of the scapula; identify the midpoint and mark it with a permanent ink felt-tip pen.

____ 8. Instruct the client to let his arm fall naturally to his side.

____ 9. Place the tapemeasure around the arm at the marked point and determine the mid-upper arm circumference (MUAC). Record.

____ 10. Pinch the skinfold parallel over the triceps at the same level as the marked point on the same arm.

____ 11. Close the arms of the calipers against the skinfold and read the measurement and release. Record.

____ 12. Repeat the skinfold measurement three times and take the average measurement.

____ 13. Calculate the arm muscle circumference (AMC) with these formula: mid-upper-arm circumference (in centimeters) − 0.314 × triceps skinfold = arm muscle circumference.

____ 14. Compare the MUAC and the AMC with standardized tables.

____ 15. Determine where the client's MUAC and AMC fall on the standardized table.

____ 16. Collect all data and compare with normal data.

____ 17. Analyze all the data to identify any nursing diagnostic category they represent.

____ 18. Refer the client to a nutritionist or dietitian if these findings are present:

- recent weight loss of more than 10 percent
- an AMC or triceps skinfold measurement less than 85 percent of the standard
- low serum albumin or lymphocyte studies

Name ______________________________ Date ______________

Observed by ____________

CHAPTER 24 HELPING THE CLIENT EAT

SKILL 24.1 Feeding the Infant

A. Preparing for feeding:

_____ 1. Assess the infant client and determine the nursing diagnostic category.

_____ 2. Plan the nursing objectives and the expected outcomes.

_____ 3. Wash hands.

_____ 4. Select the correct formula.

_____ 5. Pour the formula into the sterile bottle, never touching the rim or inside of the bottle.

_____ 6. Place the nipple on the bottle, never touching the stem or inside of the nipple. Secure tightly.

_____ 7. Set the bottle in the basin of hot water, ensuring that the water level does not reach the nipple. Wait a few minutes.

_____ 8. Remove the bottle from the water and sprinkle a few drops of formula on the inside of the nurse's wrist to ensure the correct formula temperature. Place it near a chair.

B. Bottle-feeding the infant:

_____ 9. Identify the infant by checking his name band.

_____ 10. Change the infant's diapers.

_____ 11. Wrap the infant in a soft blanket.

_____ 12. Wash hands.

_____ 13. Carry the infant to a comfortable chair and sit down.

_____ 14. Cradle the infant in one arm with his head resting on the bend of the elbow and his buttocks on your lap.

_____ 15. Tuck a bib or towel under the infant's chin.

_____ 16. Hold the bottle with the nipple down ensuring that the formula completely covers the nipple.

_____ 17. Brush the nipple tip lightly against the infant's cheek until he roots toward the nipple.

_____ 18. Place the nipple in the infant's mouth, keeping the bottle inverted at a 45° angle.

_____ 19. Allow the infant to suck for several minutes or until he has taken approximately half of the formula.

_____ 20. Position the infant so that he is sitting and leaning forward on your lap; support his head and shoulders with one hand.

_____ 21. Pat the infant's back between his scapulas or gently rub the back to encourage him to burp.

_____ 22. Continue the feeding until the infant seems satisfied (falling asleep or not sucking any longer).

_____ 23. Burp the infant by repeating steps 19 and 20.

_____ 24. Check the diaper and change it if it is wet or soiled.

_____ 25. Place the infant in his bed on his abdomen and cover as necessary.

_____ 26. Dispose of or wash bottle and nipple.

_____ 27. Wash hands.

C. Feeding the infant solid foods:

_____ 1. Assess the infant client and determine the nursing diagnostic category.

_____ 2. Plan the nursing objectives and the expected outcomes.

_____ 3. Wash hands.

_____ 4. Prepare the baby food.

_____ 5. Change the infant's diapers.

_____ 6. Wash hands.

_____ 7. Place the infant in an infant seat or a high chair.

OR

Place the infant sitting on the nurse's lap.

_____ 8. Hold the infant's hands and arms.

_____ 9. Place a small amount of solid food on the spoon and brush it against the infant's lips until he opens them.

_____ 10. Place the food well back on the tongue and remove the spoon.

_____ 11. Use the edge of the spoon to scrape away food that is pushed out of the mouth and insert it back into the mouth.

_____ 12. Repeat steps 8–10 until the infant appears satisfied (refusing further food or falling asleep).

_____ 13. Wash the infant's face with a clean cloth and remove him from the chair.

_____ 14. Change his diaper if necessary and place the infant in a comfortable place and position.

_____ 15. Clean utensils.

_____ 16. Wash hands.

Name ______________________________ Date ______________________________

Observed by ______________

SKILL 24.2 Assisting an Adult to Eat

A. Preparing the client for mealtime:

_____ 1. Assess the client to determine the nursing diagnostic category.

_____ 2. Plan the nursing objectives and the expected outcomes.

_____ 3. Remove all unpleasant objects from the client's bedside environment.

_____ 4. Assist the client to void or defecate as necessary.

_____ 5. Assist the client with washing hands, face, or doing mouth care as desired.

_____ 6. Assist the client to an upright position, either high Fowler's in bed or sitting in a chair, if he is able to eat by himself.

_____ 7. Wash hands.

_____ 8. Compare food tray with the client's name band to be sure they match; check that the diet is correct for the client.

_____ 9. Prepare the food tray in whatever manner the client desires: open cartons, remove covers, cut food, or add seasoning.

_____ 10. Place a towel under the client's chin covering his chest, if the client is likely to dribble his food or drink.

_____ 11. Position the tray on the overbed table directly in front of the client. Adjust the table's height as necessary.

_____ 12. Place the call signal within the client's reach and leave the client for a while.

_____ 13. Return after a reasonable interval to check the client's progress; remove the tray if he is finished.

_____ 14. Note the amount and type of food that the client ingested. Determine his degree of satisfaction.

_____ 15. Record fluid intake for I & O or amount of food ingested for calorie count.

_____ 16. Remove the tray and provide washcloth and towel for the client to wash his face and hands.

B. Feeding the client:

_____ 1. Assess the client to determine the nursing diagnostic category.

_____ 2. Plan the nursing objectives and the expected outcomes.

_____ 3. Remove all unpleasant objects from the client's bedside environment.

_____ 4. Assist the client to void or defecate as necessary.

_____ 5. Assist the client with washing hands, face, or doing mouth care as desired.

_____ 6. Assist the client to an upright position, either high Fowler's in bed or sitting in a chair, if he is able to eat by himself.

_____ 7. Wash hands.

_____ 8. Compare the food tray with the client's name band to be sure they match; check that the diet is correct for the client.

_____ 9. Prepare the food tray in whatever manner the client desires: open cartons, remove covers, cut food, or add seasoning.

_____ 10. Place a towel under the client's chin covering his chest, if the client is likely to dribble his food or drink.

_____ 11. Place the food tray within reach. Sit or stand next to the client's bed. Allow the client to say grace.

_____ 12. Describe the prepared food and drink and ask the client to tell you which he would like first.

_____ 13. Test food temperature by placing a small portion or a few drops on the inside of your wrist.

_____ 14. Place a medium food bite on the fork or spoon, ask the client to open his mouth, and place the food on his tongue. If the client is paralyzed on one side, place food on the functional side of his mouth.

_____ 15. Provide a drink of fluid when the client requests it. Offer a drink if he does not. Use a straw if the client is unable to sip fluid otherwise.

_____ 16. Continue to offer bites of various foods at a regular pace; alternate every few bites with a drink. Follow the client's preferences.

_____ 17. Encourage the client to direct the action. If the client is unable to talk, encourage him to communicate his desires through nods or blinks. If he is blind, describe the food to him.

_____ 18. Allow ample time between the bites if the client does not communicate when he is ready for the next one.

_____ 19. Continue until the client refuses further food or seems satisfied. Encourage him to consume the entire meal if possible.

_____ 20. Remove the tray.

_____ 21. Wash the client's face and hands. Provide mouth care as desired.

_____ 22. Record fluid intake for I & O or amount of food ingested for calorie count.

C. Setting up a food tray for the blind client:

_____ 1. Assess the client to determine the nursing diagnostic category.

_____ 2. Plan the nursing objectives and the expected outcomes.

_____ 3. Remove all unpleasant objects from the client's bedside environment.

_____ 4. Assist the client to void or defecate as necessary.

_____ 5. Assist the client with washing hands, face, or doing mouth care as desired.

_____ 6. Assist the client to an upright position, either high Fowler's in bed or sitting in a chair, if he is able to eat by himself.

_____ 7. Wash hands.

Name ________________________ Date ________________

Observed by ____________

_____ 8. Compare the food tray with the client's name band to be sure they match; check that the diet is correct for the client.

_____ 9. Place the food tray in front of the client.

_____ 10. Place a towel under the client's chin covering his chest.

_____ 11. Prepare the food tray in whatever manner the client desires: open cartons, remove covers, cut food, or add seasoning.

_____ 12. Take the client's dominant hand and place it on bowls or plates while describing the contents. Place his hand around cups with liquids, encouraging him to place a finger or thumb over the lip of the cup so that he can judge the level of the liquid. Place his hand on the utensils.

_____ 13. Encourage the client to eat while observing him. Ask if he needs assistance in any fashion.

_____ 14. Place the call signal within the client's reach and leave him to eat alone if he seems comfortable.

_____ 15. Return after a reasonable interval and assist as needed.

_____ 16. Note the amount and type of food that the client ingested. Determine his degree of satisfaction.

_____ 17. Record fluid intake for I & O or amount of food ingested for the calorie count.

_____ 18. Remove the tray and provide a washcloth and towel for the client to wash his face and hands.

_____ 19. Wash hands.

Name ______________________ Date ______________________

Observed by __________

CHAPTER 25 MANAGING THE CLIENT WITH A GASTROINTESTINAL TUBE

SKILL 25.1 Inserting a Nasogastric Tube

_____ 1. Assess the client to determine his nursing diagnostic categories.

_____ 2. Plan the expected outcomes. Determine and prepare equipment.

_____ 3. Explain the procedure to the client. Answer his questions. Offer support. Determine a signal, such as raising the hand, that the client may use to tell you if he is experiencing discomfort.

_____ 4. Wash hands.

_____ 5. Prepare the tube by placing it in the basin of hot or cold water.

_____ 6. Place the client in a high Fowler's position.

_____ 7. Drape a towel around the client's shoulders.

_____ 8. Place an emesis basin and tissues within the client's reach.

_____ 9. Stand on the right side of the bed, if right handed. Stand on the left, if left handed.

_____ 10. Remove tube from the basin and place on the towel on the client's shoulders.

_____ 11. Don clean gloves.

_____ 12. Place the internal tip of the tube on the ear; measure the distance from the earlobe to tip of nose to the xiphoid process with the tube. Mark this distance with a piece of tape. Set the tube aside.

_____ 13. Apply a small amount of anesthetic cream to the applicator; gently apply to the inside of the selected nostril.

If using a feeding tube with stylet:

_____ 14. Inject 10 cc of water into the tube.

_____ 15. Insert the stylet into the tube until it connects with the weighted tip. Secure the proximal connectors of the tube and the stylet.

_____ 16. Coil the first 5–6 inches of the distal (weighted) end of the tube around the dominant hand.

_____ 17. Lubricate about 4–5 inches of the tube with the water-soluble lubricant.

If using a self-lubricating catheter:

_____ 17. Immerse the tube tip in water.

_____ 18. Instruct the client to hold head erect, looking forward.

_____ 19. Insert curved internal end of the tube into the nostril, passing it backward along the floor of the nares, toward the ear.

_____ 20. Rotate the tube 180° toward the opposite nostril as it is advanced until it passes the nasopharyngeal corner. (It will now be pointing toward the esophagus.)

_____ 21. Remove the tube if resistance is encountered. Allow the client to rest while you relubricate the tube.

_____ 22. Instruct the client to flex his neck so that his head is pointing downward. Ask him to hold the glass of water.

_____ 23. Advance the tube toward the esophagus, instructing the client to sip and swallow the water.

_____ 24. Instruct the client to take short breaths if he is gagging at this point. If gagging continues, ask him to open his mouth. Inspect the oropharynx for coiled tubing. If the tube is coiled, withdraw it, allow the client to rest, and start again.

_____ 25. Stop the advancement of the tube when the preplaced tape marker reaches the nostril.

_____ 26. Check the placement of the tube.

- Ask the client to speak.
- Place the tip of the 50 cc syringe in the proximal end of the tube and aspirate.
- Draw approximately 10–15 cc of air into the syringe. Place the stethoscope over stomach and inject air.

_____ 27. Remove the stylet and store it in the client's room.

_____ 28. Remove gloves.

_____ 29. Anchor the tube to the client's nose.

- Split a $1\frac{1}{2}$-inch-wide tape and 2 inch long tape lengthwise from one end.
- Attach the unsplit end to the nose.
- Wrap the split ends around the tube.

_____ 30. Anchor the tube to the client's clothing with a rubber band and safety pin.

_____ 31. Attach the external end of the tube to the suction source or feeding set.

_____ 32. Provide comfort measures for the client as necessary.

_____ 33. Attach the call signal within the client's reach.

_____ 34. Wash hands.

Name ________________________________ Date ____________________

Observed by ____________

SKILL 25.2 Managing and Irrigating a Gastric Tube

A. Providing comfort measures:

_____ 1. Assess the client to determine his nursing diagnostic categories.

_____ 2. Plan the nursing objectives and expected outcomes. Determine and prepare the necessary equipment.

_____ 3. Explain to the client what will be done.

_____ 4. Wash hands.

_____ 5. Provide mouth care.

_____ 6. Remove secretions around the nares with facial tissues.

_____ 7. Soak a cotton-tip applicator in hydrogen peroxide.

_____ 8. Wipe the applicator around inside each nostril, removing secretions.

_____ 9. Apply a small amount of water-soluble lubricant to inside of each nostril.

At least once a day:

_____ 10. Remove the tape from the client's nose and the gastric tube. Hold the tube securely.

_____ 11. Remove adhesive from the client's nose with a small amount of benzene.

_____ 12. Wash the skin on the nose. Dry it.

_____ 13. Rotate the tube approximately 180°.

_____ 14. Reanchor the tube with fresh strip of tape.

B. Irrigating the nasogastric tube:

_____ 1. Explain to the client what will be done.

_____ 2. Place a protective pad on the bed under the nasogastric tubing.

_____ 3. Open the irrigating set. Pour saline into the basin.

_____ 4. Wash hands and don clean gloves.

_____ 5. Check for correct placement of the tube.

_____ 6. Fill the syringe with 30–50 cc of saline. Place on the protective pad.

_____ 7. Clamp nasogastric tube proximal to its connection to the drainage tube.

_____ 8. Disconnect nasogastric tube.

_____ 9. Elevate the drainage tubing until suction clears it. Set on the protective pad.

_____ 10. Instill irrigant into the proximal end of the nasogastric tube slowly and steadily.

_____ 11. Check tubing for kinks or evidence of drainage obstruction if resistance is met. Instruct the client to turn to one side.

_____ 12. Lower the proximal end of the tube, release the bulb of the syringe or pull back the plunger to withdraw fluid.

_____ 13. Instruct client to turn to his side if no fluid returns.

_____ 14. Instill and withdraw irrigant several times until the fluid flows in and out freely. Note the amount of fluid instilled.

_____ 15. If the NG tube has a double lumen, draw 30 cc of air into the syringe and inject it into the pigtail, which is the smaller bore tube.

_____ 16. Reclamp the nasogastric tube.

_____ 17. Reconnect the nasogastric tube to drainage tube and release clamp.

_____ 18. Remove gloves.

_____ 19. Reattach the nasogastric tube to the client's clothing.

_____ 20. Position the client comfortably and attach the call signal within reach.

_____ 21. Wash hands.

C. Measuring and emptying gastric drainage:

_____ 1. Wash hands and don clean gloves.

_____ 2. Clamp the drainage tubing.

_____ 3. Remove cover from collection container and empty drainage into a measuring container.

_____ 4. Rinse collection container with water.

_____ 5. Replace cover and unclamp tubing.

_____ 6. Observe for proper functioning of the suction and tubing.

_____ 7. Note the amount of drainage in the measuring container. Observe color, character, and odor. Discard the drainage.

_____ 8. Discard gloves and wash hands.

D. Removing the nasogastric tube:

_____ 1. Explain the procedure to the client. Answer questions.

_____ 2. Cover the bed and the client's clothing with a protective pad.

_____ 3. Turn off the suction source. Clamp the nasogastric tube.

_____ 4. Remove tape from the client's nose. Unpin the tube from his clothing.

_____ 5. Wash hands and don clean gloves.

_____ 6. Instill 20–30 cc of normal saline in the tube.

_____ 7. Disconnect the nasogastric tube from the drainage tube.

_____ 8. Instruct the client to hold his breath while the tube is being removed.

_____ 9. Pull the tube out gently and steadily. Set equipment aside.

_____ 10. Remove gloves.

_____ 11. Clean the skin around the nostrils and provide mouth care.

_____ 12. Position the client comfortably and attach the call signal within reach.

_____ 13. Measure drainage amount; dispose of equipment.

_____ 14. Wash hands.

Name ______________________________ Date ______________

Observed by __________

SKILL 25.3 Administering Enteral Nutrition

A. Preparing the formula for administration:

_____ 1. Assess the client and determine his nursing diagnostic categories.

_____ 2. Plan the nursing objectives and expected outcomes.

_____ 3. Select the correct formula, checking the physician's orders.

_____ 4. Warm the formula to room temperature by placing it in a basin of warm water if it has been refrigerated.

_____ 5. Wash hands.

_____ 6. Open the enteral administration set. Clamp the tubing.

_____ 7. Pour the desired amount of formula in the administration bag.

_____ 8. Open the tubing clamp and fill the tubing with formula. Close the clamp.

_____ 9. Place the administration set on an IV pole.

B. Checking placement of the gastric tube before an intermittent feeding:

_____ 1. Explain to the client what is being done. Answer his questions.

_____ 2. Place the client in a mid to high Fowler's position.

_____ 3. Wash hands and don clean gloves.

_____ 4. Unclamp or remove the plug to the gastric tube.

_____ 5. Place the tip of a 50 cc syringe in the proximal end of the tube and aspirate.

_____ 6. Discard aspirated fluids into the basin.

_____ 7. Draw approximately 10–15 cc of air into the syringe.

_____ 8. Place the stethoscope over stomach and listen as air is injected.

_____ 9. Reclamp the tube or pinch it between the fingers.

C. Administering formula for an intermittent feeding:

_____ 1. Prepare formula and check placement of the tube. Keep gloves in place.

_____ 2. Draw 30 cc water in the syringe.

_____ 3. Unclamp the gastric tube and inject the water slowly and steadily. Set the syringe aside.

_____ 4. Reclamp the gastric tube by pinching the tubing with the nondominant hand.

_____ 5. Connect the administration tubing to the gastric tube.

_____ 6. Unclamp the administration tube to permit a slow but steady drip of the formula.

_____ 7. Regulate the drip rate to permit the formula to infuse over 20–30 minutes:

- Adjust the height of the administration bag.
- Adjust the diameter of the tube lumen with the clamp.

_____ 8. Monitor infusion at intervals.

When infusion is complete:

_____ 9. Clamp both the administration tubing and the gastric tube. Disconnect.

_____ 10. Draw 30 cc water into the syringe; unclamp gastric tube and inject water slowly. Repeat if necessary.

_____ 11. Reclamp the gastric tube; reattach it to the client's clothing.

_____ 12. Discard gloves.

_____ 13. Place the client in comfortable position with the call signal within reach.

_____ 14. Rinse the administration bag and tubing with warm water. Hang it upside down to drain and dry.

_____ 15. Wash hands.

D. Administering and monitoring continuous tube feeding using a pump:

_____ 1. Prepare the client and formula; confirm the position of the tube.

_____ 2. Position the enteral administration bag and tubing on an IV pole with the infusion pump attached.

_____ 3. Thread the tubing through the pump as the manufacturer specifies.

_____ 4. Set the pump computer to the desired rate of administration.

_____ 5. Place the client in a mid to high Fowler's position.

_____ 6. Check placement of the tube.

_____ 7. Connect the gastric tube to the administration tubing. Open clamps on each.

_____ 8. Turn the infusion pump on.

_____ 9. Monitor the feeding rate at intervals.

_____ 10. Rinse the administration set at intervals or before adding new volume of formula.

_____ 11. Do not let formula remain in bag over six hours.

_____ 12. Change administration sets every 24 hours.

_____ 13. Discontinue continuous feeding if client must lie flat for a procedure.

To check the gastric feeding residual at intervals:

_____ 14. Clamp and disconnect gastric tube and administration tube.

_____ 15. Aspirate stomach contents with 50 cc syringe.

_____ 16. Discard syringe contents in basin and continue aspiration until no more formula returns. Note amount of residual contents. If the amount is more than the amount infused during one hour, stop the infusion and notify the physician.

Name ____ Date ____________________

Observed by ____________

CHAPTER 26 MANAGING INTRAVENOUS FLUID THERAPY

SKILL 26.1 Managing a Continuous Intravenous Infusion

A. Preparing equipment for a continuous infusion:

_____ 1. Wash hands.

_____ 2. Examine solution container for clarity and expiration date.

_____ 3. Check correctness of solution by comparing container contents and volume with the physician's order.

_____ 4. Select an infusion administration set that will deliver the volume desired. (Check the label for the drip factor.)

_____ 5. Open the administration set and tubing maintaining sterility of contents.

_____ 6. Position the tubing clamp just below the drip chamber on the administration set.

_____ 7. Screw the clamp closed.

_____ 8. Remove protective covering of the solution container and maintain sterility of container stopper or opening.

_____ 9. Remove cap from tubing of administration set and insert spike through stopper or port.

_____ 10. Add extension length of tubing (if desired) maintaining the sterility of connections.

_____ 11. Invert the solution container and hang it from the IV pole.

_____ 12. Squeeze the flexible drip chamber gently until solution is drawn into the chamber.

_____ 13. Remove tubing end protector cap and open the clamp until solution slowly fills the tubing. This is called priming the tubing.

_____ 14. Close clamp and replace end protector cap when solution has reached the distal end of the tubing.

_____ 15. Inspect tubing for air bubbles. If bubbles are present, remove the end cap, open the clamp slightly, and drain the tubing until the bubbles are expelled. Replace the end cap.

_____ 16. Label the solution container with required information.

_____ 17. Wash hands.

_____ 18. Take the prepared container and venipuncture supplies to the client's bedside.

B. Perform venipuncture:

_____ 1. Explain to the client what will be done. Check his identification bracelet.

_____ 2. Hang prepared solution and infusion set next to the client.

_____ 3. Wash hands.

_____ 4. Disinfect work surface with alcohol and arrange venipuncture supplies conveniently next to the client's bed.

_____ 5. Place tip of prepared tubing on the work surface.

_____ 6. Select the correct-size needle or catheter; maintaining the sterility of the needle, open the package, and place it with the other supplies.

_____ 7. Cut several 2-inch-long pieces of tape; attach them on the clean work surface within reach.

_____ 8. Open package of transparent dressing and place within reach.

_____ 9. Wash hands again and don clean gloves.

_____ 10. Inspect the client's arm for a suitable venipuncture site.

_____ 11. Shave excessive body hair from selected site.

_____ 12. Secure the tourniquet approximately 5–6 inches above the site; check presence of distal pulse.

_____ 13. Inspect site for suitable superficial vein that appears large enough for smooth, easy insertion of needle.

_____ 14. Instruct the client to open and clench his fist several times.

_____ 15. Select a vein that is visible and firm on palpation.

_____ 16. Cleanse site with iodine swab; follow with alcohol swab.

Using a needle:

_____ 17. Attach needle to the tip of the tubing; run fluid through needle and re-clamp the tubing.

_____ 18. Grasp the needle at the top by pinching the butterfly wings; hold the bevel up.

_____ 19. Place your thumb on the vein distal to the puncture site; press down lightly until skin over the vein is taut.

_____ 20. Insert needle at 30° angle approximately $\frac{1}{2}$ inch distal to the vein puncture site.

_____ 21. Watch tubing for blood return.

_____ 22. Advance needle carefully through the course of the vein. Hold steady.

_____ 23. Release tourniquet with free hand.

Using a venous catheter:

_____ 17. Remove cover from needle and catheter.

_____ 18. Grasp the catheter tubing with your fingers; hold the bevel up.

_____ 19. Place your thumb on the vein distal to the puncture sites; press down lightly until skin over vein is taut.

_____ 20. Insert catheter and needle at a 30° angle approximately $\frac{1}{2}$ inch from vein puncture site.

_____ 21. Note blood return through catheter hub; insert catheter and needle into the vein another $\frac{1}{4}$ inch.

Name ________________ Date ________________

Observed by ________________

_____ 22. Release the tourniquet with free hand.

_____ 23. Place a fingertip firmly against the catheter tip and withdraw needle from inside the catheter.

_____ 24. Advance the catheter gently into the vein until the hub is next to the puncture site or resistance is felt; connect hub to IV tubing.

For both needle and catheter:

_____ 25. Open clamp on IV tubing and monitor drip chamber for dripping solution.

_____ 26. Inspect the puncture site for swelling or discoloration.

_____ 27. Place a piece of tape with adhesive side up, under the needle or catheter hub; wrap around hub and secure to skin.

OR

Place folded gauze pad under the hub to hold it at the exact angle of insertion; apply tape across the hub and anchor to skin.

_____ 28. Place iodine ointment at puncture site.

_____ 29. Place tape or transparent dressing over needle hub and distal end of the tubing (if agency policy).

_____ 30. Monitor site for swelling around the site or blood return in the tubing for 5–10 minutes.

_____ 31. Secure tubing, hub, and dressing with a length of loose-weave stockinette, if available.

_____ 32. Write time and date of venipuncture on the venipuncture site label; secure to the site.

_____ 33. Adjust flow rate.

_____ 34. Secure the client's wrist or arm to an arm board, if IV site is in a flexion area.

_____ 35. Discard used equipment; gather unused supplies.

_____ 36. Discard gloves and wash hands.

C. Adjusting the flow rate of the infusion:

_____ 1. Identify the volume of solution for infusion in one hour.

_____ 2. Place timing strip on side of the infusion bottle or bag; mark it at the correct increments with hourly intervals.

_____ 3. Check the drop factor in milliliters per cubic centimeter delivered by the IV administration set.

_____ 4. Identify the number of drops per minute.

_____ 5. Time the number of drops in the drip chamber in one minute by using watch.

_____ 6. Adjust the rate of drops by opening or closing the tubing clamp; match the rate with the calculated minute rate.

_____ 7. Monitor at frequent intervals checking the volume of solution that has infused and the drip rate.

D. Adjusting drip rate using infusion controller or pump:

_____ 1. Mount the machine on the IV pole.

_____ 2. Ensure that infusion pump has a power source (electric or battery).

_____ 3. Prepare solution container and administration. Fill drip chamber one-third full; prime the tubing and close the clamp. Hang the container on the IV pole.

For a controller device:

_____ 4. Attach the IV drop sensor to the container drip chamber above the solution level.

For an infusion pump:

_____ 5. Thread the tubing through the machine according to the manufacturer's instructions.

_____ 6. Perform venipuncture and attach primed tubing.

_____ 7. Open the tubing clamp completely.

_____ 8. Calculate the correct drip rate.

_____ 9. Set the dials to the correct infusion rate and volume; follow the manufacturer's instructions.

_____ 10. Turn on the power and set the alarm signal.

_____ 11. Count the drops for a full minute.

_____ 12. Monitor at regular intervals; count the drops and check the volume infused for accuracy.

E. Managing a continuous intravenous infusion:

_____ a. Check the physician's orders for type and amount of solutions given during the management time period.

_____ b. Check the nursing care plan for further instructions on rate of flow and suggested infusion schedule.

_____ c. Examine the infusion equipment and IV flowsheet to identify IV status at regular intervals.

_____ d. Inspect the infusion site for evidence of infiltration.

_____ e. Inspect the infusion site for evidence of inflammation.

_____ f. Troubleshoot if the solution is not dripping as expected.

_____ g. Monitor for signs of circulatory overload.

_____ h. Discontinue the IV if signs of inflammation, infiltration, or circulatory overload are present.

F. Changing the solution container:

_____ 1. Monitor amount of solution infused until less than 50 cc remain.

Name ______________________________ Date ______________

Observed by __________

_____ 2. Check the physician's orders for the correct solution and amount.

_____ 3. Obtain a new container; compare it with physician's orders for accuracy.

_____ 4. Take the container to the bedside; explain to the client what will be done; reassure him that this will not be painful.

_____ 5. Wash hands.

_____ 6. Remove protective cover from the new solution container; maintain sterility of the top.

_____ 7. Remove used container from pole; clamp tubing; invert the container and remove spike of the administration set.

_____ 8. Insert spike through stopper or opening of new container without twisting the tubing.

_____ 9. Hang new container immediately.

_____ 10. Open clamp and regulate the flow rate.

_____ 11. Monitor system to ensure proper functioning,

_____ 12. Attach correct label and timing strip on the new bottle.

G. Changing the solution container and tubing:

_____ 1. Check venipuncture site label for time and date of venipuncture; check tubing label for time and date of next tubing change.

_____ 2. Monitor amount of solution infused until less than 50 cc remain.

_____ 3. Check the physician's orders for the correct solution and amount.

_____ 4. Obtain a new container; compare it with physician's orders for accuracy.

_____ 5. Wash hands.

_____ 6. Attach a new administration set and extra tubing to container; prime the tubing, clamp, and replace protective end cap.

_____ 7. Take new set-up to the bedside and hang on IV pole next to used container.

_____ 8. Clamp used tubing.

_____ 9. Don clean gloves.

_____ 10. Place an antiseptic swab under the connecting hub of the needle or catheter.

_____ 11. Hold the hub of the needle or catheter in one hand to steady it.

_____ 12. Twist old tubing gently and remove from the hub; hold the hub steady.

_____ 13. Remove protective cap from new tubing and insert tip into the needle hub quickly.

_____ 14. Open the tubing clamp.

_____ 15. Clean the venipuncture site of any blood or solution that leaked during the change.

_____ 16. Reapply venipuncture dressing at this time if agency policy dictates.

_____ 17. Attach new venipuncture site label with updated information.

_____ 18. Regulate the flow rate of the new bottle.

_____ 19. Discard gloves and wash hands.

H. Discontinuing an infusion:

_____ 1. Explain to the client what will be done.

_____ 2. Wash hands and don clean gloves.

_____ 3. Clamp the infusion tubing.

_____ 4. Hold the needle or catheter firmly and loosen the tape or transparent dressing from the venipuncture site.

_____ 5. Place an antiseptic swab above the puncture site.

_____ 6. Pull the needle or catheter gently in the direction of insertion until it is removed.

_____ 7. Press against the site firmly for 2–3 minutes or until bleeding stops.

_____ 8. Apply a bandage or dressing to the site.

_____ 9. Inspect the needle or catheter for intactness; if it is broken, report to the physician immediately.

_____ 10. Indicate the amount of solution infused on the IV record.

_____ 11. Discard the solution container and attachments.

_____ 12. Provide comfort measures for the client as needed.

_____ 13. Discard gloves and wash hands.

Name ______________________________ Date ______________________

Observed by ____________

CHAPTER 27 MANAGING TOTAL PARENTERAL NUTRITION

SKILL 27.1 Managing Total Parenteral Nutrition

A. Assisting the physician with the insertion of the subclavian catheter:

_____ 1. Assess the client to determine his nursing diagnosis.

_____ 2. Plan the nursing objectives and expected outcomes.

_____ 3. Gather and prepare the necessary supplies and equipment.

_____ 4. Explain to the client exactly what will be done and why. Answer his questions.

_____ 5. Draw the curtains around the client's bed or close door to his room.

_____ 6. Wash hands.

_____ 7. Cleanse surface of the overbed table with a 4 × 4 inch gauze pad soaked with isopropyl alcohol. Allow the surface to dry.

_____ 8. Place supplies and equipment on the overbed table.

_____ 9. Prepare an isotonic IV infusion and hang on an IV pole at the client's bedside.

_____ 10. Raise the bed height to a comfortable working level.

_____ 11. Place client in a supine position.

_____ 12. Change any dressings that the client may have.

_____ 13. Wash hands using an antiseptic soap.

_____ 14. Wash the client's anterior neck and upper chest with an antiseptic soap. Dry.

_____ 15. Fold a bath towel in half and roll it.

_____ 16. Place the rolled towel under the client's thoracic vertebrae, between the scapulas.

_____ 17. Shave the skin around the proposed insertion site. Remove all hairs and dry carefully.

_____ 18. Don gown and mask and clean gloves.

_____ 19. Instruct the client to turn his head away from the insertion site. Place a mask over his nose and mouth, if possible.

_____ 20. Saturate three 4 × 4 inch gauze pads, one with acetone, one with alcohol, and one with iodine solution.

_____ 21. Grasp acetone 4 × 4 with forceps and scrub skin area from shoulder to shoulder, ear to chin to nipples. Discard the 4 × 4.

_____ 22. Repeat scrub with alcohol 4 × 4 and with iodine 4 × 4. Discard them.

_____ 23. Open the sterile drapes and place them on the client from shoulder to waist on either side and from nipples to hips.

_____ 24. Discard gloves and wash hands.

_____ 25. Place the client in Trendelenberg position.

The physician prepares to insert catheter by donning gown and mask, opening sterile equipment, donning sterile gloves, arranging drapes, and preparing sterile needle and syringe, catheter.

_____ 26. Open a 6 inch length of sterile tubing and place it on the sterile field using aseptic technique.

_____ 27. Cleanse the rubber stopper on the lidocaine vial and invert the vial.

The physician inserts the sterile needle and syringe and withdraws the desired amount of lidocaine. This is inserted intradermally (beneath the skin) over the proposed insertion site.

_____ 28. Talk with the client; explain what is happening.

_____ 29. Assess client for signs or symptoms of insertion complications.

_____ 30. Instruct the client to turn his head away from the insertion site as the physician works. Instruct him to avoid any movement.

The physician inserts needle and syringe into the subclavian vein; venous blood is withdrawn.

_____ 31. Instruct the client to perform the Valsalva maneuver (hold breath and bear down) while the physician detaches the syringe and inserts the cannula. Tell him to breathe when the catheter is attached.

The physician removes needle, attaches the catheter to the insertion site with a single silk suture, and attaches the 6 inch length of tubing to the catheter.

_____ 32. Attach 6 inch length of tubing to IV tubing and open the clamp.

_____ 33. Lower the bottle below the client's heart level.

_____ 34. Raise the bottle and adjust the flow rate to 30–40 ml/hour.

_____ 35. Reposition client in supine horizontal position. Remove the rolled towel.

_____ 36. Don sterile gloves.

_____ 37. Cleanse around the insertion site with alcohol swabs, beginning at the site and moving the swab in a circular path outward from the site. Repeat two times.

_____ 38. Apply iodine-povidone ointment around the insertion site with a sterile applicator.

_____ 39. Apply the clear adhesive dressing over the site.

_____ 40. Cut a slit in a 1 × 3 inch piece of tape and place the uncut end under the catheter just at the edge of the adhesive dressing.

_____ 41. Press the cut ends of the tape against the top of the adhesive dressing on either side of the catheter.

_____ 42. Remove gloves and drapes.

_____ 43. Wash hands.

Name ______________________________ Date ______________________________

Observed by ______________

_____ 44. Assist with chest x-ray.

_____ 45. Position client comfortably; open drapes or door.

_____ 46. Dispose of used equipment.

_____ 47. Wash hands.

_____ 48. Prepare TPN for administration.

B. Preparing the TPN solution for administration:

_____ 1. Gather supplies in a clean, low-traffic area.

_____ 2. Wash hands.

_____ 3. Allow refrigerated solutions to warm to room temperature before administration.

_____ 4. Inspect the bottle or bag for cracks or openings.

_____ 5. Examine the solutions for clarity.

_____ 6. Compare the information on the bottle label with the physician's orders for the client.

_____ 7. Ensure that additives are compatible with the solution.

_____ 8. Remove cap from additive vial and cleanse stopper with alcohol swab.

_____ 9. Inject the correct size sterile syringe and needle into the vial; withdraw the correct amount of additive.

_____ 10. Inject additive into the TPN bottle.

_____ 11. Label the bottle with the additive.

_____ 12. Wash hands.

_____ 13. Attach the IV administration set to the bottle.

When the location of the catheter tip has been verified by x-ray examination:

_____ 14. Hang the bottle on the IV pole at the client's bedside.

_____ 15. Open the clamp and remove protective cap at the end of tubing and allow the solution to run through. Reclamp.

_____ 16. Prime the filter in the tubing, if filter is required by agency policy.

_____ 17. Attach tubing to infusion pump and regulate pump to desired flow rate.

_____ 18. Turn off infusion that is running and remove tape from the tubing connections.

_____ 19. Instruct the client to perform Valsalva maneuver.

_____ 20. Hold catheter hub with clamp and quickly detach old tubing and connect new tubing.

_____ 21. Instruct client to breathe.

_____ 22. Observe infusion and adjust pump if necessary.

_____ 23. Apply tape around all junctions of the tubings.

_____ 24. Remove gloves and wash hands.

_____ 25. Monitor infusion process periodically.

C. Monitoring the infusion of TPN:

_____ 1. Adjust the infusion rate according to the physician's orders.

_____ 2. Check the line and the catheter site every hour.

_____ 3. Check the accuracy of the amount of solution infused by monitoring the actual amount given during a time period.

_____ 4. Weigh the client daily.

_____ 5. Monitor intake and output.

_____ 6. Measure urine sugar and acetone every six hours or according to agency policy.

_____ 7. Assess client for signs or symptoms of infection.

_____ 8. Assess client for signs or symptoms of circulatory overload.

_____ 9. Assess client for his response to TPN therapy. Revise the nursing care plan according to stated problems.

D. Changing the TPN site dressing:

_____ 1. Explain the procedure to the client.

_____ 2. Cleanse overbed table with 4 × 4 inch gauze pad soaked with alcohol.

_____ 3. Gather supplies and place on overbed table.

_____ 4. Draw curtains around the bed or close door to room.

_____ 5. Wash hands.

_____ 6. Raise bed to working height.

_____ 7. Position client supine.

_____ 8. Remove bedclothing from dressing site.

_____ 9. Inspect dressing for drainage. Loosen the edges.

_____ 10. Wash hands with antiseptic soap.

_____ 11. Prepare a sterile field with these items:

- 4 × 4 inch gauze pads saturated with acetone
- 4 × 4 pads saturated with iodine
- 4 × 4 pads saturated with alcohol
- transparent adhesive dressing

_____ 12. Don a face mask; instruct client to don a mask or turn his head away from the catheter site.

_____ 13. Don clean gloves.

_____ 14. Remove old dressing; stabilize the catheter with one hand. Discard the old dressing.

Name ______________________ Date ______________________

Observed by ____________

_____ 15. Inspect site for redness, swelling, or exudate.

_____ 16. Inspect catheter for intact sutures and no kinking.

_____ 17. Change tubing and extension set, if ordered.

_____ 18. Remove and discard gloves.

_____ 19. Don sterile gloves.

_____ 20. Cleanse around catheter site with 4 × 4 inch gauze pad saturated with acetone, using an outward, circular motion. Cleanse 3 inches around the site. Discard the pad.

_____ 21. Repeat with a 4 × 4 saturated with iodine. Discard it.

_____ 22. Repeat with a 4 × 4 saturated with alcohol. Discard it.

_____ 23. Cleanse the catheter site with a 4 × 4 saturated with iodine. Discard it.

_____ 24. Apply iodine ointment to a 4 × 4 and lay it over insertion site.

_____ 25. Remove and discard gloves.

_____ 26. Apply a skin prep to the skin around the site. Allow it to dry until sticky.

_____ 27. Apply the clear adhesive dressing over the site.

_____ 28. Cut a slit in a 1 × 3 inch piece of tape and place the uncut end under the catheter just at the edge of the adhesive dressing.

_____ 29. Press the cut ends of the tape against the top of the adhesive dressing on either side of the catheter.

_____ 30. Label the dressing with date and initials.

_____ 31. Wrap a piece of tape around the catheter about 10–12 inches from the dressing and secure with a safety pin to the client's gown.

_____ 32. Position the client comfortably. Open the bedside curtains or the door.

_____ 33. Wash hands.

Name ______________________________ Date ______________

Observed by ____________

CHAPTER 28 ASSESSING GENITOURINARY FUNCTION

SKILL 28.1 Assessing Genitourinary Function

A. Physically examining the male client's external genitourinary organs:

_____ 1. Explain to the client what will be examined. Answer his questions.

_____ 2. Close the door to the room or draw the curtains around his bed.

_____ 3. Instruct the client to empty his bladder, remove his lower clothing, and lie supine on the bed or examining table with his chest, abdomen, and lower body draped.

_____ 4. Wash hands and don gloves while client is preparing.

If the client is the opposite sex of the nurse, ask another nurse or health care worker of the same sex as the client to be present during the examination.

_____ 5. Lower the drape so that only the genitalia are exposed.

_____ 6. Inspect the penis for skin color, intactness, edema, inflammation, lesions.

_____ 7. Retract foreskin, if present, and observe for lesions on the glans, inflammation, edema, or discharge. Note the location and appearance of meatus.

_____ 8. Replace foreskin in natural position.

_____ 9. Palpate the shaft of the penis for tenderness or induration if client has subjective complaints.

_____ 10. Inspect the scrotum for

- excoriation, ulcers, color uniformity
- presence, shape, and symmetry of two testes

_____ 11. Palpate scrotum for

- shape and size of two testes
- tenderness or nodules
- spermatic cord as it runs from epididymis to inguinal ring

_____ 12. Instruct the client to perform testicular self-examination regularly after his bath or shower.

_____ 13. Inspect inguinal areas for swelling or bulging.

_____ 14. Palpate inguinal area for lymph node size, shape, swelling, or tenderness.

Perform rectal exam at this time, if desired (see skill 31.1B.)

_____ 15. Replace drape over the client's genitalia and instruct him to get dressed.

_____ 16. Remove gloves and wash hands.

B. Physically examining the female client's external genitalia:

_____ 1. Explain to the client what will be examined. Answer her questions.

_____ 2. Close the door to the room or draw the curtains around her bed.

_____ 3. Instruct the client to empty her bladder, remove her lower clothing, and lie supine on the bed or examining table with her chest, abdomen, and lower body draped.

_____ 4. Wash hands and don gloves while client is preparing.

If the client is the opposite sex of the nurse, ask another nurse or health care worker of the same sex as the client to be present during the examination.

_____ 5. Position the drape in a triangular fashion over the client's lower body.

_____ 6. Instruct the client to flex her knees and hips, relax her thighs, and allow her legs to rotate laterally from her body. (If she is on an examining table, place her feet in stirrups.)

_____ 7. Wrap the outer corners of the drape around the legs.

_____ 8. Lift the corner of the drape that covers the genitals and fold it back over the client's abdomen.

_____ 9. Direct the examination light on the perineum for illumination.

_____ 10. Inspect the external genitalia for

- hair growth and distribution
- size and shape of labia

_____ 11. Place forefinger and thumb between labia and retract gently. Inspect for

- size and color of clitoris
- presence of inflammation, edema, excoriation, urethral or vaginal discharge, or masses

_____ 12. Instruct the client to "bear down" and inspect opening of vagina and surrounding tissues.

_____ 13. Place index finger just inside opening of vagina and with the thumb, palpate Bartholin's glands on either side of the vaginal orifice. Perform rectal exam at this time, if desired. (See Skill 31.1B.)

_____ 14. Replace drape over the client's genitalia and instruct her to get dressed.

_____ 15. Remove gloves and wash hands.

Name ____________________ Date ____________________

Observed by ____________

CHAPTER 29 TOILETING

SKILL 29.1 Toileting

____ 1. Assess the client and determine the nursing diagnosis.

____ 2. Plan the expected outcomes.

____ 3. Wash hands and don clean gloves.

____ 4. Draw the curtains around the client's bed or close the door.

____ 5. Remove the bedpan from the bedside table and warm it by running warm water around the rim, being careful not to overheat a metal pan.

____ 6. Lower the client's pajamas or underclothing or raise gown above buttocks.

If client is alert, able to assist, and can move in bed:

____ 7. Instruct the client to lie supine, flex the knees, and raise the hips.

____ 8. Slide the bedpan under the client's hips with the open lip end toward the buttocks.

____ 9. Visually determine that the urethra or anus is directly over opening in the bedpan. Raise the bed to a Fowler's position.

If client is unable to raise hips:

____ 7. Instruct the client to turn over on the bedpan so that open lip end is directed toward the foot of the bed and the rim of pan fits securely over the buttocks.

____ 8. Instruct the client to turn back on the bedpan or assist client in this turn. Hold the bedpan firmly against the buttocks while the client is turning.

____ 9. Visually determine that the urethra or anus is directly over the bedpan opening. Raise the bed to a Fowler's position.

If a urinal is being used:

____ 7. Place urinal between the client's thighs, inserting the client's penis into the opening.

____ 10. Instruct the client to void.

____ 11. Place call signal within the client's reach.

____ 12. Place toilet tissues within the client's reach if the client is able to perform own toileting hygiene.

____ 13. Step outside of the curtained area or room if the client prefers to be alone for elimination.

____ 14. Return to the client's bedside as soon as he signals that he is ready for help.

If the client is alert, able to assist, and can move in bed:

_____ 15. Lower the bed. Instruct the client to raise his hips and immediately remove the bedpan.

If client is unable to raise his hips:

_____ 15. Lower the bed. Holding the bedpan flat to the bed, turn the client away and off the bedpan.

If client is using a urinal:

_____ 15. Remove urinal from between the client's thighs.

_____ 16. Place bedpan or urinal on nearby table or low chair, NOT the overbed table.

_____ 17. Wipe and clean the perineal area as necessary.

_____ 18. Assist client into a position of comfort.

_____ 19. Offer soap, washcloth, and water for handwashing to the client.

_____ 20. Place bedpan cover on the bedpan and remove to bathroom or utility room.

_____ 21. Collect specimen of stool or urine as necessary.

_____ 22. Measure urine output.

_____ 23. Empty and clean bedpan or urinal with fresh running water or disinfectant.

_____ 24. Return bedpan or urinal to bedside table.

_____ 25. Remove gloves and wash hands.

Name ______________________________ Date ______________

Observed by ____________

CHAPTER 30 INSERTING AND MANAGING URINARY CATHETERS

SKILL 30.1 Catheterizing the Client

A. Inserting a straight catheter into a female client:

_____ 1. Assess the client and determine the nursing diagnosis.

_____ 2. Plan the expected outcomes.

_____ 3. Explain to the client what is going to happen and why.

_____ 4. Pull curtains around the client's bedside and close the door to the room.

_____ 5. Bring the necessary equipment to the client's bedside.

_____ 6. Wash hands thoroughly.

_____ 7. Place the bed at a comfortable working height.

_____ 8. Position the client on her back with knees flexed and legs laterally rotated. Place a flat pillow or folded bath blanket just under the coccyx. (If client is unable to assume this position, place her on her side with upper leg flexed at the hip and knee.)

_____ 9. Drape the client with a bath blanket or sheet so that only the perineum is exposed.

_____ 10. Position light directly on the exposed perineum.

_____ 11. Stand at the client's right side if you are right-handed; stand at the client's left side if you are left-handed.

_____ 12. Wash perineum with plain water using clean gloves on hands.

_____ 13. Examine the perineum with clean gloved hands and identify the urethra.

_____ 14. Remove gloves and wash hands again.

_____ 15. Place a waste receptable close to the working area at the bedside.

_____ 16. Remove the outer wrap from the catheterization set, maintaining sterility of the inner contents.

_____ 17. Don the sterile gloves (see step 19).

_____ 18. Pick up the underdrape by the corners, unfold it, and wrap the corner around the gloved hands.

_____ 19. Place the underdrape under the patient's buttocks between the abducted thighs. (If underdrape is on top of the set, place it under the client's buttocks without touching the sterile upper surface, and then don the sterile gloves.)

_____ 20. Place the perineal drape with the center opening over the perineum so that only the labia are exposed (or discard drape).

_____ 21. Lift the plastic tray and place it between the client's thighs within easy reach.

_____ 22. Pour the cleansing antiseptic solution over the five cotton balls or gauze squares.

_____ 23. Open a small specimen container and set it aside for later use.

_____ 24. Open the lubricant pack and place the lubricant container on the sterile field near the working area. Discard outer wrapper in waste receptacle.

_____ 25. Lubricate the tip of the catheter and place drainage end of the catheter in the collecting basin.

_____ 26. Using your nondominant hand, place forefinger and thumb together into the opening of the client's vagina, between the labia majora and minora.

_____ 27. Separate both labia minora and labia majora in an upward and outward direction. Leave your nondominant hand in this position.

_____ 28. Pick up a saturated cotton ball with the sterile forceps and clean the distal labia majora from the anterior of the perineum to the posterior. Wipe only once and discard the ball in the disposal container. Pick up a second ball, clean the proximal labia majora; discard. Pick up a third ball, clean the distal labia minora; discard. Pick up another ball, clean the proximal labia minora; discard. Clean the midline of the perineum directly over the meatus of the urethra with the final cotton ball, discard.

_____ 29. Ask the client to take a deep breath and release it slowly just as you begin insertion of catheter.

_____ 30. Keeping the labia separated, grasp the lubricated catheter about 3 inches from the tip with the dominant hand and insert the tip through the meatus into the bladder about 2–3 inches, or until urine flows through the catheter into the collecting tray.

_____ 31. Remove your nondominant hand from the labia, and grasp the catheter.

_____ 32. Allow urine to flow from the catheter into the collecting basin until the flow stops. If a specimen is required, carefully fill the provided container and then replace catheter end in the collecting basin.

_____ 33. Remove the catheter about 1 cm at a time with the dominant hand until any remaining urine empties from the bladder.

_____ 34. Remove catheter completely from the bladder.

_____ 35. Wash the perineum gently to remove lubricant or antiseptic solution that remains on the mucous membranes.

_____ 36. Remove equipment from the bed.

_____ 37. Wash hands. Discard gloves.

_____ 38. Label the specimen container.

B. Inserting a straight catheter into a male client:

_____ 1. Assess the client and determine the nursing diagnosis.

_____ 2. Plan the expected outcomes.

_____ 3. Explain to the client what is going to happen and why.

_____ 4. Pull curtains around the bedside and close the door to the room.

Name ________________________________ Date ________________

Observed by ____________

_____ 5. Bring the necessary equipment to the client's bedside.

_____ 6. Wash hands thoroughly.

_____ 7. Place the bed at a comfortable working height.

_____ 8. Position client in a dorsal recumbent position with legs straight and slightly abducted.

_____ 9. Drape the client's upper body with a bath blanket or sheet so that only the genital area is exposed.

_____ 10. Stand at the client's right side if you are right-handed; stand at the client's left side if you are left-handed.

_____ 11. Wash the penis with plain water using clean gloves on hands.

_____ 12. Remove gloves and wash hands again.

_____ 13. Place a waste receptable close to the working area at the bedside.

_____ 14. Place the overbed table adjacent to the bedside. Place catheterization tray on it.

_____ 15. Open the catheterization set.

_____ 16. Don the sterile gloves. (If underdrape is on top of the set, see step 17.)

_____ 17. Pick up the underdrape by the corners, unfold it, and place it on the client's thighs near the penis. (If drape is on top of the set, place it on the client's thighs without touching the sterile upper side of the drape. Then don the sterile gloves.)

_____ 18. Unfold the perineal drape and position it with the penis in the opening.

_____ 19. Lift the plastic tray and place it in the middle of the protective drape, on the patient's thighs.

_____ 20. Pour the cleansing antiseptic solution over the five cotton balls or gauze squares.

_____ 21. Open a small specimen container and set it aside for later use.

_____ 22. Open the lubricant pack and place its container on the sterile field near the working area. Discard outer wrapper in the waste receptacle.

_____ 23. Lubricate the tip of the catheter.

_____ 24. Place drainage end of the catheter in the collecting basin.

_____ 25. Grasp the penis firmly behind the glans with your nondominant hand.

_____ 26. Retract the foreskin with the thumb and forefinger of the nondominant hand and spread the meatus open.

_____ 27. Pick up a cotton ball with the forceps and, starting at the meatus, gently clean the glans in a circular motion outward. Repeat this motion twice, using a fresh cotton ball each time.

_____ **28.** Hold the penis at a 90° angle from the body and gently pull upward.

_____ **29.** Pick up the catheter about 3–4 inches from the tip and gently insert it into the urethra for 8 inches or until urine drains. (If resistance occurs, have the client take a deep breath or bear down as if he is urinating. If resistance continues, remove the catheter and report to the physician.)

_____ **30.** Lower the collecting container and allow urine to flow freely by gravity until it ceases.

_____ **31.** Remove the catheter gently about 1 cm at a time.

_____ **32.** Gently wash the penis.

_____ **33.** Remove the equipment from the bed and bedside. Discard gloves.

_____ **34.** Remove drapes, replace the bedcovers, and return the client to a position of comfort.

_____ **35.** Measure the amount of urine drained and record in the desginated area. Label the specimen container.

_____ **36.** Wash hands.

Name ______________________________ Date ______________

Observed by ____________

SKILL 30.2 Inserting an Indwelling Catheter

A. Inserting an indwelling catheter into a female client:

_____ 1. Assess the client and determine the nursing diagnosis.

_____ 2. Plan the expected outcomes.

_____ 3. Explain to the client what is going to happen and why.

_____ 4. Pull curtains around the bedside and close the door to the room.

_____ 5. Bring the necessary equipment to the client's bedside.

_____ 6. Wash hands thoroughly.

_____ 7. Place the bed at a working height.

_____ 8. Position the client on her back with knees flexed and legs laterally rotated. Place a flat pillow or folded bath blanket just under the coccyx. (If client is unable to assume this position, place her on her side with the legs flexed exposing the perineum.)

_____ 9. Drape the client with a bath blanket or sheet so that only the perineum is exposed.

_____ 10. Shine a light directly on the exposed perineum.

_____ 11. Stand at the client's right side if you are right-handed; position self at the client's left side if you are left-handed.

_____ 12. Wearing clean gloves, wash the perineum with plain water.

_____ 13. Examine the perineum with clean gloved hands and identify the urethra.

_____ 14. Remove gloves and wash hands again.

_____ 15. Place a waste receptacle close to the working area at the bedside.

_____ 16. Remove the outer wrap from the catheterization set, maintaining sterility of the inner contents. (If catheterization set is enclosed in a plastic bag, place this bag on the bedside near the working area and use as a disposal receptacle.)

_____ 17. Don the sterile gloves if they are on the top of the set (see step 19).

_____ 18. Pick up the underdrape by the corners, unfold it, and wrap the corner around the gloved hands.

_____ 19. Place the underdrape under the client's buttocks between the abducted thighs. (If the underdrape is on top of the set, place it under the client's buttocks without touching the sterile upper side of the drape. Then don the sterile gloves.)

_____ 20. Place the perineal drape with the center opening over the perineum so that only the labia are exposed (*or* discard drape).

_____ 21. Lift the plastic tray and place it in the middle of the underdrape, between the client's thighs, within easy reach.

_____ 22. Pour the cleansing antiseptic solution over the five cotton balls or gauze squares.

_____ 23. Remove the drainage tube and collecting bag from the kit. If it is not connected to the catheter, connect it at this time.

_____ 24. Test the balloon of the catheter by connecting the syringe to the balloon port and inserting fluid to inflate the balloon. Deflate it by removing the fluid. Leave the syringe connected to the connecting port and position the catheter, tubing, and bag so that the catheter is ready for insertion.

_____ 25. Open a small specimen container and set it aside for later use.

_____ 26. Open the lubricant package and place the lubricant container on the sterile field near the working area. Discard outer wrapper in waste receptacle.

_____ 27. Lubricate the tip of the catheter. Place drainage end of the catheter in the collecting basin.

_____ 28. Using your nondominant hand, place forefinger and thumb together into the opening of the vagina, between the labia majora and minora.

_____ 29. Separate both labia minora and labia majora in an upward and outward direction. Leave the nondominant hand in this position.

_____ 30. Pick up a saturated cotton ball with the sterile forceps and clean the distal labia majora from the anterior of the perineum to the posterior. Wipe only once and discard in disposing receptacle. Pick up a second ball and clean the proximal labia majora; discard. Pick up a third ball, clean the distal labia minora; discard. Pick up another ball, clean the proximal labia minora; discard. With the final cotton ball, clean the midline of the perineum directly over the meatus of the urethra; discard.

_____ 31. Ask client to take a deep breath.

_____ 32. Keeping the labia separated, grasp the lubricated catheter about 3 inches from the tip with the dominant hand and insert the tip through the meatus into the bladder about 2–3 inches, or until urine flows through the catheter into the drainage tube.

_____ 33. Remove the nondominant hand from the labia, and grasp the catheter. Insert another inch.

_____ 34. Grasp the syringe connected to the balloon port, and insert 5–30 cc of water or air (depending on size) into the balloon.

_____ 35. Tug gently on the catheter to make sure it is properly positioned in the bladder.

_____ 36. Anchor the catheter to the medial aspect of the client's thigh with tape.

_____ 37. Attach the collecting bag on the side of the bed, keeping the bag at or below bladder level at all times.

_____ 38. Coil extra tubing and lay it on the bedside. Secure it to the bottom sheet.

_____ 39. Wash the perineum gently to remove lubricant or antiseptic solution that remains on the mucous membranes.

_____ 40. Remove equipment from the bed and bedside. Discard gloves.

_____ 41. Remove drapes, replace the bedcovers, and return the client to a position of comfort.

_____ 42. Wash hands.

Name ______________________________ Date ______________________

Observed by ____________

B. Inserting an indwelling catheter in a male client:

_____ 1. Assess the client and determine the nursing diagnosis.

_____ 2. Plan the expected outcomes.

_____ 3. Explain to the client what is going to happen and why.

_____ 4. Pull curtains around the bedside and close the door to the room.

_____ 5. Bring the necessary equipment to the bedside.

_____ 6. Wash hands thoroughly.

_____ 7. Place the bed at a comfortable working height.

_____ 8. Position client in a dorsal recumbent position with legs straight and slightly abducted.

_____ 9. Drape the client's upper body with a bath blanket and cover the lower body with the bedsheets so that only the genital area is exposed.

_____ 10. Stand at the client's right side if you are right-handed; stand at the client's left side if you are left-handed.

_____ 11. Wearing clean gloves, wash the penis with plain water.

_____ 12. Remove gloves and wash hands again.

_____ 13. Place a waste receptacle close to the working area at the bedside.

_____ 14. Place the overbed table adjacent to the bed.

_____ 15. Open the catheterization set. (If catheterization set is enclosed in a plastic bag, place this bag on the bed near the working surface to use as a waste receptacle.)

_____ 16. Don the sterile gloves. If they are not on top of the set, see step 18.

_____ 17. Pick up the underdrape by the corners, unfold it, and wrap the corner around the gloved hands.

_____ 18. Place the underdrape on the client's thighs just distal to the exposed genitals. (If underdrape is on top of the set, place it on the client's thighs without touching the sterile upper side of the drape. Then don the sterile gloves.)

_____ 19. Unfold the perineal drape and place over the perineum so that the penis is placed in the opening (or discard drape).

_____ 20. Lift the plastic tray and place it on the middle of the protective drape on the client's thighs.

_____ 21. Pour the cleansing antiseptic solution over the five cotton balls or gauze squares.

_____ 22. Remove the drainage tube and collecting bag from the kit. If it is not connected to the catheter, connect it at this time.

_____ 23. Test the balloon by connecting the syringe to the balloon port and insert the fluid, inflating the balloon. Deflate it by removing the fluid. Leave the syringe connected to the connecting port and position the catheter, tubing, and bag so that the catheter is ready for insertion.

_____ 24. Open a small specimen container and set it aside for later use.

_____ 25. Open the lubricant pack and place the lubricant container on the sterile field near the working area. Discard outer wrapping in waste receptacle.

_____ 26. Lubricate the tip of the catheter. Place drainage end of the catheter in the collecting basin.

_____ 27. Grasp the penis firmly behind the glans with your nondominant hand.

_____ 28. Retract the foreskin with the thumb and forefinger and spread the meatus open.

_____ 29. Pick up a cotton ball with the forceps and, starting at the meatus, gently clean the glans in a circular motion outward. Repeat this motion twice, using a fresh cotton ball each time.

_____ 30. Hold the penis at a 90° angle from the body and gently pull upward.

_____ 31. Pick up the catheter about 3–4 inches from the tip and gently insert it into the urethra for 8 inches or until urine drains. Insert another inch. (If resistance occurs, have the client take a deep breath or bear down as if he is urinating.)

_____ 32. Grasp the syringe connected to the balloon port, and insert 5–30 cc of water or air (depending on size) into the balloon.

_____ 33. Tug gently on the catheter to make sure it is properly positioned in the bladder.

_____ 34. Anchor the catheter to the lower outer quadrant of the abdomen.

_____ 35. Attach the collecting bag on the side of the bed, keeping the bag at or below bladder level at all times.

_____ 36. Coil extra tubing and lay it on the bedside. Secure it to bottom sheet.

_____ 37. Wash the penis gently around the urethra to remove lubricant or antiseptic solution that remains on the glans.

_____ 38. Remove equipment from the bed and bedside. Discard gloves.

_____ 39. Remove drapes, replace the bedcovers, and return the client to a position of comfort.

_____ 40. Wash hands.

Name ______________________________ Date ______________

Observed by ____________

SKILL 30.3 Removing an Indwelling Catheter

_____ 1. Assess the client and determine the nursing diagnosis.

_____ 2. Plan the expected outcomes.

_____ 3. Explain to the client what is going to be done.

_____ 4. Bring necessary equipment to the client's bedside.

_____ 5. Pull the curtains around the bed and close the door to the client's room.

_____ 6. Wash hands.

_____ 7. Lower the upper bedcovers, exposing the catheter.

_____ 8. Place a protective pad under client's hips.

_____ 9. Remove anchoring tape from thigh or abdomen and catheter.

_____ 10. Don clean gloves.

_____ 11. Clamp the catheter.

_____ 12. Insert hub of syringe into the inflation port of the catheter and draw back, withdrawing water or air.

_____ 13. Gently pull the catheter out from the urethra.

_____ 14. Cleanse and dry the perineal area.

_____ 15. Remove the protective pad, catheter, drainage tubing, and collecting bag. Remove gloves.

_____ 16. Explain to client that he may have dysuria and urgency and that he should notify the nurse when he urinates.

_____ 17. Encourage client to increase fluid intake.

_____ 18. Wash hands.

Name ____________________ Date ____________________

Observed by ____________

SKILL 30.4 Applying an External Catheter

_____ 1. Assess the client and determine the nursing diagnosis.

_____ 2. Plan the expected outcomes.

_____ 3. Explain the procedure to the client.

_____ 4. Close the curtains around the bed and close the door to the room.

_____ 5. Bring equipment to the bedside.

_____ 6. Wash hands and don clean gloves.

_____ 7. Place the bed at a comfortable working height.

_____ 8. Expose the client's genital area by lowering the covers.

_____ 9. Gently wash the penis and surrounding perineum.

_____ 10. Wipe around the penis in a circular fashion with the alcohol prep.

_____ 11. Attach the collection bag to the bed or leg.

_____ 12. Grasp the penis along the shaft, beneath the glans, with your nondominant hand.

_____ 13. Place the rolled condom sheath at the tip of the glans with the dominant hand. Gently and smoothly unroll the sheath onto the penile shaft.

_____ 14. Allow about 1 inch (2–3 cm) between the urethra meatus and the end of the condom that empties into the tubing.

_____ 15. Anchor the end of the sheath by encircling the adhesive strip around the penis so that the adhesive does not touch the skin or constrict the opening and securely fasten the sheath in place.

_____ 16. Attach the condom tubing to the drainage tubing.

_____ 17. Coil excess tubing on the bed and attach to the bottom bedsheet.

_____ 18. Replace the top bedcovers, place the client in a position of comfort.

_____ 19. Discard gloves and wash hands.

Name ____________________ Date ____________________

Observed by ____________

SKILL 30.5 Managing Urinary Drainage Systems

A. Guidelines for managing drainage systems:

_____ a. The collection bag is hung from the *frame* of the bed when the client is in bed.

In the home:

_____ b. Hang the collection bag on the seat or rung of a chair at the client's bedside if the bag cannot be hung on the client's bed.

_____ c. The bag is hung on the side of the bed away from the door.

_____ d. The drainage tubing hangs straight from the end of the bed to the collecting bag.

_____ e. Excess drainage tubing is coiled on the bed.

_____ f. The tubing is never kinked or clamped unless specifically ordered.

_____ g. The tubing is fastened in place with a clamp or safety pin attached to tape secured to the tubing.

_____ h. The client is never positioned on top of the drainage tubing.

_____ i. The collecting bag is kept below the bladder level at all times when the client is moving or ambulating.

_____ j. The bag is never placed on the floor.

_____ k. The system is never opened to obtain a specimen or empty urine.

_____ l. Empty the collection bag only

- when it is nearly full
- at designated intervals to record output, a minimum of every eight hours
- when the client is ambulating

_____ m. Do not allow the spigot or drain to touch a contaminated object, such as the floor. If it does, cleanse it with an antiseptic swab.

B. Providing catheter care:

_____ 1. Explain the procedure to the client.

_____ 2. Wash hands.

_____ 3. Place catheter care kit on the bedside table and open it.

_____ 4. Lower the upper bedcovers and expose the perineum and catheter.

_____ 5. Place the drape under the catheter by holding it by the corners only.

_____ 6. Remove tape securing catheter to the client's thigh.

_____ 7. Don gloves.

_____ 8. Saturate cotton balls or gauze sponges with antiseptic solution or soap.

_____ 9. Pick up the catheter with your nondominant hand.

_____ 10. Wipe in a circular fashion around the meatus with the cotton or gauze using the dominant hand.

_____ 11. Repeat step 10.

_____ 12. Wrap a cotton ball or gauze sponge around the catheter at the meatus and wipe from the meatus to the juncture of the drainage tubing.

_____ 13. Repeat step 12.

_____ 14. Discard equipment and remove gloves.

_____ 15. Resecure catheter to the client's thigh with tape.

_____ 16. Remove drapes and replace top covers.

_____ 17. Wash hands.

Name ____________________ Date ____________________

Observed by ____________

SKILL 30.6 Irrigating or Instilling into a Bladder or Catheter

A. Irrigating an open system:

_____ 1. Explain what is going to be done and why.

_____ 2. Arrange the curtains around the client's bed or close the door to his room.

_____ 3. Bring the necessary equipment to the bedside.

_____ 4. Wash hands and don clean gloves.

_____ 5. Place the bed at a comfortable working height.

_____ 6. Fold back the top bed linens to expose the junction of the catheter and drainage tubing.

_____ 7. Remove the tape from the catheter and from client's thigh or abdomen.

_____ 8. Place the irrigating set on the overbed table adjacent to the bed.

_____ 9. Open the irrigating set using sterile technique.

_____ 10. Place the protective pad under the juncture of the catheter and the drainage tubing.

_____ 11. Pour irrigating solution into the solution basin.

_____ 12. Disconnect catheter from the drainage tubing holding each tube approximately $1\frac{1}{2}$ inches from the end.

_____ 13. Place the protective cap on the proximal end of the drainage tubing and coil the tubing on the bed so that it will not fall onto the floor.

_____ 14. Place tip of the catheter securely into the collecting basin.

_____ 15. Discard contaminated gloves and don sterile gloves.

_____ 16. Draw 30 cc of solution into the syringe.

_____ 17. Insert syringe into tip of the catheter and slowly inject solution into the bladder.

_____ 18. Remove syringe and replace catheter tip into the collecting basin.

_____ 19. Lower the basin and allow solution to return by gravity flow.

_____ 20. Repeat steps 16–19 until solution flows freely from the catheter.

_____ 21. Wipe the tip of the catheter and the proximal end of the drainage tubing with an antiseptic swab.

_____ 22. Reconnect the catheter with the drainage tubing.

_____ 23. Remove and discard gloves.

_____ 24. Remove protective pad from under the catheter and replace bedcovers.

_____ 25. Remove equipment from bedside.

_____ 26. Wash hands.

_____ 27. Leave the client in a comfortable position.

B. Instilling solutions or medication into an open urinary drainage system:

_____ 1. Explain what is going to be done and why.

_____ 2. Arrange the curtains around the client's bed or close the door to his room.

_____ 3. Bring the necessary equipment to the bedside.

_____ 4. Wash hands and don clean gloves.

_____ 5. Place the bed at a comfortable working height.

_____ 6. Fold back the top bed linens to expose the junction of the catheter and drainage tubing.

_____ 7. Remove the tape from the catheter and client's thigh or abdomen.

_____ 8. Place the irrigating set on the overbed table adjacent to the bed.

_____ 9. Open the irrigating set using sterile technique.

_____ 10. Place the protective pad under the juncture of the catheter and the drainage tubing.

_____ 11. Pour irrigating solution into the solution basin.

_____ 12. Disconnect catheter from the drainage tubing holding each tube approximately $1\frac{1}{2}$ inches from the end.

_____ 13. Place the protective cap on the proximal end of the drainage tubing and coil the tubing on the bed so that it will not fall onto the floor.

_____ 14. Place tip of the catheter securely into the collecting basin.

_____ 15. Discard contaminated gloves and don sterile gloves.

_____ 16. Draw 30 cc of solution into the syringe.

_____ 17. Insert syringe into tip of the catheter and slowly inject solution into the bladder.

_____ 18. Place clamp on catheter and tighten it.

_____ 19. Remove the syringe.

_____ 20. Wipe the tip of the catheter and the proximal end of the drainage tubing with an antiseptic swab.

_____ 21. Reconnect the catheter with the drainage tubing.

_____ 22. Remove and discard gloves.

_____ 23. Remove protective pad from under the catheter and replace bedcovers.

_____ 24. Remove equipment from bedside.

_____ 25. Wash hands.

_____ 26. Note time of instillation.

_____ 27. Leave the client in a comfortable position.

_____ 28. Return at designated interval and unclamp the catheter.

Name ______________________________ Date ______________

Observed by ____________

C. Intermittently irrigate or instill solutions into a closed system:

_____ 1. Explain what is going to be done and why.

_____ 2. Arrange the curtains around the client's bed or close the door to his room.

_____ 3. Bring the necessary equipment to the bedside.

_____ 4. Wash hands.

_____ 5. Place the bed at a comfortable working height.

_____ 6. Fold back the top bed linens to expose the junction of the catheter and drainage tubing.

_____ 7. Remove the tape from the catheter and client's thigh or abdomen.

_____ 8. Place the irrigating set on the overbed table adjacent to the bed.

_____ 9. Open the irrigating set using sterile technique.

_____ 10. Place the protective pad under the juncture of the catheter and the drainage tubing.

_____ 11. Pour irrigating solution into the solution basin.

_____ 12. Locate the irrigation port or irrigation channel in the indwelling catheter and cleanse with disinfectant.

_____ 13. Don the sterile gloves.

If irrigating:

_____ 14. Draw 30 cc of solution into the syringe.

_____ 15. Insert tip of syringe into the irrigation channel or port and slowly insert solution into the bladder.

_____ 16. Remove syringe and lower the catheter below the level of the bladder.

_____ 17. Repeat steps 14–16 until solution flows freely from the catheter.

If instilling:

_____ 14. Clamp the drainage tubing just below the junction with the catheter.

_____ 15. Draw 30 cc of solution into the syringe.

_____ 16. Insert tip of syringe into the irrigation channel or port and slowly insert solution into the bladder.

_____ 17. Repeat steps 15 and 16 until all solution is instilled in the bladder.

For both irrigating and instilling:

_____ 18. Cleanse port with the disinfectant.

_____ 19. Remove and discard gloves.

_____ 20. Remove protective pad from under the catheter and replace bedcovers.

_____ 21. Remove equipment from bedside.

_____ 22. Wash hands.

_____ 23. Leave the client in a comfortable position.

Name ______________________ Date ______________________

Observed by ____________

SKILL 30.7 Assembling and Maintaining a Closed Three-Way Bladder Irrigation System

_____ 1. Explain the purpose of the equipment and irrigation.

_____ 2. Assemble the equipment at the bedside.

_____ 3. Close the curtains around the bed or close the door to the room.

_____ 4. Wash hands. If not already in place, insert 3-lumen indwelling Foley. Correctly hang the collection bag from the client's bed frame.

_____ 5. Remove protective packaging from the irrigation equipment.

_____ 6. Clamp and attach tubing to irrigation container.

_____ 7. Position the container on the IV pole at the foot of the client's bed.

_____ 8. Place the correct amount of irrigant in the irrigation container and elevate to 2–3 feet above the bladder level.

_____ 9. Open the tubing camp, fill the drip chamber on the irrigation container and flood the tubing with irrigant, removing all air bubbles, and close the clamp.

_____ 10. Fold back the upper bed linens, exposing the indwelling catheter.

_____ 11. Place the end of the irrigation tubing on the bed, close to the indwelling catheter.

_____ 12. Open or prepare antiseptic swabs for use.

_____ 13. Don sterile gloves.

_____ 14. Pick up the irrigation lumen or Y-connector with your nondominant hand and cleanse it with an antiseptic swab using the dominant hand.

_____ 15. Remove the protective cap from the end of the irrigation tubing.

_____ 16. Attach tubing to the irrigation lumen or Y-connector using gloved hands.

_____ 17. Open the clamp on the tubing and adjust flow rate to the amount of irrigant ordered for a given period of time.

_____ 18. Position the catheter so that it freely receives irrigant and maintains straight drainage.

_____ 19. Replace the top bedcovers and place the client in a position of comfort.

_____ 20. Remove gloves and discard packaging.

_____ 21. Wash hands.

Name ______________________________ Date ______________________

Observed by ____________

CHAPTER 31 ASSESSING BOWEL ELIMINATION FUNCTION

SKILL 31.1 Assessing Bowel Elimination Function

A. Examining the abdomen:

_____ 1. Explain to the client what will be examined. Answer his questions.

_____ 2. Close the door to the room or draw the curtains around his bed.

_____ 3. Instruct the client to empty his bladder.

_____ 4. Instruct the client to remove his lower clothing and lie supine on the bed or examining table with the drape over his body. OR Remove the client's lower clothing and cover his lower body with the drape.

_____ 5. Wash hands.

_____ 6. Instruct the client to lie with hands at his sides. Encourage him to relax abdominal muscles and breathe quietly during exam.

_____ 7. Reposition the drape so that the abdomen is exposed but not the genitalia.

_____ 8. Inspect the abdomen.

a. Divide abdomen into four quadrants by drawing an imaginary line from xiphoid to pubis; cross that line with one drawn through the umbilicus.

b. Observe shape and symmetry. Note presence of lesions, protrusions, rashes.

c. Observe skin for scars, striae, dilated veins.

d. Note visible peristaltic waves.

e. Observe position, shape, and color of umbilicus.

_____ 9. Auscultate the abdomen.

a. Place the bell of the stethoscope on each quadrant and listen for bowel sounds. Note frequency and character in each quadrant.

b. Place bell over midline of abdomen and listen for bruits (vascular noises like blowing or swishing sounds indicating changes in the hemodynamics in the major vessels).

_____ 10. Percuss the abdomen.

a. Percuss in each of the four quadrants.

b. Percuss in the right midclavicular line, beginning below the umbilicus and moving toward the liver.

c. Percuss right midclavicular line from below the clavicles toward the liver.

_____ 11. Palpate the abdomen.

a. Observe the client's face for reactions while palpating.

b. Palpate lightly over each quadrant with palmar surfaces of fingers, using a smooth but firm movement. Press surface approximately 1 cm. Note presence of masses or tenderness.

c. Check for rebound tenderness by pressing firmly and deeply into area of tenderness and then releasing abruptly.

_____ 12. Palpate the liver.

a. Place your left hand under client's posterior thorax at eleventh and twelfth ribs; press upward.

b. Place your right hand on the client's right abdomen with fingertips pointing toward the costal margin.

c. Instruct the client to take a deep breath.

d. Press your right hand gently in and up.

_____ 13. Palpate the kidney region.

a. Instruct the client to turn laterally so that his back faces you.

b. Locate the costovertebral angle and deeply palpate. Note tenderness.

_____ 14. Replace drape over the abdomen.

_____ 15. Instruct the client to replace his lower clothing; or assist him to dress.

_____ 16. Return client to a position of comfort.

_____ 17. Wash hands.

B. Examining the rectum and anus:

_____ 1. Explain to the client what will be examined. Answer his questions.

_____ 2. Close the door to the room or draw the curtains around the client's bed.

_____ 3. Instruct the client to empty his bladder.

_____ 4. Instruct the client to remove his lower clothing and lie supine on the bed or examining table with the drape over his body. OR Remove the client's lower clothing and cover the lower body with the drape.

_____ 5. Wash hands.

_____ 6. Assist the client to a left Sims' or lateral position.

_____ 7. Arrange the drapes to expose the buttocks.

_____ 8. Direct lighting to the exposed body area.

_____ 9. Don clean gloves. Open package of lubricant and place it within reach.

_____ 10. Place your left hand on the upper (right) buttocks and pull upward with thumb.

_____ 11. Inspect the area around the anus and between the buttocks for redness, lumps, rashes, excoriation, ulcers, or other abnormal appearance.

_____ 12. Lubricate the index finger of your right hand.

Name ____ Date ____________________

Observed by ____________

_____ 13. Instruct the client to bear down; observe for lesions protruding from the anus.

_____ 14. Place pad of lubricated finger over the anus as the client bears down.

_____ 15. Insert fingertip into the anus as the sphincter relaxes.

_____ 16. Instruct the client to relax if the sphincter tightens.

_____ 17. Note the sphincter tone, tenderness, or abnormalities of the anus.

_____ 18. Insert finger into the rectum as far as possible.

_____ 19. Rotate finger around the rectal wall, noting nodules or lumps.

_____ 20. Withdraw finger and wipe fecal matter from glove on tissues. Note color.

_____ 21. Remove lubricant or fecal material from anal area with tissues or provide tissues for the client to do so.

_____ 22. Remove and discard gloves.

_____ 23. Replace drape and assist client to supine position.

_____ 24. Wash hands.

_____ 25. Assist the client to a position of comfort; open drapes or door.

Name ____ Date ____________________

Observed by ____________

CHAPTER 32 REMOVING FECES AND FLATUS

SKILL 32.1 Removing Feces or Flatus

A. Preparing a large-volume enema using disposable enema equipment:

_____ 1. Wash hands and gather equipment.

_____ 2. Open the enema administration package and remove items.

_____ 3. Run the desired amount of solution (water or saline) into the clean pitcher.

_____ 4. Check the water temperature with a thermometer. If using saline, place saline container in a basin of hot water.

_____ 5. Adjust solution temperature as necessary.

_____ 6. Add soap (if soap suds enema is ordered) and stir into the solution.

_____ 7. Clamp the tubing.

_____ 8. Pour the solution into the administration container.

_____ 9. Secure the top of the container.

B. Administering a large-volume enema from a container:

_____ 1. Assess the client to determine the nursing diagnosis.

_____ 2. Plan the nursing objectives and expected outcomes.

_____ 3. Explain to the client that he is to have an enema. Inform him that he will achieve maximum benefit if he is able to hold the enema for 10–15 minutes. Answer his questions.

_____ 4. Bring the prepared enema to the bedside and hang the bag or container on the IV pole next to the client.

_____ 5. Draw the curtains around the bed or close the door to the room.

_____ 6. Raise the bed to a comfortable working level and raise the siderails.

_____ 7. Wash hands.

_____ 8. Assist the client into a left Sims' position and drape him so that his buttocks are exposed.

_____ 9. Place a protective pad under the client's buttocks and thighs.

_____ 10. Place a bedpan adjacent to the client on the bed if uncertain about his ability to retain the enema.

_____ 11. Don the disposable gloves.

_____ 12. Remove protective cap from nozzle, open the tubing clamp and allow solution to flow through tubing into the bedpan. Reclamp.

_____ 13. Lubricate 3–4 inches of nozzle, if not prelubricated.

_____ 14. Remove the solution container from the IV pole and hold it at the same height as the client's rectum.

_____ 15. Separate buttocks and locate the anus.

_____ 16. Instruct the client to take a deep breath; simultaneously insert the nozzle into the anus pointing toward the umbilicus for about 3–4 inches.

_____ 17. Unclamp the tubing and hold in position while raising the container until the solution flows into the rectum.

_____ 18. Inform the client that the solution is going in; ask him to signal if he cannot hold the solution any longer.

_____ 19. Clamp tubing and remove the nozzle when all of the solution is instilled or the client cannot hold it. Remove nozzle.

_____ 20. Wipe the anal area with toilet tissue.

_____ 21. Set aside enema equipment for later disposal or cleansing. Remove gloves inside out and discard.

_____ 22. Place client on bedpan, or assist to commode or bathroom as necessary when he signals his desire for defecation.

_____ 23. Ensure that the call signal is within the client's reach and leave him in private. If the client is using the toilet, ask him to not flush it.

_____ 24. Put on clean gloves, and assist the client to wash and dry the perianal area after he finishes defecation.

_____ 25. Return the client to a position of comfort. Leave the protective pad in place or replace if it was soiled.

_____ 26. Examine the expelled enema and feces before emptying bedpan, commode, or flushing toilet.

_____ 27. Wash hands.

_____ 28. Wash, rinse, and hang the enema equipment to dry.

C. Administering a small-volume prepackaged enema:

_____ 1. Assess the client to determine the nursing diagnosis.

_____ 2. Plan the nursing objectives and expected client outcomes.

_____ 3. Explain to the client that he is to have an enema. Inform him that he will achieve maximum benefit if he is able to hold the enema for 10–15 minutes. Answer his questions.

_____ 4. Bring the prepared enema to the bedside.

_____ 5. Draw the curtains around the bed or close the door to the room.

_____ 6. Raise the bed to a comfortable working level and raise the siderails.

_____ 7. Wash hands.

_____ 8. Assist the client into a left Sims' position and drape him so that his buttocks are exposed.

_____ 9. Place a protective pad under the client's buttocks and thighs.

_____ 10. Place a bedpan adjacent to the client on the bed if uncertain about his ability to retain the enema.

_____ 11. Don the disposable gloves.

Name ______________________________________ Date ____________________

Observed by ____________

_____ 12. Remove the protective cap from the nozzle.

_____ 13. Inspect the nozzle for lubricant. Add if necessary.

_____ 14. Squeeze the container gently to expel air.

_____ 15. Separate buttocks and locate anus.

_____ 16. Instruct the client to take a deep breath; simultaneously insert the nozzle into the anus pointing toward the umbilicus for about 3–4 inches.

_____ 17. Inform the client that the solution is going in; ask him to signal if he cannot hold the solution any longer.

_____ 18. Squeeze the container until all enema solution is instilled in the rectum.

_____ 19. Remove container and discard.

_____ 20. Wipe the anal area with toilet tissue.

_____ 21. Remove gloves inside out and discard.

_____ 22. Place client on bedpan, or assist to commode or bathroom as necessary when he signals his desire for defecation.

_____ 23. Ensure that the call signal is within the client's reach and leave him in private. If the client is using the toilet, ask him to not flush the toilet.

_____ 24. Assist the client to wash and dry the perianal area after he finishes defecation.

_____ 25. Return the client to a position of comfort. Leave the protective pad in place or replace if it was soiled.

_____ 26. Examine the expelled enema and feces before emptying bedpan, commode, or flushing toilet.

_____ 27. Wash hands.

C. Inserting a rectal tube:

_____ 1. Assess the client to determine the nursing diagnosis.

_____ 2. Plan the nursing objectives and expected outcomes.

_____ 3. Explain to the client that a tube will be placed in his rectum to help remove flatus and relieve his discomfort.

_____ 4. Gather equipment.

_____ 5. Prepare the rectal tube by placing the distal end in a plastic bag and securing with a rubber band.

OR

Insert the distal end of the tube through a small opening punctured in the lid of a cardboard or plastic specimen container. Secure with tape.

_____ 6. Cut two lengths of tape approximately 6 inches long. Place within reach.

_____ 7. Wash hands.

_____ 8. Draw the bedside curtains or close the door to the room.

_____ 9. Assist the client into a left Sims' position and drape him so that his buttocks are exposed.

_____ 10. Place a protective pad under the client's buttocks and thighs.

_____ 11. Don clean gloves.

_____ 12. Lubricate the proximal tip of the rectal tube.

_____ 13. Separate the buttocks and locate the anus.

_____ 14. Insert the lubricated tip approximately 4–6 inches into the rectum, directing the tube toward the umbilicus.

_____ 15. Secure the tube in position with the lengths of tape.

_____ 16. Remove gloves inside out and discard.

_____ 17. Cut a small slit in the top of the collecting bag or container on its upper aspect.

_____ 18. Replace the client's top bedcovers.

_____ 19. Attach the client's call signal within his reach.

_____ 20. Leave the client with the rectal tube in place for 20–30 minutes.

_____ 21. Ask the client if he expelled flatus. Don gloves and remove rectal tube and set aside.

_____ 22. Remove protective pad. Wash and dry the anal area if necessary.

_____ 23. Return the client to a position of comfort. Attach call signal.

_____ 24. Take the rectal tube and collecting container to the bathroom; inspect the contents, if present.

_____ 25. Discard tube and container.

_____ 26. Discard gloves and wash hands.

D. Digitally removing feces:

_____ 1. Assess the client to determine the nursing diagnosis.

_____ 2. Plan the nursing objectives and expected outcomes.

_____ 3. Explain to the client that the nurse is going to do a rectal exam, during which any feces found within reach will be removed. Tell the client that this may be uncomfortable for him; ask him to tell you when he feels the discomfort.

_____ 4. Gather equipment.

_____ 5. Draw the bed curtains and close the door to the room.

_____ 6. Raise the bed to a working level and raise the siderails.

_____ 7. Wash hands.

_____ 8. Assist the client into a left Sims' position and drape so that his buttocks are exposed.

_____ 9. Place a protective pad under the client's buttocks and thighs.

_____ 10. Place a bedpan adjacent to the client on the bed.

_____ 11. Don the disposable gloves.

Name ______________________________ Date ______________

Observed by ____________

_____ 12. Separate the buttocks and locate the anus.

_____ 13. Lubricate the forefinger and middle finger of the dominant hand.

_____ 14. Place the hand on the client's hip and insert the lubricated fingers through the anus toward the umbilicus.

_____ 15. Loosen the fecal mass from the rectal walls.

_____ 16. Manipulate the mass with fingers, breaking it into small parts.

_____ 17. Move the mass toward the anus and remove small pieces. Place in bedpan or wipe gloved fingers on protective pad.

_____ 18. Monitor the client's response; assess for fatigue or pain; stop the procedure if the client's heart slows.

_____ 19. Repeat steps 16–18 until all fecal material within easy reach is removed.

_____ 20. Remove fingers from rectum; remove gloves inside out and discard.

_____ 21. Don clean gloves and wash perianal area with washcloth; dry thoroughly.

_____ 22. Remove bedpan and empty. Remove and dispose of protective pad.

_____ 23. Assist client to bathroom, commode, or on a bedpan if he feels he must defecate.

_____ 24. Wash hands.

Name ______________________________ Date ______________

Observed by __________

CHAPTER 33 MANAGING THE OSTOMY

SKILL 33.1 Managing a Colostomy or Ileostomy

A. Teaching the client how to manage his fecal diversion ostomy independently:

_____ 1. Determine what the client needs to know to manage his ostomy safely and independently.

_____ 2. Identify what the client and his caregivers know by interviewing them.

_____ 3. Identify learning objectives (with the client and his caregivers, when appropriate and when they are able to participate).

_____ 4. Explain what is being done and why as the ostomy is managed as all care measures are given.

_____ 5. Encourage the client to observe and ask questions.

_____ 6. Encourage the client to participate in any way that he seems interested or able.

_____ 7. Observe the client's emotional responses and acceptance of the ostomy.

_____ 8. Increase the amount of client participation as he gains comfort and skill.

_____ 9. Reinforce new information and skills as the client learns.

_____ 10. Observe as the client does his own care completely; correct him *only* when he does something that is potentially harmful.

_____ 11. Make suggestions for changes in technique when client has completed his tasks.

_____ 12. Empathize and demonstrate caring throughout the teaching episodes.

B. Placing a skin barrier on the postoperative peristomal skin:

_____ 1. Explain to the client what will be done.

_____ 2. Close the door to the room or draw the curtains.

_____ 3. Wash hands.

_____ 4. Raise the client's bed.

_____ 5. Assist the client to a low Fowler's position.

_____ 6. Position the client's bedclothes away from the stoma site.

_____ 7. Place a protective pad under the client's side next to the stoma.

_____ 8. Donning disposable gloves, remove dressing and discard it in a plastic bag.

_____ 9. Inspect the stoma for: color, moisture, effluent, and intact suture line.

_____ 10. Inspect peristomal skin for redness, irritation, and intactness.

_____ 11. Note the client's facial expression and verbal comments.

_____ 12. Remove any effluent that is discharging from the stoma with tissues. Discard the soiled tissues. Repeat as necessary.

If placing a barrier wafer or sheet on the skin:

_____ 13. Measure the size of the stoma with a stoma template; if none is available, draw a proximal stoma size on a paper held near the stoma; cut out the stoma and compare. Adjust size as needed.

_____ 14. Place the correct template size against the wafer; cut the wafer to match the size.

_____ 15. Remove protective backing (if present) from the wafer. Set aside with the adhesive side upright.

_____ 16. Squirt liquid barrier onto a sterile sponge or open a liquid barrier packet. Set it aside.

_____ 17. Wash the peristomal skin gently with warm water on washcloth.

_____ 18. Pat dry gently.

_____ 19. Coat the peristomal skin with the liquid barrier. Move in concentric circles outward from the stoma until all the skin from the stoma to about 2 inches beyond the anticipated wafer is covered.

_____ 20. Allow liquid barrier to dry for several minutes. Test it with fingers; the surface will feel sticky or tacky.

_____ 21. Place the wafer sticky side down on the skin around the stoma.

_____ 22. Press down gently against the wafer to ensure that it is adhered to the skin around the stoma edges outward to the wafer edges.

_____ 23. Remove effluent from the stoma with tissues periodically throughout the procedure.

_____ 24. Discard gloves and wash hands.

C. Placing a barrier paste around the stoma:

_____ 1. Explain to the client what will done.

_____ 2. Close the door to the room or draw the curtains.

_____ 3. Wash hands.

_____ 4. Raise the client's bed.

_____ 5. Assist the client to a low Fowler's position.

_____ 6. Position the client's bedclothes away from the stoma site.

_____ 7. Place protective pad under the client's side next to the stoma.

_____ 8. Don disposable gloves and remove dressing and discard in plastic bag.

_____ 9. Inspect the stoma for: color, moisture, effluent, and intact suture line.

_____ 10. Inspect peristomal skin for redness, irritation, and intactness.

_____ 11. Note the client's facial expression and verbal comments.

_____ 12. Remove any effluent that is discharging from the stoma with tissues. Discard the soiled tissues. Repeat as necessary.

Name ______________________________ Date ______________

Observed by ____________

_____ 13. Place a container with tepid water on the nurse's work area.

_____ 14. Open the paste tube and squeeze out a small amount and discard it.

_____ 15. Squeeze a ribbon of paste directly onto the peristomal skin•approximately $\frac{1}{2}$ inch from the stoma. Make a complete circle.

_____ 16. Repeat: Place other paste ribbons in concentric circles outward from the stoma.

_____ 17. Dip fingers in water and smooth paste until peristomal skin is entirely covered; dip fingers in water if paste begins to stick to them.

_____ 18. Ensure that skin surface is covered from edge of stoma to 3–4 inches outward.

_____ 19. Discard gloves and wash hands.

D. Placing an appliance on the protective skin barrier:

_____ 1. Select the appliance and pouch that best suits the effluent and client.

_____ 2. Measure the size of the stoma with a stoma template; if none is available, draw a proximal stoma size pattern on a paper held near the stoma; cut out the stoma pattern and compare. Adjust size as needed.

_____ 3. Place the correct template size against the appliance faceplate; match stoma opening size.

_____ 4. Cut opening in paper faceplate to match stoma size if needed. Set aside.

_____ 5. Prepare skin surface with protective barrier (as above).

_____ 6. Remove protective backing from paper faceplate.

_____ 7. Don disposable gloves and reach inside of the pouch from the distal end; hold faceplate against fingers.

_____ 8. Place the faceplate against the skin barrier, centering the stoma opening accurately over the stoma.

_____ 9. Press gently against the faceplate from inside the pouch; remove hand.

_____ 10. Press against the faceplate outer circumference from the outside of the pouch.

_____ 11. Ensure there are no gaps between the faceplate and the skin barrier.

_____ 12. Place several strips of tape around the edges of the faceplate (if desired).

_____ 13. Insert 10–15 cc of mineral oil into the pouch; milk the outside of pouch to distribute it evenly.

_____ 14. Squirt a small amount of ostomy deodorizer into the pouch.

_____ 15. Fold the distal edges of the pouch and secure clamp.

_____ 16. Reposition the client's bedclothing; remove protective pad.

_____ 17. Discard gloves and all used materials.

_____ 18. Open curtains or door to room.

_____ 19. Wash hands.

E. Emptying the pouch when the client must remain in bed:

_____ 1. Explain to the client what will be done.

_____ 2. Close door to room or draw bedside curtains.

_____ 3. Raise bed to working height.

_____ 4. Wash hands.

_____ 5. Fill a large syringe (Asepto or 50 cc) with warm water; place it in a small basin next to the bedside.

_____ 6. Place protective pad under the client's hips on the side of the stoma.

_____ 7. Position covers at the foot of bed.

_____ 8. Rearrange clothing to expose pouch.

_____ 9. Assist the client to a semilateral position, with the stoma and pouch positioned toward the bed surface.

_____ 10. Don disposable gloves.

_____ 11. Place bedpan next to the client, just under the pouch.

_____ 12. Unclamp the pouch and drain effluent into the bedpan.

_____ 13. Milk the pouch from the faceplate toward the distal end to expel all contents.

_____ 14. Hold distal end of the pouch above the bedpan at approximately the level of the stoma.

_____ 15. Insert syringe into distal end and rinse inside of the pouch with water.

_____ 16. Place distal end of pouch in the bedpain to drain.

_____ 17. Insert 10–15 cc of mineral oil into the pouch; milk the outside of pouch to distribute it evenly.

_____ 18. Squirt a small amount of deodorizer into distal end of pouch.

_____ 19. Wipe the end of the pouch; fold it and reattach the clamp.

_____ 20. Remove the bedpan and protective pad.

_____ 21. Note effluent characteristics: color, odor, consistency, and amount. Discard the effluent and cleanse the bedpan.

_____ 22. Remove and discard gloves.

_____ 23. Assist client to resume position of comfort.

_____ 24. Wash hands.

F. Emptying the pouch in the toilet:

_____ 1. Explain to the client what will be done.

_____ 2. Wash hands.

_____ 3. Assist the client to the bathroom.

_____ 4. Close the door.

Name ______________________________ Date ______________

Observed by ____________

_____ 5. Assist the client to sit on the commode with thighs abducted.

_____ 6. Fill a large syringe (Asepto or 50 cc) with warm water; place in small basin next to the toilet.

_____ 7. Arrange client's gown or clothing so that it is not near the pouch.

_____ 8. Don gloves.

_____ 9. Place the distal end of the pouch between the client's thighs, above the commode.

_____ 10. Unclamp the pouch or direct the client to unclamp it.

_____ 11. Milk the pouch from the stoma toward the open end of the pouch.

_____ 12. Hold the distal end of the pouch above the toilet at approximately the level of the stoma.

_____ 13. Insert syringe into distal end and rinse inside of the pouch with water.

_____ 14. Replace distal end of pouch in the toilet to drain.

_____ 15. Insert 10–15 cc of mineral oil into the pouch; milk the outside of pouch to distribute it evenly.

_____ 16. Squirt a small amount of deodorizer into the distal end of pouch.

_____ 17. Wipe the end and replace the clamp when the bag is emptied.

_____ 18. Remove gloves.

_____ 19. Assist the client to return to bed or a chair.

_____ 20. Examine effluent in toilet for character. Flush toilet.

_____ 21. Wash hands.

G. Changing an appliance and pouch:

_____ 1. Explain to the client what will be done.

_____ 2. Wash hands.

_____ 3. Assist the client to the bathroom or position him comfortably in bed.

_____ 4. Close the door.

_____ 5. Assist the client in the bathroom to sit on the commode with thighs abducted.

_____ 6. Arrange client's gown or clothing so that it is not near the pouch.

_____ 7. Prepare a new appliance and pouch. Set it aside.

_____ 8. If the client remains in bed, place a plastic-bag-lined trash container at the bedside or place a bedpan at the client's side.

_____ 9. Don disposable gloves.

_____ 10. Peel back the faceplate from skin barrier until it is separated completely.

_____ 11. Apply solvent to remove any adhesive if necessary.

_____ 12. Place the entire appliance and bag with effluent in the collecting container. Set the container aside.

_____ 13. Wipe any effluent from the stoma.

_____ 14. Cleanse the peristomal skin with warm water and dry it thoroughly.

_____ 15. Apply the new appliance.

_____ 16. Remove bedpan; inspect effluent for characteristics; empty in toilet.

_____ 17. Discard gloves.

_____ 18. Replace bedclothing and reposition the client.

_____ 19. Wash hands.

H. Draining the continent ileostomy:

_____ 1. Explain to the client what will be done.

_____ 2. Assist the client to a sitting position at the bedside or on the toilet.

_____ 3. Wash hands and don disposable gloves.

_____ 4. Arrange bedclothes to expose the stoma. Remove dressing, if present.

_____ 5. Place a collecting container (bedpan or large cup) next to the client if he is not on the toilet.

_____ 6. Lubricate the tip of the irrigating catheter.

_____ 7. Insert catheter about 2 inches through the stoma gently, placing the distal end in the container or toilet.

_____ 8. Instruct client to take a deep breath and gently push catheter tip through the nipple valve. Effluent will flow through the catheter.

_____ 9. Monitor effluent returns, which will contain feces and flatus.

_____ 10. Withdraw catheter when drainage stops.

_____ 11. Wash peristomal area with soap and water; dry and apply dressing, if desired.

_____ 12. Wash catheter with soap and water; rinse it and store it in a clean place.

_____ 13. Discard gloves.

_____ 14. Assist the client to comfortable position.

_____ 15. Wash hands.

Name ______________________________ Date ______________________________

Observed by ______________

SKILL 33.2 Irrigating the Colostomy

_____ 1. Explain to the client what will be done.

_____ 2. Wash hands.

_____ 3. Prepare the irrigating bag with approximately 1,000 cc of warm water.

_____ 4. Hang the bag on an IV pole so that the bottle hangs approximately 12–18 inches above the client's colostomy.

_____ 5. Run solution through the bag's tubing and clamp.

If doing the procedure in the bathroom:

_____ 6. Assist the client to the bathroom. Close the door.

If the client is in bed:

_____ 7. Close the door to the room or draw the bed curtains.

_____ 8. Place the client in a high Fowler's position.

_____ 9. Place a protective pad under the client's hips.

_____ 10. Place a bedpan between the client's thighs (if possible) or place it outside of his thigh nearest the colostomy.

In both bathroom and bedside procedures:

_____ 11. Reposition the client's bedclothing to expose the colostomy.

_____ 12. Remove the appliance and pouch from the colostomy (if used by the client); set aside or discard.

_____ 13. Inspect the stoma.

_____ 14. Don disposable gloves.

_____ 15. Center the irrigation bag directly over the stoma; secure in place with a belt or tie.

_____ 16. Place the distal end of the bag between the client's legs into the bedpan or toilet.

_____ 17. Lubricate little finger and dilate the stoma if ordered by the physician.

_____ 18. Lubricate the tip of the stoma cone or the colon catheter.

_____ 19. Open the tubing clamp to permit a gentle flow of water through the tip.

_____ 20. Insert the catheter tip 3–4 inches through the irrigation port into the stoma using a gentle, rotating motion as the water flows out.

_____ 21. Let water flow in slowly over four or five minutes with the cone preventing backflow.

_____ 22. Clamp the tubing if the client experiences severe cramping.

_____ 23. Continue water flow. Use the least amount of water possible to stimulate peristalsis and stool evacuation.

_____ **24.** Remove the tubing from the stoma and gently wash stoma with water flow. Withdraw tubing and irrigation bag; set aside.

_____ **25.** Remove gloves and wash hands.

_____ **26.** Leave the irrigation bag in place; instruct the client to gently massage his abdomen around the stoma.

_____ **27.** Have the client remain in place for 10–15 minutes or until all irrigating solution has drained.

_____ **28.** Wipe dry the base of the irrigation bag and clamp it.

_____ **29.** Wash hands.

_____ **30.** Encourage the client to walk if he can.

_____ **31.** Remove and empty irrigation bag after 45–60 minutes; cleanse bag and hang to dry.

_____ **32.** Cleanse peristomal skin as needed. Replace the colostomy appliance if one is used by the client.

_____ **33.** Wash hands.

Name ______________________ Date ______________________

Observed by ____________

SKILL 33.3 Managing a Urinary Ostomy

A. Teaching the client how to manage his urinary diversion ostomy independently:

_____ 1. Determine what the client needs to know to manage his ostomy safely and independently.

_____ 2. Identify what the client and his caregivers know by interviewing them.

_____ 3. Identify learning objectives (with the client and his caregivers, when appropriate and when they are able to participate).

_____ 4. Explain what is being done and why during all care measures for ostomy management.

_____ 5. Encourage the client to observe and ask questions.

_____ 6. Encourage the client to participate in any way that he seems interested or able.

_____ 7. Observe the client's emotional responses and acceptance of the ostomy.

_____ 8. Increase the amount of client participation as he gains comfort and skill.

_____ 9. Reinforce new information and skills as the client learns.

_____ 10. Observe as the client does his own care completely; correct him *only* when he does something that is potentially harmful.

_____ 11. Make suggestions for changes in technique when client has completed his tasks.

_____ 12. Empathize and demonstrate caring throughout the teaching episodes.

B. Placing a skin barrier on the postoperative peristomal skin:

_____ 1. Explain to the client what will be done.

_____ 2. Close the door to the room or draw curtains.

_____ 3. Wash hands.

_____ 4. Raise the client's bed.

_____ 5. Assist the client to a low Fowler's position.

_____ 6. Position the client's bedclothes away from the stoma site.

_____ 7. Place protective pad under the client's side next to the stoma.

_____ 8. Tear facial tissues into smaller segments; twist each segment into a 2-inch wick; repeat until 15–20 wicks are created. If the client is well enough, have him participate.

_____ 9. Donning disposable gloves, remove the dressing, and discard it in a plastic bag.

_____ 10. Place tissue wick against the stoma opening; hold in place. Discard when the wick is saturated and replace with a dry wick. Continue this until the appliance is placed.

_____ 11. Inspect the stoma for: color, moisture, effluent, and intact suture line.

_____ 12. Inspect peristomal skin for redness, irritation, and intactness.

_____ 13. Note the client's facial expression and verbal comments.

If placing a barrier wafer or sheet on the skin:

_____ 14. Measure the size of the stoma with a stoma template; if none is available, draw a proximal stoma size on a paper held near the stoma; cut out the stoma pattern and compare. Adjust size as needed.

_____ 15. Place the correct template size against the wafer; cut the wafer to match the size.

_____ 16. Remove protective backing (if present) from the wafer. Set the wafer aside with the adhesive side upright.

_____ 17. Squirt liquid barrier onto a sterile sponge or open a liquid barrier packet. Set it aside.

_____ 18. Wash the peristomal skin gently with warm water on washcloth.

_____ 19. Pat dry gently.

_____ 20. Coat the peristomal skin with the liquid barrier. Move in concentric circles outward from the stoma until all the skin from the stoma to about 2 inches beyond the anticipated wafer is covered.

_____ 21. Allow liquid barrier to dry for several minutes. Test it with your fingers; the surface will feel sticky or tacky.

_____ 22. Place the wafer sticky side down on the skin around the stoma.

_____ 23. Press down gently against the wafer around the stoma edges outward to the wafer edges.

If placing a barrier paste around the stoma:

_____ 1. Explain to the client what will be done.

_____ 2. Close the door to the room or draw curtains.

_____ 3. Wash hands.

_____ 4. Raise the client's bed.

_____ 5. Assist the client to a low Fowler's position.

_____ 6. Position the client's bedclothes away from the stoma site.

_____ 7. Place a protective pad under the client's side next to the stoma.

_____ 8. Tear facial tissues into smaller segments; twist each segment into a 2-inch wick; repeat until 15–20 wicks are created. If the client is well enough, have him participate.

_____ 9. Donning disposable gloves, remove the dressing and discard it in a plastic bag.

_____ 10. Place tissue wick against the stoma opening; hold in place. Discard when the wick is saturated and replace with a dry wick. Continue this until the appliance is placed.

Name ______________________ Date ______________________

Observed by ____________

_____ 11. Inspect the stoma for color, moisture, effluent, and intact suture line.

_____ 12. Inspect peristomal skin for redness, irritation, and intactness.

_____ 13. Note the client's facial expression and verbal comments.

_____ 14. Place a container (cup or basin) with tepid water on the nurse's work area.

_____ 15. Open the paste tube and squeeze out a small amount; discard. Set tube aside.

_____ 16. Don disposable gloves (if desired).

_____ 17. Squeeze a ribbon of paste directly into the peristomal skin approximately $\frac{1}{2}$ inch from the stoma. Make a complete circle.

_____ 18. Repeat, placing other paste ribbons in concentric circles outward from the stoma.

_____ 19. Dip fingers in water and smooth the paste until the peristomal skin is entirely covered; dip fingers in water if paste begins to stick to them.

_____ 20. Ensure that skin surface is covered from edge of stoma to 3–4 inches outward with a $\frac{1}{4}$–$\frac{1}{2}$ inch layer of paste.

_____ 21. Discard gloves and wash hands.

C. Placing an appliance on the protective skin barrier:

_____ 1. Select the appliance and pouch that best suits the effluent and client.

_____ 2. Measure the size of the stoma with a stoma template; if none is available, draw a proximal stoma size on a paper held near the stoma; cut out the stoma and compare. Adjust size as needed.

_____ 3. Place the correct template size against the appliance faceplate; match stoma opening size.

_____ 4. Cut opening in paper faceplate to match stoma size if needed. Set aside.

_____ 5. Prepare skin surface with protective barrier (as above). Continue to place wicks against the stoma to absorb urine.

_____ 6. Remove protective backing from paper faceplate.

_____ 7. Reach inside of the pouch from the distal end; hold faceplate against fingers.

_____ 8. Place the faceplate against the skin barrier, centering the stoma opening exactly over the stoma.

_____ 9. Press gently against the faceplate from inside the pouch; remove hand.

_____ 10. Press against the faceplate's outer circumference from the outside of the pouch.

_____ 11. Ensure there are no gaps between the faceplate and the skin barrier.

_____ 12. Place several strips of tape around the edges of the faceplate (if desired).

_____ 13. Fold the distal edges of the pouch and secure clamp; or close the spigot.

_____ 14. Reposition the client's bedclothes; remove protective pad.

_____ 15. Discard all used materials.

If attaching the pouch to a urinary collection bag:

_____ 16. Hang collection bag on the bedrail.

_____ 17. Connect collecting tubing to the spigot. Firmly secure.

_____ 18. Open curtains or door to room.

_____ 19. Discard gloves and wash hands.

D. Emptying the pouch when the client must remain in bed:

_____ 1. Explain to the client what will be done.

_____ 2. Close door to room or draw bedside curtains.

_____ 3. Raise bed to working height.

_____ 4. Wash hands.

_____ 5. Place protective pad under the client's hips on the side of the stoma.

_____ 6. Position covers at the foot of bed.

_____ 7. Rearrange clothing to expose pouch.

_____ 8. Assist the client to a semilateral position, with the stoma and pouch positioned toward the bed surface.

_____ 9. Don disposable gloves.

_____ 10. Place bedpan or urine beaker next to the client, just under the pouch.

_____ 11. Unclamp the pouch, direct the end into the container, and drain the urine.

_____ 12. Wipe the end of pouch; fold it and reattach the clamp.

_____ 13. Remove the container and protective pad.

_____ 14. Note urine characteristics: color, odor, and amount. Discard the effluent and cleanse the container.

_____ 15. Remove and discard gloves.

_____ 16. Wash hands.

_____ 17. Assist client to resume a position of comfort.

_____ 18. Wash hands.

E. Emptying the pouch in the toilet:

_____ 1. Explain to the client what will be done.

_____ 2. Wash hands.

_____ 3. Assist the client to the bathroom.

_____ 4. Close the door.

_____ 5. Assist the client to sit on the commode (toilet) with thighs abducted.

_____ 6. Arrange client's gown or clothing so that it is not near the pouch.

Name ____________________ Date ____________________

Observed by ____________

_____ 7. Don gloves.

_____ 8. Place the distal end of the pouch between the client's thighs, above the commode.

_____ 9. Unclamp or direct the client to unclamp the pouch; empty.

_____ 10. Wipe end and replace the clamp when the pouch is emptied.

_____ 11. Remove gloves and wash hands.

_____ 12. Assist the client to return to bed or chair of his choice.

_____ 13. Examine urine in toilet for character. Flush toilet.

_____ 14. Wash hands.

F. Changing an appliance and pouch:

_____ 1. Explain to the client what will be done.

_____ 2. Wash hands.

_____ 3. Assist the client to the bathroom.

_____ 4. Close the door.

_____ 5. Assist the client to sit on the commode with thighs abducted.

_____ 6. Arrange client's gown or clothing so that it is not near the pouch.

_____ 7. Tear facial tissues into smaller segments; twist each segment into 2-inch wicks; repeat until 15–20 wicks are created. If the client is well enough, have him participate.

_____ 8. Prepare a new appliance and pouch. Set aside.

_____ 9. If the client remains in bed, place a plastic-bag-lined trash container at the bedside or place a bedpan at the client's side.

_____ 10. Place tissue wicks against the stoma until saturated; replace as necessary until new appliance is secured.

_____ 11. Don disposable gloves.

_____ 12. Peel back the faceplate from skin barrier until it is separated completely.

_____ 13. Apply solvent to remove any remaining adhesive from the skin.

_____ 14. Place entire appliance and bag with urine in the collecting container. Set the container aside.

_____ 15. Cleanse the peristomal skin with warm water.

_____ 16. Apply the new appliance (Skill 33.3 B and C).

_____ 17. Remove bedpan; inspect the effluent for characteristics; empty the bedpan into toilet.

_____ 18. Discard gloves.

_____ 19. Wash hands.

_____ 20. Replace bedclothes and reposition client.

_____ 21. Wash hands.

G. Emptying and irrigating a continent urostomy:

_____ 1. Explain to the client what will be done.

_____ 2. Provide privacy.

_____ 3. Wash hands and don disposable gloves.

_____ 4. Assist the client to sit in Fowler's position (if he cannot leave his bed) or to sit on a toilet or stand facing the toilet.

_____ 5. Place a bedpan or urine-collecting cup in the client's lap if he is in bed.

_____ 6. Set aside client's clothing and remove dressing from stoma, if present.

_____ 7. Fill an Asepto or other large syringe with 50 cc of saline. Set it aside.

_____ 8. Lubricate the tip of catheter with water-soluble lubricant.

_____ 9. Insert catheter into stoma very gently until urine drains; direct end of catheter into toilet or container.

_____ 10. Leave catheter in place after urine has drained.

_____ 11. Place tip of syringe in distal end of catheter and instill saline gently into the catheter.

_____ 12. Remove the syringe and allow saline to drain into toilet or container.

OR

Draw saline back with the syringe.

_____ 13. Repeat if drainage contains a lot of mucus.

_____ 14. Remove catheter and place dressing over stoma, if desired. Reposition clothes.

_____ 15. Assist client to a comfortable position, if necessary.

_____ 16. Assess urine for color, clarity, odor, and amount.

_____ 17. Wash catheter with soap and water and rinse; dry with paper towels.

_____ 18. Store the catheter in a clean area.

_____ 19. Wash hands.

Name ________________________________ Date ____________________

Observed by ____________

CHAPTER 34 ASSESSING RESPIRATORY FUNCTION

SKILL 34.1 Assessing Respiratory Function

A. Preparing for each physical examination:

_____ 1. Explain to the client that his nose, sinuses, throat, chest, and lungs will be examined to determine his overall ability to breathe.

_____ 2. Wash hands.

_____ 3. Close the door to the room or draw the curtains around the bed.

B. Physically assessing the nose and sinuses:

_____ 1. Prepare for the examination.

_____ 2. Assist the client to a sitting or semi-Fowler's position.

_____ 3. Inspect the external nose for its general appearance: placement, symmetry, alignment, skin condition.

_____ 4. Inspect the mucosa inside the nostril (using a penlight) for color and dryness.

_____ 5. Place the tip of the nasal speculum in one nostril and inspect the interior nasal cavity for septal deviation, congestion, inflammation, mucosal excoriation.

_____ 6. Palpate the frontal sinus by placing thumb on the bony ridge under the eyebrow and press upward. Repeat on other side.

_____ 7. Palpate the maxillary sinus by placing fingertips on the maxillary ridge lateral to the nose and press upward. Repeat on the other side.

C. Physically assessing the pharynx and tonsils:

_____ 1. Prepare for the examination.

_____ 2. Instruct the client to tilt his head back and open his mouth as wide as possible.

_____ 3. Place the tongue depressor against the superior tongue surface and instruct the client to say "Ah."

_____ 4. Illuminate the posterior pharynx with the penlight.

_____ 5. Inspect the posterior pharynx for color, hydration, presence or absence of palantine tonsils, exudate.

_____ 6. Remove and discard tongue blade.

D. Physically assessing the external neck:

_____ 1. Prepare for the examination.

_____ 2. Instruct the client to tilt his head back and turn his face from side to side. Ask him to swallow.

_____ 3. Inspect the throat, while the client swallows, for symmetry of shape and movement; observe the movement of the thyroid cartilage. Inspect for unusual features such as masses or wounds.

_____ 4. Stand directly behind the patient.

_____ 5. Place your fingers along the angle of the jaw and gently palpate for lymph nodes along the normal node chains.

_____ 6. Palpate the thyroid.

- Place both hands around the client's neck so that the fingertips rest on the trachea.
- Palpate gently for the thyroid isthmus. Instruct the client to swallow.

_____ 7. Place thumb and fingertip on either side of the trachea just above the substernal notch.

E. Physically assessing the thorax and lungs:

_____ 1. Prepare for the examination.

_____ 2. Assist the client to remove his clothing so that his upper body is entirely exposed.

_____ 3. Assist the client into a sitting or semi-Fowler's position.

To examine the posterior thorax:

_____ 4. Stand directly behind the client.

_____ 5. Inspect the posterior chest, observing for

- symmetry of thorax shape
- normal alignment of the spine and scapula
- symmetry of respiratory movement
- retraction or bulging of the intercostal spaces

_____ 6. Using the bony landmarks, imagine the placement of the internal organs.

_____ 7. Palpate the intercostal spaces, noting presence, location, and characteristics of tender or painful areas or masses.

_____ 8. Palpate for respiratory excursion.

- Place hands on lower third of the rib cage, with thumbs pointing toward each other and fingers pointing laterally.
- Press thumbs together so that a fold of skin is formed between them.
- Instruct client to take a deep breath.
- Note the movement of the area between thumbs.

_____ 9. Place palm of dominant hand over the chest wall and instruct the client to say "ninety-nine." Palpate for fremitus.

_____ 10. Place palm symmetrically around the posterior chest and repeat step 8.

_____ 11. Percuss the chest wall using indirect technique, moving the hands symmetrically up and down the rib cage.

_____ 12. Auscultate breath sounds by placing the diaphragm of the stethoscope over the intercostal spaces, beginning above the scapula and moving down to the base of the lungs.

Name ______________________ Date ______________

Observed by __________

To examine the lateral thorax:

_____ **13.** Instruct the client to raise his arms above his head.

_____ **14.** Inspect both lateral chest walls in the same manner as the posterior wall.

_____ **15.** Palpate for fremitus as in step 9.

_____ **16.** Percuss the lateral chest wall as in step 11.

_____ **17.** Auscultate breath sounds as in step 12, moving from the axilla to the base of the rib cage.

To examine the anterior chest:

_____ **18.** Stand directly in front of the client.

_____ **19.** Inspect the anterior chest, observing for

- symmetry of thorax shape
- normal alignment of the clavicles and costal margins
- symmetry of respiratory movement
- retraction or bulging of the supraclavicular, intercostal, or substernal spaces

_____ **20.** Using the bony landmarks, imagine the placement of the internal organs.

_____ **21.** Locate the intercostal spaces.

- Palpate the sternal notch.
- Move fingers down to the bony horizontal ridge that is the junction of the manubrium and sternum.
- Move fingers laterally to the second intercostal space.
- Move fingers down the ribs, counting each space.

_____ **22.** Palpate the intercostal space, noting presence, location, and characteristics of tender or painful areas or masses.

_____ **23.** Palpate for respiratory excursion.

- Place hands on lateral rib cage with thumbs along the costal margins.
- Press thumbs together so that a fold of skin is formed between them.
- Instruct client to take a deep breath.
- Note the movement of the area between thumbs.

_____ **24.** Place palm of dominant hand over the chest wall and instruct the client to say "ninety-nine." Palpate for fremitus.

_____ **25.** Place palm symmetrically around the posterior chest and repeat step 9.

_____ **26.** Percuss the chest wall using indirect technique, moving the hands symmetrically up and down each side of the rib cage.

_____ **27.** Auscultate breath sounds by placing the diaphragm of the stethoscope over the intercostal spaces, moving from the clavicles to the costal margins.

_____ **28.** Instruct client to take deep breaths through the mouth while auscultating.

_____ **29.** Assist the client to replace his clothing; assist him to a position of comfort.

_____ **30.** Open the curtains or doors to the room.

_____ **31.** Wash hands.

Name ______________________ Date ______________

Observed by __________

CHAPTER 35 PROVIDING PULMONARY PHYSIOTHERAPY

SKILL 35.1 Providing Pulmonary Physiotherapy

A. Teaching the client to deep breathe:

_____ 1. Assess the client to determine his nursing diagnostic category.

_____ 2. Plan the nursing objectives and expected outcomes.

_____ 3. Explain to the client the rationale for deep breathing techniques.

_____ 4. Instruct the client to assume or assist him into one of these positions:

- sitting so that chest is upright, legs are dangling or feet are on the floor, and arms are resting on overbed table
- high Fowler's with head supported on a pillow and legs slightly flexed

_____ 5. Place palms of hands on the ribs just above the costal margins.

_____ 6. Instruct the client to breathe in slowly and deeply, expanding the chest and raising the rib cage.

_____ 7. Instruct the client to exhale.

_____ 8. Repeat steps 6 and 7 while evaluating the effectiveness of the breathing.

B. Teaching the client to breathe with pursed lips:

_____ 1. Assess the client to determine his nursing diagnostic category.

_____ 2. Plan the nursing objectives and expected outcomes.

_____ 3. Explain to the client the rationale for using this technique.

_____ 4. Position the client in an upright position.

_____ 5. Instruct the client to take a deep breath.

_____ 6. Instruct the client to purse his lips (a "kissing" position) and exhale fully.

_____ 7. Instruct the client to pause briefly and repeat steps 5 and 6.

_____ 8. Encourage the client to continue to breathe with pursed lips until he uses this mode of breathing continually.

C. Teaching the client to breathe with his diaphragm:

_____ 1. Assess the client to determine his nursing diagnostic category.

_____ 2. Plan the nursing objectives and expected outcomes.

_____ 3. Explain to the client the rationale for this breathing technique.

_____ 4. Place the client in the standing position.

_____ 5. Place palms of your hands on his ribs just above the costal margins.

_____ 6. Instruct the client to take a deep breath.

_____ 7. Instruct the client to purse his lips and slowly exhale while tightening his abdominal muscles.

_____ 8. Push down and outward against the ribs as the client exhales.

_____ 9. Instruct the client to pause briefly and repeat steps 6 and 7.

_____ 10. Instruct the client to practice this technique until he is able to breathe with his diaphragm up to 10 minutes at a time.

D. Teaching the client to breathe deeply and cough:

_____ 1. Assess the client to determine his nursing diagnostic category.

_____ 2. Plan the nursing objectives and expected outcomes.

_____ 3. Explain to the client that he will learn how to cough deeply so that he can remove collected excretions from his airways (or lungs).

_____ 4. Close the door to the room or draw the curtains around the client's bed.

_____ 5. Wash hands.

_____ 6. Instruct the client to assume or assist him to assume one of these positions:

- sitting so that chest is upright, legs are dangling or feet are on the floor, and arms are resting on overbed table
- high Fowler's with head supported on a pillow and legs slightly flexed

_____ 7. Place the tissues within the client's reach.

_____ 8. Splint the client's abdomen with one of three methods:

- Place a pillow against the abdomen and instruct the client to hold it firm.
- Fold a towel, bath blanket, or drawsheet so that it has a width of approximately 12–15 inches; place it around the client's abdomen and hold the ends securely behind his back.
- Stand behind the client and hold hands firmly against his abdomen.

_____ 9. Instruct the client to take two or three deep breaths, fully expanding the chest on inhalation and slowly exhaling.

_____ 10. Instruct the client to lean forward, take another breath, hold it for a second, and contract the abdominal and thigh muscles for two seconds.

_____ 11. Direct the client to cough deeply, expelling air and secretions forcefully.

_____ 12. Instruct the client to pause and breathe normally for 10–15 seconds.

_____ 13. Repeat steps 9–12 until the client expectorates secretions.

_____ 14. Encourage the client to rest and breathe normally for several minutes.

_____ 15. Auscultate the major airways for evidence of retained secretions.

If retained secretions are present:

_____ 16. Repeat steps 9–12 until airways are clear.

_____ 17. Return the client to a position of comfort.

_____ 18. Dispose of tissues.

_____ 19. Wash hands.

_____ 20. Encourage or assist the client to wash his hands.

Name ______________________ Date ______________

Observed by __________

_____ 21. Provide mouth care as necessary.

_____ 22. Encourage the client to drink fluids.

E. Teaching the client to use an incentive spirometer:

_____ 1. Assess the client to determine his nursing diagnostic category.

_____ 2. Plan the nursing objectives and expected outcomes.

_____ 3. Explain to the client the purpose of the spirometer and how often he will use it.

_____ 4. Wash hands.

For a flow spirometer:

_____ 5. Instruct the client to hold the spirometer so that it is upright.

For a volume spirometer:

_____ 5. Set a predetermined volume on the spirometer. Place within the client's reach.

For both spirometers:

_____ 6. Instruct the client to exhale slowly and completely.

_____ 7. Instruct the client to place the mouthpiece in his mouth with his lips forming a seal.

_____ 8. Instruct the client to take a deep breath and hold it for three seconds.

For a flow spirometer:

_____ 9. Instruct the client to watch the gauge (or ball) rise in the spirometer. Encourage him to note the flow rate.

For a volume spirometer:

_____ 9. Instruct the client to observe the gauge to determine if the set goal is achieved.

For both spirometers:

_____ 10. Direct the client to remove the mouthpiece and exhale slowly.

_____ 11. Instruct the client to repeat steps 6–10 about four or five times, attempting to increase the flow rate with each inhalation.

_____ 12. Instruct the client to cough when he has completed five cycles.

_____ 13. Remove the mouthpiece and rinse it with cold water; store it in the client's bedside unit.

_____ 14. Wash hands.

_____ 15. Encourage the client to use the spirometer every hour.

_____ 16. Instruct the client to drink fluids.

F. Performing percussion, vibration, and postural drainage (PVD):

_____ 1. Assess the client to determine his nursing diagnostic category.

_____ 2. Plan the nursing objectives and expected outcomes.

_____ 3. Explain the procedure to the client. Answer his questions.

_____ 4. Schedule the procedure so that it doesn't conflict with meals.

_____ 5. Encourage the client to drink fluids frequently.

_____ 6. Wash hands.

_____ 7. Close the door to the client's room or draw curtains around his bed.

_____ 8. Place the client in the proper position to drain the congested lung segment.

_____ 9. Apply pillows or folded bath blankets around the client's body.

_____ 10. Place tissues within the client's reach.

_____ 11. Have the client maintain the position for 10–15 minutes.

_____ 12. Instruct the client to deep breathe and cough while in the position.

_____ 13. Keep suctioning equipment available if client has tenacious secretions that he cannot expel without help.

To perform percussion:

_____ 14. Cover the chest area with a towel or the client's gown.

_____ 15. Cup hands and alternately clap hands over the lung segment. Keep wrists and elbows relaxed.

_____ 16. Percuss for three to five minutes.

To perform vibration:

_____ 17. Place hands flat on the client's chest. Keep arms and shoulders straight.

_____ 18. Instruct the client to inhale through the nose and exhale slowly through the mouth.

_____ 19. Vibrate hands by quickly contracting and relaxing arms and shoulders for 8–10 seconds during the client's exhalation.

_____ 20. Relax arms and shoulders while the client inhales.

_____ 21. Repeat steps 18 and 19 for two to five minutes, depending on the client's tolerance and amount of secretions.

_____ 22. Position the client upright after completing PVD in each lung segment.

_____ 23. Instruct client to deep breathe and cough.

_____ 24. Auscultate lung segment for abnormal sounds.

_____ 25. Position the client to drain other lung segments, repeating steps 8–20.

_____ 26. Return the client to a position of comfort.

_____ 27. Provide mouth care for the client.

_____ 28. Open bedside curtains or door to the room.

_____ 29. Offer fluids to the client.

_____ 30. Remove used tissues from the bedside.

_____ 31. Wash hands.

Name ______________________________ Date ______________

Observed by __________

CHAPTER 36 ADMINISTERING OXYGEN

SKILL 36.1 Administering Oxygen

A. Preparing for each type of oxygen delivery device:

_____ 1. Assess the client to determine his nursing diagnostic category.

_____ 2. Plan the nursing objectives and expected outcomes.

_____ 3. Explain to the client the reasons why he is to receive oxygen. Explain and demonstrate the method of administration. Answer his questions.

_____ 4. Place signs on the client's room door and above his bed indicating "OXYGEN IN USE" and "NO SMOKING."

_____ 5. Wash hands.

_____ 6. Open distilled water and pour into humidifier reservoir; close water.

_____ 7. Attach the humidifier to the oxygen flow meter and secure.

_____ 8. Insert the flow meter and humidifier into the oxygen source wall outlet.

_____ 9. Turn the knob on the flow meter to open the oxygen flow. Adjust to approximately 5 liters/minute.

_____ 10. Turn the oxygen flow to "Off."

_____ 11. Attach the oxygen tubing to the flow meter. Lay aside.

B. Administering oxygen via a nasal cannula:

_____ 1. Prepare for oxygen administration.

_____ 2. Remove packaging from the cannula and discard.

_____ 3. Attach distal end of the cannula to the oxygen tubing.

_____ 4. Open the oxygen flow to the prescribed rate, usually in the range 1–6 liters/minute. If rate is not indicated in the physician's orders, set it at 2 liters/minute.

_____ 5. Examine humidifier to note bubbling as oxygen flows through water.

_____ 6. Place the nasal prongs in the client's nostrils.

_____ 7. Slip the elastic band around the client's head above the ears.

OR

Adjust the tubing around the client's ears and slip the plastic holder to secure the tubing under the client's chin.

_____ 8. Secure the oxygen tubing to the client's clothing or bed linens, allowing slack for movement.

_____ 9. Check the flow meter at intervals to ensure the correct flow rate.

_____ 10. Inspect the client's nostrils every four hours; lubricate with water-soluble lubricant as required if skin is dry or irritated.

_____ 11. Encourage the client to increase his fluid intake if this is not contraindicated for therapeutic reasons.

_____ 12. Monitor the client's vital signs, level of awareness, degree of anxiety, and other signs of hypoxia at frequent intervals.

C. Inserting and administering oxygen via a nasal catheter:

_____ 1. Prepare for oxygen administration.

_____ 2. Place the client in a semi-Fowler's position.

_____ 3. Cut approximately 4–5 inches length of tape; make a vertical cut about 2 inches from one end. Set the strip within reach.

_____ 4. Remove packaging from the catheter and discard.

_____ 5. Hold the tip of the catheter near the client's nostril and measure the distance to the earlobe.

_____ 6. Mark the measured length with an indelible pen or piece of tape.

_____ 7. Attach the distal end of the catheter to the oxygen tubing.

_____ 8. Open the oxygen flow to the prescribed rate, usually 1–6 liters/minute. If no rate is indicated in the physician's orders, set it at 2 liters/minute.

_____ 9. Lubricate the tip of the catheter with water-soluble lubricant.

_____ 10. Insert the catheter gently into one nostril, guiding it medially along the floor of the nasal cavity until the marked point is at the vestibule of the nostril.

_____ 11. Hold the catheter in position with one hand.

_____ 12. Instruct the client to open his mouth wide.

_____ 13. Illuminate the posterior oral cavity with a penlight; observe for the catheter tip on the side of uvula.

_____ 14. Place the uncut end of adhesive lengthwise on the client's nose; wrap the two ends around the catheter, securing it in place.

_____ 15. Secure the oxygen tubing to the client's clothing or bed linens, allowing slack for movement.

_____ 16. Check the flow meter at intervals to ensure the correct flow rate.

_____ 17. Inspect the client's nostrils every four hours; lubricate with water-soluble lubricant as required if skin is dry or irritated.

_____ 18. Encourage the client to increase his fluid intake if this is not contraindicated for therapeutic reasons.

_____ 19. Monitor the client's vital signs, level of awareness, degree of anxiety, and other signs of hypoxia at frequent intervals.

D. Administering oxygen by a simple face mask, face tent, or a venturi mask:

_____ 1. Prepare for oxygen administration.

_____ 2. Remove packaging from the mask and discard.

_____ 3. Attach mask to the oxygen tubing.

_____ 4. Open the oxygen flow to the prescribed rate.

Name ______________________________ Date ______________

Observed by ____________

On a venturi mask:

____ 5. Adjust the venturi control device to deliver the prescribed O_2 percentage.

____ 6. Examine the humidifier to note bubbling as oxygen flows through water. Look for visible mist coming from the face tent.

____ 7. Place the mask or tent in position on the client's face.

____ 8. Fasten the mask's elastic band over the client's ears and tighten so that the mask fits snugly against the face. Check for leaks around the edge of the mask.

____ 9. Check the controls for oxygen flow rate and oxygen delivery percentage to ensure accuracy.

____ 10. Attach the oxygen tubing to the client's clothing or bed linens.

____ 11. Check the ports on the venturi device at intervals to ensure patency.

____ 12. Monitor the client every hour for discomfort. Check the skin under the mask for pressure necrosis.

____ 13. Remove mask briefly; bathe and dry the facial skin every two to four hours.

____ 14. Monitor the client's vital signs, level of awareness, degree of anxiety, and other signs of hypoxia at frequent intervals.

____ 15. Raise the mask slightly above the face when the client eats or drinks.

E. Administering oxygen by a partial rebreather or nonrebreather mask:

____ 1. Prepare to administer oxygen.

____ 2. Remove packaging from the mask and discard.

____ 3. Attach mask to the oxygen tubing.

____ 4. Open the oxgyen flow to 8–10 liters/minute.

____ 5. Examine the humidifier to note bubbling as oxygen flows through water.

____ 6. Place mask on the client's face.

____ 7. Pull mask back and slip thumb over the reservoir bag outlet. Allow the bag to fill completely.

____ 8. Remove thumb quickly and readjust the mask over the client's face.

____ 9. Observe the reservoir bag to ensure that it deflates slightly with inspiration.

____ 10. Attach tubing to the client's clothing or bed linens; ensure that tubing does not become kinked.

____ 11. Monitor the client every hour for discomfort. Check for pressure necrosis under the mask.

_____ **12.** Remove mask briefly; bathe and dry the facial skin every two to four hours.

_____ **13.** Monitor the client's vital signs, level of awareness, degree of anxiety, and other signs of hypoxia at frequent intervals.

_____ **14.** Raise the mask slightly above the face when the client eats or drinks.

Name ______________________________ Date ______________

Observed by ____________

CHAPTER 37 MANAGING THE CLIENT WITH A CHEST TUBE

SKILL 37.1 Managing the Client with a Chest Tube

A. Assisting with the insertion of chest tubes:

_____ 1. Explain the procedure to the client.

_____ 2. Ensure that an informed consent form is signed by the client.

_____ 3. Gather the necessary equipment.

_____ 4. Wash hands.

_____ 5. Set up the water seal system.

_____ 6. Position the client.

_____ 7. Assist the physician with sterile technique.

_____ 8. Provide emotional support to the client.

_____ 9. Assist with the application of an occlusive dressing around the stable wound site after insertion of the chest tube.

_____ 10. Connect the tube to the water seal drainage system and tape all connections.

_____ 11. Assess breath sounds by auscultating the chest.

_____ 12. Wash hands.

_____ 13. Prepare the patient for a postinsertion chest x-ray.

_____ 14. Observe the client for symptoms. Observe the water seal drainage for proper functioning.

B. Assessing the client and chest tubes:

_____ 1. Explain the procedures and observations you are making to the client.

_____ 2. Wash hands.

_____ 3. Assess the client using interview, inspection, and auscultation.

_____ 4. Assess the equipment including tubing, water seal bottle, suction control bottle, and the position of the entire unit.

_____ 5. Position the client to allow maximal lung expansion.

_____ 6. Encourage the client to move side to side and be mobile.

_____ 7. Encourage the client to deep breathe and cough.

_____ 8. Observe the color, rate of accumulation, and volume of drainage at least hourly and record the output from the chest tube at the end of each shift.

_____ 9. Measure and note drainage output at the end of each shift, but do not empty bottle.

Name ____________________ Date ____________

Observed by ________

CHAPTER 38 MAINTAINING AN AIRWAY

SKILL 38.1 Clearing the Airway

A. Clearing an obstructed airway by using back blows:

If the client is standing or sitting:

____ 1. Stand behind the client and place one hand on his sternum.

____ 2. Instruct the client to lean forward against your arm until his head is lower than his shoulders.

If the client is lying down:

____ 1. Turn the client to a lateral position facing you with his chest braced against your thighs.

____ 2. Deliver four sharp blows between the client's scapula with the heel of your hand.

If client is a young child:

____ 1. Place client face down across your knees with head lower than the shoulders.

____ 2. Deliver four sharp blows between the client's scapula with the heel of your hand. Use less force with the blow to avoid injuring the child.

For each position:

____ 3. Assess for expulsion of foreign body and return of respiration. If present, assess the client for evidence of further injury. If absent, proceed to next technique.

B. Clearing an obstructed airway with abdominal thrusts (the Heimlich maneuver):

If the client is standing or sitting:

____ 1. Stand behind the client and wrap your arms around the waist.

____ 2. Make a fist with one hand, with the thumb tucked in the fist; place thumb against the client's epigastrium just below the xiphoid process.

____ 3. Wrap the other hand around the fist.

____ 4. Press upward with a firm but quick thrust.

If the client is lying down:

____ 1. Kneel next to client and roll him to his back.

____ 2. Turn the client's face away from you.

____ 3. Place the heel of your hand against the epigastrium; place your other hand over it; keep elbows straight.

____ 4. Press heel of the hand firmly toward the client's head with a quick thrust.

For each position:

_____ 5. Assess for expulsion of foreign body and return of respiration. If respiration resumes, assess the client for evidence of further injury. If it does not, call for emergency assistance. Monitor pulse; if pulse is absent, initiate CPR.

C. Digitally removing a foreign object from the mouth:

_____ 1. Open the client's mouth by grasping the tongue and lower jaw with your finger and thumb; lift up.

_____ 2. Remove dentures.

_____ 3. Insert index finger of other hand inside the cheek to the back of the mouth.

_____ 4. Attempt to dislodge objects at the back of the oral cavity with a sweeping motion of the fingers; pull it forward to the mouth.

_____ 5. If object is removed, assess client's pulse and respiration. If the object is not expelled, call for emergency assistance; if pulse is absent, initiate CPR.

D. Inserting an artificial oral airway:

_____ 1. Select the appropriate size airway for the client.

_____ 2. Wash hands.

_____ 3. Open client's mouth with a tongue blade; hyperextend the neck if necessary.

_____ 4. Turn the airway upside down or sideways and insert into the mouth until the flange touches the client's lips.

_____ 5. Turn the airway quickly so that the curve fits over the tongue.

_____ 6. Tape the airway in position if the client is likely to spit it out.

Name ______________________________ Date ______________

Observed by ____________

SKILL 38.2 Suctioning the Airway

A. Performing oropharyngeal suctioning:

_____ 1. Assess the client to identify the nursing diagnostic category and need for suctioning.

_____ 2. Plan the nursing goals and identify the expected outcomes of the suctioning procedure.

_____ 3. Explain exactly what will occur to the client; encourage him to ask questions (if he is alert).

_____ 4. Gather the equipment.

_____ 5. Draw bedside curtains or close the door to the room.

_____ 6. Elevate the client to a mid-Fowler's position (about 45°).

_____ 7. Place a towel or disposable pad around the client's shoulders and over the chest.

_____ 8. Wash hands.

_____ 9. Unfold a sterile towel on a table near the client's head.

_____ 10. Connect the extra length of plastic tubing to the suction source. Place the distal end near the overbed table work area.

_____ 11. Remove the cap from the sterile water or saline solution; set the bottle on the overbed table.

_____ 12. Place a cup on sterile field and pour 100 cc water or saline in it.

_____ 13. Attach a tonsillar tip to the connecting tubing.

_____ 14. Turn on the suction source.

_____ 15. Don clean gloves.

_____ 16. Instruct the client to open his mouth (if the client is conscious and cooperative).

OR

Grasp the client's lower jaw and pull down, opening the mouth.

_____ 17. Insert the tonsillar tip on the outside of the lower gums and remove secretions.

_____ 18. Move the tonsillar tip to the inside of the lower gums, under the tongue, and remove secretions.

_____ 19. Insert the tonsillar tip along the top of the tongue to the posterior oral cavity while removing secretions.

_____ 20. Encourage the alert and cooperative client to cough.

_____ 21. Remove the tonsillar tip and immerse it in cup to draw water through tip and tubing.

_____ 22. Wait one minute and repeat steps 17–21 until all secretions are cleared from the mouth and pharynx.

_____ 23. Cleanse the client's mouth and face with tissues or moist washcloth after completing suctioning.

_____ 24. Position the client comfortably.

_____ 25. Disconnect the tonsillar tip from tubing and turn off suction source.

_____ 26. Clean the tonsillar tip with solution of water and hydrogen peroxide; rinse it with water and air dry.

_____ 27. Cleanse or discard other equipment.

_____ 28. Remove and discard gloves. Wash hands.

B. Preparing for suctioning with a sterile catheter:

_____ 1. Assess the client to identify the nursing diagnostic category and need for suctioning.

_____ 2. Plan the nursing goals and identify the expected outcomes of the suctioning procedure.

_____ 3. Explain exactly what will occur to the client; encourage him to ask questions (if he is alert).

_____ 4. Draw bedside curtains or close the door to the room.

_____ 5. Gather the needed equipment.

_____ 6. Elevate the client to a mid-Fowler's position (about 45°).

_____ 7. Place a towel or disposable pad around the client's shoulders and over the chest.

_____ 8. Wash hands.

_____ 9. Connect the extra length of plastic tubing to the suction source. Place the distal end near the overbed table work area.

_____ 10. Remove the cap from the sterile water or saline; set the bottle on the overbed table.

_____ 11. Open a tube or package of lubricant; set it on the table.

_____ 12. Open the suction tray kit on overbed table using correct sterile technique.

_____ 13. Place the sterile glove from the kit on dominant hand. (If two gloves: don both. During the remainder of this technique, the "gloved hand" is the dominant hand.)

_____ 14. Set up the irrigant cup with gloved hand.

_____ 15. Pour water or saline in the cup using the ungloved hand.

_____ 16. Squeeze small amount of water-soluble lubricant on tray with ungloved hand.

_____ 17. Pick up the catheter with the gloved hand and coil it around the hand so that the distal end is between fingers and thumb.

_____ 18. Pick up the connecting tubing with ungloved hand and attach to catheter in gloved hand.

Name ______________________ Date ______________

Observed by ____________

_____ 19. Turn on the suction source with the ungloved hand.

_____ 20. Place the tip of the catheter in the saline with the gloved hand and place thumb over the port near the distal end.

_____ 21. Observe the saline draw through the catheter and tubing and enter the collection bottle.

_____ 22. Turn off suction source with the ungloved hand.

_____ 23. Dip the end of the catheter in the lubricant.

_____ 24. Lay the catheter on the packaging paper if other client preparations are necessary.

C. Suctioning the nasotrachea:

_____ 1. Place the client in semi-Fowler's with pillow behind shoulders and neck extended.

_____ 2. Explain to the client what will occur during suctioning; direct him to signal nonverbally if he wishes the procedure stopped.

_____ 3. Prepare the catheter.

_____ 4. Pick up the catheter with the gloved hand and coil it around the hand so that the tip is between the thumb and forefinger.

_____ 5. Hold the distal end of the catheter with the ungloved hand; place thumb in position near the suction port but not on it.

_____ 6. Insert catheter through the nares, quickly directing it medially and inferiorly until approximately 6–8 inches are inserted.

_____ 7. Place thumb of the ungloved hand over catheter port for 10–15 seconds; gently rotate and withdraw catheter. Encourage the client to cough.

_____ 8. Immerse the catheter in water and apply suction.

_____ 9. Wait two minutes and repeat steps 4–8 until no secretions are removed.

_____ 10. Auscultate the client's breath sounds.

_____ 11. Disconnect catheter from suction tubing; coil in the palm of gloved hand.

_____ 12. Remove the glove inside out so that the catheter is wrapped inside.

_____ 13. Discard the glove and catheter.

_____ 14. Position the client comfortably.

_____ 15. Clean or discard equipment, according to agency policy.

_____ 16. Wash hands.

D. Suctioning through a nasopharyngeal airway:

_____ 1. Prepare the suctioning catheter and equipment.

_____ 2. Open a packaged, sterile nasopharyngeal airway on the open sterile packaging paper *before* donning sterile glove while preparing the catheter.

_____ 3. Turn on oxygen source to 2 liters/minute.

_____ 4. Place the oxygen delivery mask over the client's mouth only.

_____ 5. Explain to the client what will occur during suctioning; direct him to signal nonverbally if he wishes the procedure stopped.

_____ 6. Lubricate the blunt end of the nasopharyngeal airway.

_____ 7. Insert airway into nostril, directing the blunt end medially and inferiorly until the flanged end rests against the opening of the nares.

_____ 8. Pick up the catheter with the gloved hand and coil it around the hand so that the tip is between the thumb and forefinger.

_____ 9. Hold the distal end of the catheter with the ungloved hand; place thumb in position near suction port but not on it.

_____ 10. Insert the tip of catheter through the airway quickly as the client inhales; keep thumb away from suction port.

_____ 11. Advance the catheter tip until resistance is met or the client coughs vigorously; pull it back about a half inch.

_____ 12. Encourage the client to take slow, deep breaths. Tell him to swallow.

_____ 13. Place thumb over the suction port and direct the client to cough.

_____ 14. Rotate catheter and withdraw while occluding suction port for 10–15 seconds. Do not withdraw catheter entirely from airway.

_____ 15. Observe secretions moving through the suction tubing to verify their removal from pharynx.

_____ 16. Wait 15–30 seconds before suctioning a second time if the client has more secretions.

_____ 17. Repeat steps 10–15.

_____ 18. Remove the catheter from the airway when secretions are no longer withdrawn.

_____ 19. Immerse the catheter in the water and draw water through it by applying suction.

_____ 20. Disconnect the catheter from suction tubing; coil it in the palm of gloved hand.

_____ 21. Remove the glove inside out so that the catheter is wrapped inside.

_____ 22. Discard the glove and catheter.

_____ 23. Place the oxygen device over the client's nose; encourage him to relax. Evaluate his breathing.

_____ 24. Turn off suction source.

_____ 25. Auscultate the client's breath sounds.

_____ 26. Leave airway in place if the client will be suctioned again within a few hours; otherwise withdraw.

_____ 27. Remove oxygen device if the client does not receive continual therapy.

_____ 28. Clean or discard equipment, according to agency policy.

Name ________________________________ Date ____________________

Observed by ____________

_____ 29. Position the client comfortably.

_____ 30. Wash hands.

E. Suctioning through an endotracheal or tracheostomy tube:

_____ 1. Attach the manual ventilator bag (Ambu) to the oxygen flow meter to deliver 100 percent oxygen and place next to the client's head.

_____ 2. Elevate the head of the bed between 35° and 45°.

_____ 3. Explain to the client what will be done.

_____ 4. Assess for baseline data.

- Auscultate the lungs for quality of the breath sounds.
- Determine heart rate and rhythm.

_____ 5. Prepare the suctioning catheter.

_____ 6. Attach the ventilator (Ambu) bag to the distal tube opening and pump the bag two or three times.

_____ 7. Detach the bag and set it aside.

_____ 8. Instill prescribed amount of saline into tube opening with nondominant hand.

_____ 9. Open the endotracheal tube adapter's suction port.

_____ 10. Introduce the catheter into the suction port or distal tracheostomy tube opening gently during inspiration; advance it until resistance is felt. Do NOT apply suction.

_____ 11. Withdraw catheter about a half inch.

_____ 12. Place thumb over the catheter's suction port.

_____ 13. Rotate and withdraw the catheter smoothly within 10–15 seconds.

_____ 14. Remove catheter from the tube and close the endotracheal adapter's port.

_____ 15. Encourage the client with a tracheostomy to cough. Wipe expelled secretions from the tube with a clean tissue.

_____ 16. Attach the resuscitation bag to the tube opening and pump the bag two or three times. Remove.

_____ 17. Immerse the catheter in the water and apply suction.

_____ 18. Wait two to three minutes and repeat steps 9–16 if the client continues to have secretions as determined by audible bubbling.

_____ 19. Observe the client's responses throughout the suctioning procedure.

_____ 20. Disconnect the catheter from suction tubing; coil it in the palm of gloved hand.

_____ 21. Remove the glove inside out so that the catheter is wrapped inside; discard the glove and catheter.

_____ **22.** Reattach the client's oxygen source.

_____ **23.** Auscultate the client's lungs and note his heart rate and rhythm.

_____ **24.** Position the client comfortably.

_____ **25.** Clean or discard equipment according to agency policy.

_____ **26.** Wash hands.

Name ______________________________ Date ______________

Observed by ____________

SKILL 38.3 Managing the Tracheostomy

A. Communicating with the client with a tracheostomy:

_____ 1. Explain to the client that he cannot speak because the tracheostomy has changed the way sound is produced by his larynx.

_____ 2. Explain that you will demonstrate how he can speak or signal for help.

_____ 3. Place one gloved fingertip over the tracheostomy tube opening and ask the client to speak a few words.

_____ 4. Instruct the client to place his fingertip over the opening and speak.

_____ 5. Instruct the client to signal with his hands or head if he cannot speak because of shortness of breath.

_____ 6. Keep a pad of paper and pen or pencil within the client's reach for him to write longer messages.

_____ 7. Keep the client's call signal within reach at all times; be sure the client knows exactly where it is.

B. Cleaning the tracheostomy cannula:

_____ 1. Assess the client to determine his nursing diagnostic categories.

_____ 2. Plan the nursing objectives and expected outcomes, and prepare the necessary supplies and equipment.

_____ 3. Explain exactly what will be done to the client. Assure him that he will be able to breathe throughout the procedure. Arrange a nonverbal signal for him to use if he feels uncomfortable or can't breathe.

_____ 4. Draw the curtains around the bed or close the door to the room.

_____ 5. Place the client in a mid- to high Fowler's position.

_____ 6. Perform tracheostomy suctioning. Leave equipment available for use.

_____ 7. Wash hands.

_____ 8. Open the plastic disposal bag and fold the top edges downward. Set it on the client's bed or another surface other than the work surface.

_____ 9. Open the tracheostomy care kit on a work table next to the client's bed.

If kit is not used:

_____ 10. Prepare sterile field by opening a sterile drape on work table. Open and place necessary equipment on it.

_____ 11. Pour hydrogen peroxide in one of the basins and sterile saline in the other.

_____ 12. Saturate two 4 × 4 gauze pads with hydrogen peroxide. Keep others dry.

_____ 13. Pick up the sterile drape in the kit by the corners.
OR
Open sterile drape package.

_____ 14. Unfold the drape and lay it on the client's chest just under the tracheostomy.

_____ 15. Remove the oxygen mist collar from the tracheostomy opening, if present, and set it next to the client's head.

_____ 16. Don clean gloves and hold the soiled dressing by a dry corner; remove from under the tracheostomy opening; place in the disposal bag. Discard gloves.

_____ 17. Wash hands.

_____ 18. Don clean gloves.

To clean the double-cannula tracheostomy tube:

_____ 19. Remove the inner cannula with nondominant hand and place it in a basin of hydrogen peroxide.

_____ 20. Replace oxygen collar over the stoma with nondominant hand.

_____ 21. Don sterile gloves.

_____ 22. Pick up inner cannula with nondominant hand and quickly brush the outside and inside surface with brush or pipe cleaners using the dominant hand.

_____ 23. Rinse with peroxide using the dominant hand.

_____ 24. Transfer cannula to the basin of saline solution and rinse thoroughly.

_____ 25. Dry inside cannula of cannula tube with dry pipe cleaner.

_____ 26. Lay cannula on sterile field to dry.

To clean the outer cannula or a single-cannula tracheostomy tube:

_____ 27. Saturate an applicator with peroxide.

_____ 28. Remove oxygen collar.

_____ 29. Wipe the applicator around the stoma, skin, and cannula opening, loosening secretions.

_____ 30. Wipe 4 × 4 gauze saturated with peroxide around areas that are heavily crusted. Avoid dislodging the cannula.

_____ 31. Repeat steps 26–29 until all secretions are removed.

_____ 32. Saturate an applicator with saline or a 4 × 4 gauze and rinse areas that were cleansed with peroxide.

_____ 33. Pat dry with clean, dry 4 × 4.

_____ 34. Prepare tracheostomy dressing if one is not available.

_____ 35. Pick up the tracheostomy dressing with the forceps and slip it under the flanges of the tube, arranging it flat and smooth against the skin. Discard forceps.

_____ 36. Suction the outer cannula.

_____ 37. Reinsert an inner cannula and lock into position.

Name ______________________________ Date ______________

Observed by ____________

_____ 38. Replace oxygen collar.

_____ 39. Remove and discard gloves in disposal bag.

_____ 40. Position client comfortably.

_____ 41. Wash hands.

C. Replacing tracheostomy ties:

_____ 1. Wash hands.

_____ 2. Cut two pieces of tape or ties about 15–16 inches long.

_____ 3. Fold one end of each strip over about 1 inch.

_____ 4. Cut a small slit in the corner of the fold. Unfold and set within reach.

_____ 5. Remove oxygen collar.

_____ 6. Slip the slit end of the tie through the opening in the flange with forceps tips until the end is visible; draw through the opening with the forceps. If old ties and secretions occlude the opening, remove them with forceps in one hand while holding the tube in place with the other.

_____ 7. Thread the opposite end of the tape through the slit and draw it tight.

_____ 8. Repeat steps 6 and 7 on the other side.

_____ 9. Bring the ties around the client's neck.

_____ 10. Slip one finger under the ties and secure them with a square knot at the side of the neck.

_____ 11. Cut the used, soiled tapes from the tracheostomy flange and discard.

_____ 12. Replace the oxygen collar.

_____ 13. Wash hands.

D. Measuring the cuff pressure:

_____ 1. Wash hands.

_____ 2. Attach a three-way stopcock to the test valve of the cuff.

_____ 3. Attach a blood pressure manometer to one stopcock port.

_____ 4. Draw 2–3 cc of air into a syringe; attach the end of syringe into the remaining stopcock port. Inject air.

_____ 5. Turn stopcock on to manometer and read the cuff pressure.

_____ 6. Remove air from cuff by pulling back on the syringe plunger if pressure is greater than 15 mm Hg.

_____ 7. Decrease pressure to less than 15 mm Hg.

_____ 8. Remove syringe, stopcock, and manometer. Cuff is now inflated at the desired pressure.

To deflate cuff:

_____ 9. Attach syringe to cuff port and withdraw air.

_____ 10. Provide tracheostomy care or suctioning as desired.

To inflate cuff:

_____ 11. Draw 2–3 cc air into the syringe and attach to the inflation port.

_____ 12. Inject air; withdraw syringe.

_____ 13. Wash hands.

E. Teaching the client and caregiver to suction and care for the tracheostomy at home with these steps:

_____ 1. Gather necessary equipment in a clean setting near a sink (kitchen may be best if client is ambulatory.)

_____ 2. Wash hands.

_____ 3. Prepare suctioning equipment by attaching suction catheter to machine and testing for patency by drawing distilled water through it. (Water is placed in a small receptacle, perhaps a small bowl or a coffee cup.)

_____ 4. Insert suction catheter as far as possible into the opening; place finger on catheter port and withdraw while rotating the catheter.

_____ 5. Rinse the catheter by suctioning water through the distilled water. Wipe the outside of the catheter on a clean paper or hand towel.

_____ 6. Pause for a minute or until the client breathes comfortably; repeat the suctioning.

_____ 7. Detach catheter from machine when finished; rinse the catheter thoroughly and allow to drain dry.

To clean the stoma:

_____ 8. Prepare equipment: pour hydrogen peroxide and saline into two receptacles (cups will do).

_____ 9. Seat the client in a high Fowler's in front of a portable mirror.

_____ 10. Suction the tracheostomy and remove the inner cannula; place in solution.

_____ 11. Clean the inner cannula as in a hospital.

_____ 12. Discard stoma dressing, if present.

_____ 13. Soak a 4 × 4 gauze in peroxide and clean around stoma to remove secretions; pat dry with clean 4 × 4.

_____ 14. Replace stoma dressing if excess secretions are present.

_____ 15. Remove tracheostomy ties and replace. (Explain to the client that another person may have to hold the tube in place.)

_____ 16. Replace inner cannula.

_____ 17. Discard used materials in a paper or plastic bag; secure shut and discard.

_____ 18. Rinse receptacles thoroughly; wash in hot water or a dishwasher.

_____ 19. Wash hands.

Name ______________________________ Date ______________________

Observed by ____________

CHAPTER 39 ASSESSING CARDIOVASCULAR FUNCTION

SKILL 39.1 Assessing Cardiovascular Function

_____ 1. Explain to the client that you are examining his heart and blood vessels to determine how they are working.

_____ 2. Wash hands.

_____ 3. Examine the client in a closed room or quiet area if at all possible.

_____ 4. Close the door to the room or draw curtains around the client's bed.

_____ 5. Assist the client or direct him to a semi-Fowler's or supine position.

To assess the heart:

_____ 6. Inspect the client's chest for symmetry of size and respiratory movement.

_____ 7. Locate the heart using anatomic landmarks: from the sternal notch, locate the manubrium and second intercostal space. The client's right is the aortic area; the client's left is the pulmonic area. The fifth intercostal space is the tricuspid area; laterally at the midclavicular line. Epigastric area is at the tip of the xiphoid.

_____ 8. Inspect the chest for pulsations. Note location.

_____ 9. Palpate aortic, pulmonic, tricuspid, apical, and epigastric areas for vibrations with the ball of your hand and with the fingertips. Note location.

_____ 10. Locate the PMI by palpating the apical area at the fourth or fifth intercostal space in the midclavicular line.

_____ 11. Percuss the chest wall from the fourth or fifth intercostal space along the anterior axillary line toward the sternum.

_____ 12. Auscultate the heart by placing the stethoscope diaphragm at the apex. Identify the first (S_1) and second (S_2) heart sounds. Next listen with bell of the stethoscope.

_____ 13. Count the heart rate at the apical site (Skill 12.2). Be alert to irregularities. If you note a dysrhythmia, palpate the radial pulse for deficits. If deficits are present, take an apical-radial rate with another health worker (Skill 12.2).

_____ 14. Auscultate heart sounds at aortic, pulmonic, tricuspid, and apical areas, using both the diaphragm and the bell of the stethoscope. Listen for pitch, intensity, rhythm; be alert for extra sounds or a blowing sound over the lub-dub sound.

To assess vascular circulation:

_____ 15. Inspect the skin and mucous membranes for color. (Chapter 9 describes normal and variations from normal skin color.)

_____ 16. Inspect extremities for edema. If edema is present, gently press against the edematous area for 15 seconds. Upon release, note if the skin remains indented.

_____ 17. Inspect extremities for reduced hair growth, tight or shiny skin, changes in pigmentation, or thick nail growth.

_____ 18. Palpate skin temperature of extremities with the back of your hand.

_____ 19. Inspect the jugular veins for distention or collapse.

To assess arterial circulation:

_____ 20. Inspect carotid arteries for pulsations. Palpate each artery for pulse rate, rhythm, strength, and elasticity.

_____ 21. Auscultate each carotid artery for bruits.

_____ 22. Palpate peripheral arteries for rate, rhythm, strength, and elasticity: radial, brachial, femoral, popliteal, dorsalis pedis, and posterior tibial. (See Chapter 12.)

_____ 23. Return the client to a position of comfort.

_____ 24. Wash hands.

Name ______________________ Date ______________________

Observed by ______________

SKILL 39.2 Measuring Central Venous Pressure

A. Setting up the equipment:

_____ 1. Explain to the client what you are going to do.

_____ 2. Prepare the intravenous solution container, administration set, and tubing; prime the tubing and clamp it.

_____ 3. Attach a stopcock to the bottom of the manometer.

_____ 4. Attach an IV extension set to one stopcock connector.

_____ 5. Attach the end of the primed tubing to the other stopcock connector.

_____ 6. Turn the stopcock so that the IV tubing and manometer are connected and open. This is the *IV to manometer route.*

_____ 7. Unclamp the IV tubing and fill the manometer with IV solution to approximately 18–20 cm. Clamp tubing.

_____ 8. Turn the stopcock to open the connection to the IV extension set. This is the *manometer to vein route.*

_____ 9. Unclamp tubing and fill extension set with fluid; clamp.

_____ 10. Attach extension tubing to the central catheter in the client.

_____ 11. Open the tubing clamp so that IV solution is flowing into the client's vein. This is the *IV to vein route.*

_____ 12. Position the client supine without a pillow.

_____ 13. Locate the midaxillary line at the fourth intercostal space and mark. (This is the right atrium.)

_____ 14. Attach the manometer to the IV pole so that the zero level is at the client's right atrium.

B. Measuring the central venous pressure:

_____ 15. Turn the stopcock to open the IV to manometer route.

_____ 16. Increase the amount of fluid in the manometer, but do not allow it to flow out of the top.

_____ 17. Turn the stopcock to open the manometer to vein route.

_____ 18. Monitor the manometer as the fluid level falls and stabilizes.

_____ 19. Read the fluid level at the highest level in the manometer column.

_____ 20. Turn the stopcock to open the IV to client route and regulate IV as required.

_____ 21. Position the client comfortably.

_____ 22. Place the client in the flat supine position for subsequent pressure readings.

Name ______________________ Date ______________

Observed by __________

CHAPTER 40 PROVIDING CARDIOPULMONARY RESUSCITATION

SKILL 40.1 Providing Cardiopulmonary Resuscitation

_____ 1. Call for help when cardiac arrest is identified.

_____ 2. Place the client on a flat, firm surface. Use a bedboard or cardiac board; if none is available, place the client on the floor.

_____ 3. Stand facing the client parallel to his sternum.

_____ 4. Clear the airway if foreign body obstruction is suspected.

_____ 5. Hyperextend the neck by placing one hand on the forehead and the other behind the neck. Lift the neck and apply pressure to the forehead. (*Caution:* Do NOT hyperextend the neck if spinal cord injury is suspected. Use jaw thrust maneuver: kneel at the top of the client's head; place thumbs on maxilla and fingers under mandible; pull mandible upward toward you. Avoid hyperextending the neck.)

_____ 6. Assess for breathing; if not restored, insert oral airway if available and continue:

If ventilator bag is available:

_____ 7. Place face mask in position over the nose and mouth; secure in place by holding with one hand. Compress the bag fully with other hand for four breaths.

Using mouth-to-mouth technique:

_____ 7. Pinch client's nose closed with thumb and index finger.

_____ 8. Take a deep breath and place your wide-open mouth around the client's mouth until an airtight seal is obtained. For an infant or child, cover both the nose and mouth with your mouth.

_____ 9. Blow four quick, full breaths into the client's lungs. For an infant or child, blow short puffs using cheeks only, once every three seconds.

_____ 10. Observe the client's chest for rising and falling. If chest does not rise and fall, check for airway obstruction, and remove it, or reposition the client's head and repeat.

_____ 11. Continue to administer one breath every five seconds.

_____ 12. Check carotid or femoral artery for five seconds; if no pulse is present, continue as follows.

To begin chest compressions on an older child or adult:

_____ 13. Locate the xiphoid process at the end of the sternum by following the costal margins to where they join.

_____ 14. Place the heel of one hand about 2 inches (4–5 cm) above xiphoid on sternum; place the heel of other hand on top of it. Keep hands parallel with fingers pointed away from yourself and interlocked.

_____ 15. Lean forward to position your shoulders directly over the client's thorax; keep elbows extended.

_____ 16. Press downward against the client's sternum with body weight, depressing the sternum about 1.5–2 inches (4–5 cm).

_____ 17. Keep hands in place and release pressure; repeat.

To begin compression on an infant or child:

_____ 13. For an infant up to one year of age: Place two fingers in the middle of the child's sternum, or encircle the chest with hands, placing your thumbs on the sternum. Deliver 100–200 compressions per minute.

_____ 14. For a child one to four years old, place the heel of your hand at the junction of the middle and lower thirds of the sternum. Deliver 80–100 compressions per minute.

_____ 15. For a child over age four, place the heels of the hands in the same position as for an adult. Apply compressions at the same rate as for an adult but with less force.

For all clients:

_____ 18. Establish a rhythm of pressing and releasing approximately once a second. To monitor rhythm and rate, count to self, "One one-thousand, two one-thousand, three one-thousand, ..."

_____ 19. Inflate the lungs with two deep breaths after 15 compressions; continue.

_____ 20. Check the carotid or femoral pulse after one full minute of compressions. If no pulse is present, continue. Check every four or five minutes thereafter.

_____ 21. If pulse is present, observe for respiration and discontinue CPR if present.

_____ 22. Continue CPR until help arrives, the client regains spontaneous breathing and circulation, or a physician declares the client clinically dead.

When help arrives:

_____ 23. Signal when you wish to change positions by verbalizing, "Change one-thousand, two one-thousand, ..." When you reach "five one-thousand," move to the client's head and check the carotid pulse. The second person then ventilates the client and begins compressions.

_____ 24. Stand by to assist and support in whatever way needed.

Name ____________________ Date ____________________

Observed by ____________

CHAPTER 41 MEDICATION ADMINISTRATION

SKILL 41.1 Preparing for Medication Administration

A. Determining that the medication order is complete and legal:

_____ 1. Check the order for each of the required seven parts: name of client, name of drug, dose, route and time of administration, date of the order, and the physician's signature.

_____ 2. Evaluate the dose, route of administration, and time of administration to be sure they are within recommended ranges.

B. Becoming knowledgeable about the medications that are to be given:

_____ 1. Determine the actions and effects of the drug ordered for the client by researching the information in a pharmacology book or by asking the physician or pharmacologist.

_____ 2. Determine that the drug ordered is within safe medical practice for the client.

3. Evaluate other medications ordered for the client for interactions with this drug.

C. Preparing for the administration of the medication:

_____ 1. Obtain the medication administration record (MAR) for the client.

_____ 2. Examine the MAR to determine where and how each drug is listed and how the individual dose is recorded.

_____ 3. Determine the day and time the drug is scheduled to be given.

_____ 4. Select the correct medication card (if this system is used) for the client, drug, and time from the storage area. Match the "five rights" on the card with the MAR *at least three times.*

_____ 5. Assess the client to determine if he meets the criterion for giving a p.r.n. medication.

_____ 6. Determine the last time the client received the drug.

_____ 7. Place the MAR or medication card at the medication supply and storage area.

_____ 8. Wash hands.

_____ 9. Prepare the drug for administration with the five rights checked at least three times each:

a. Check the MAR or medication card to determine that the right medication card matches the *right* client.

b. Select the *right* drug from the storage area. Compare the drug label with the MAR or card three times to check accuracy.

c. Select or prepare the *right* dose of the drug. Compare drug label with the MAR or card three times to check accuracy.

d. Compare the present time with the ordered *right* time of administration on the MAR or card.

e. Note the *right* route of administration and prepare the drug correctly.

_____ 10. Place the prepared medication on a small tray with a method of identification if several medications are prepared.

_____ 11. Take the prepared medications and the MAR or medication card to the client's bedside.

_____ 12. Identify the client by inspecting his identification name band. Compare the name on the band with name on the MAR or card.

_____ 13. Inform the client about his medications and determine what he knows.

_____ 14. Administer the medication correctly.

D. Calculating the desired dose of the drug when the dose on hand is different:

_____ 1. Determine if the dose on hand and the desired dose are in the same system and units of measurement.

Calculate dose in the same system and units by following these steps:

_____ 2. For solid medications, divide the desired dose by the dose on hand and multiply this by the quantity of the unit dose to determine the number of unit doses to give. The formula is:

$$\frac{DD}{DH} \times Q = N$$

_____ 3. For solutions, divide the desired dose by the dose on hand and multiply this by the volume of the drug solution to determine the amount of the solution to give. The formula is:

$$\frac{DD}{DH} \times V = A$$

OR

Use this proportion to determine the amount of solution to give:

$$\frac{DH}{V} = \frac{DD}{A}$$

To convert from one unit to another unit in the same system:

_____ 4. Let K represent the known unit; let U represent the unknown unit.

_____ 5. Select the conversion factor from the Equivalents Charts.

_____ 6. Determine if the unknown unit is larger or smaller than the known unit. If the unknown is smaller, use this formula:

$$K \text{ (Known)} \times C \text{ (Conversion factor)} = U \text{ (Unknown)}$$

If the unknown is larger, use this formula:

$$\frac{K}{C} = U$$

To convert from one system of measurement to another:

_____ 7. Select the conversion factor from the Conversion Equivalents Table 41.5.

Name ______________________ Date ______________________

Observed by ____________

_____ 8. Multiply the conversion factor times the dose on hand to convert the dose on hand to the same measurement system as the desired dose. The formula is:

$$C \times DH = DH$$

in same system as the desired dose (DD).

_____ 9. Next calculate the desired dose by using the formula to calculate within the same measuring system.

$$\frac{DD}{DH} \times Q = N$$

E. Teaching the client (or his caregivers) the reasons for and effects of his medications:

_____ 1. Determine what the client and his caregivers know by interviewing them.

_____ 2. Determine what information is essential for safe self-administration of the medications prescribed for the client.

_____ 3. Identify learning objectives with the client (and his caregivers) when appropriate and when they are able to participate.

_____ 4. Explain the actions and effects of the drugs in terms that are understandable to the client.

_____ 5. Tell the client about any adverse effects or known interactions with other drugs or foods.

_____ 6. Encourage the client to ask questions.

_____ 7. Observe the client's emotional responses and acceptance of the need for the medications.

_____ 8. Empathize and demonstrate acceptance and caring throughout the teaching sessions.

F. Guiding the home care client and caregiver to manage medication administration:

_____ a. Suggest using a series of envelopes labeled with the name of the drug, day, and time of administration for all medications. Place the correct doses of each drug in the envelopes. Arrange the envelopes in a time-order sequence so one is opened after the other for self-administration.

_____ b. Label an empty egg carton with dates and times for administration. Place the correct doses in the egg pockets. The client can tell at a glance if he has taken his medications for the day or the time.

_____ c. Color code pill containers if the client has a visual impairment but no memory loss or confusion. An example is placing a red tag on all medication containers for drugs taken morning, noon, and night and a yellow tag on the containers for drugs taken only in the morning.

_____ **d.** Prepare a simple calendar if drugs are to be taken for a limited time period (for example, 10 days of antibiotics). The client crosses off the day as he takes that day's dose.

_____ **e.** Advise these ways to properly store medications:
- Keep medications away from children or pets by placing them in a locked or out-of-reach storage area.
- Never store medications in direct sunlight or a very damp environment.
- Refrigerate those medications that require cold storage.

_____ **f.** Discard all medications that are no longer prescribed or are out of date.

Name ____________________ Date ____________________

Observed by ____________

CHAPTER 42 ADMINISTERING ORAL, TOPICAL, INSTILLED, AND PARENTERAL MEDICATIONS

SKILL 42.1 Administering Oral Medications

A. Administering a solid oral medication:

_____ 1. Determine that the medication order is complete and legal.

_____ 2. Be knowledgeable about the pharmacology of the medication that will be administered.

_____ 3. Calculate the desired dose when the drug on hand is not the ordered dose.

_____ 4. Prepare for the administration of the medication.

_____ 5. Assess the client and determine the nursing diagnosis.

_____ 6. Plan the expected outcomes and gather the equipment needed to administer oral medications.

_____ 7. Wash hands.

_____ 8. Place a medication paper cup on a small tray next to the MAR, medication Kardex, or drug card in the medication storage area. If giving more than one drug or if giving drugs to more than one client, mark the medication cup with the client's name and room number.

If the drug is stored in a central stock supply:

_____ 9. Select the storage container that contains the right drug and right dose.

_____ 10. Remove the cap from the bottle and place it upright next to the bottle.

_____ 11. Gently shake or tap the correct number of pills, tablets, or capsules from the bottle into the bottle cap.

_____ 12. Pour the units from the bottle cap into the medication cup.

_____ 13. Check three times to determine that the name of the drug and the dose match the ordered drug and dose for the client:

- when taking the container from the storage area
- before placing the drug in the cup
- when replacing the storage container or after placing the unit dose in the cup

If the drug is stored as a single-unit dose in the client's own drug supply:

_____ 14. Select the correct unit dose from among client's stock of drugs.

_____ 15. Place the wrapped unit dose in the medicine cup.

_____ 16. Check three times to determine that the name of the drug and the dose match the ordered drug and dose for the client.

_____ 17. Prepare any remaining medications that are ordered for the same client at the same time.

_____ 18. Sign for any controlled substances in the narcotic or controlled registry.

_____ 19. Place the medication cup with the unit dose on the tray.

_____ 20. Take the medication tray to the client's bedside.

_____ 21. Confirm the client's identity by matching his name and room number on the identification bracelet with the same information on the client's MAR, medication Kardex, or card, and by asking the client to tell you his name.

_____ 22. Perform any nursing assessments that may be required prior to administering the drug.

_____ 23. Explain to the client that he will now take his medication. Identify the medication by name and determine if he has any questions about it. Remind him of the purpose of the medication.

_____ 24. Place the client in an upright position if necessary.

_____ 25. Pour an adequate amount of water or juice of the client's choosing. Hand the cup to the client.

_____ 26. Read the label on the packaged unit dose to determine that it contains the right drug and dose. Remove the wrap.

_____ 27. Ask the client to hold out his hand and pour the pill, capsule, or tablet into his hand from the cup.

_____ 28. Instruct the client to take the medication into his mouth, take a drink of water, and swallow.

_____ 29. Observe the client as he takes and swallows the medication.

_____ 30. Offer any assistance the client needs.

_____ 31. Offer the client more liquid to drink after he has ingested the medication.

_____ 32. Discard the used medication cup.

_____ 33. Return the client to a position of comfort and ensure that his call signal is within reach.

_____ 34. Wash hands.

_____ 35. Return to the MAR and immediately record, according to agency policies, that the medication was given.

B. Administer a liquid oral medication:

_____ 1. Determine that the medication order is complete and legal.

_____ 2. Be knowledgeable about the pharmacology of the medication that will be administered.

_____ 3. Calculate the desired dose when the drug on hand is incorrect.

_____ 4. Prepare for the administration of the medication.

_____ 5. Assess the client and determine the nursing diagnosis.

_____ 6. Plan the expected outcomes and gather the equipment needed to administer oral medications.

Name ______________________ Date ______________________

Observed by ____________

_____ 7. Wash hands.

_____ 8. Select a graduated measuring medication cup that will hold the correct amount of liquid. If giving drugs to more than one client, mark the medication cup with the client's name and room number.

_____ 9. Place the medication cup next to the MAR, medication Kardex, or medication card.

_____ 10. Select the storage container that holds the liquid medication. If the container holds a unit dose and is the exact dose of the drug, pour the entire contents into the medication cup unless the liquid can be drunk from the container itself.

_____ 11. Remove the cap from the multidose medication bottle and hold the bottle so that the label faces you.

_____ 12. Check the label of the medication bottle three times to determine that the name and dose of the drug matches the name and dose of the drug that is ordered.

- when taking the medication container from the storage area
- before pouring the medication into the measuring cup
- when replacing the medication container in the storage area

_____ 13. Place the medication cup on a firm surface and pour the correct volume of medication into the cup. Check the fluid line at eye level. If a meniscus forms, measure the amount of fluid at its lowest point.

_____ 14. Place the medication cup on the tray in the correct slot or next to the medication card.

_____ 15. Wipe the lip of the medication bottle with the paper towel and replace the cap tightly.

_____ 16. Replace the multidose bottle in its storage area with the label facing outward.

_____ 17. Take the medication tray to the client's bedside.

_____ 18. Correctly identify the client by matching his name and room number on the identification bracelet with the same information on the client's MAR, medication Kardex, or card.

_____ 19. Explain to the client that he will now take his medication. Identify the medication by name and ask if he has any questions about it. Remind him of the purpose of the medication.

_____ 20. Place the client in an upright position.

_____ 21. Perform any nursing assessments that may be required prior to administering the drug.

_____ 22. Prepare an adequate amount of water or juice of the client's choosing if added liquid is not contraindicated when administering this medication.

_____ 23. Hand the cup to client and instruct him to drink all of the liquid.

OR

Place the cup to the client's lips and pour the medication into his mouth.

_____ 24. Offer the client a drink if liquid is not contraindicated.

_____ 25. Offer assistance in whatever manner the client requires.

_____ 26. Discard the used medication cup.

_____ 27. Return the client to a position of comfort and be sure that his call signal is within reach.

_____ 28. Wash hands.

_____ 29. Return to the MAR and immediately record that the medication was given according to agency policies.

Name ______________________________ Date ______________________

Observed by ____________

SKILL 42.2 Administering Topical Medications

A. Applying a liquid or semisolid medication on the skin:

_____ 1. Assess the client and determine the nursing diagnosis.

_____ 2. Plan the expected outcomes of the medication administration.

_____ 3. Prepare to administer the drug.

_____ 4. Identify the client by comparing the information on the MAR, medication Kardex, or card with the information on the client's identification band.

_____ 5. Explain the procedure to the client.

_____ 6. Wash hands.

_____ 7. Draw the curtains around the client's bed or close the door to the room.

_____ 8. Lower the top bedcovers and expose the designated area of the client's skin.

_____ 9. Gently clean the skin using the cleansing agent designated by the physician.

_____ 10. Open the medication container.

_____ 11. Don clean gloves if desired.

_____ 12. Apply the medication to your hands or clean gloves, a gauze pad or sponge, a medication applicator, or directly to the client's skin.

_____ 13. Apply the medication to the designated skin area and spread it smoothly and evenly.

_____ 14. Close the medication container, remove and discard the gloves, and discard the medication applicator.

_____ 15. Observe the skin closely for signs of an allergic response.

_____ 16. Cover the applied medication with a dressing or covering if indicated by the physician's order or the instructions with the medication.

_____ 17. Instruct the client to inform the nurse if unusual itching, pain, or swelling occurs in the area of the application.

_____ 18. Replace the client's clothing and bedcovers.

_____ 19. Open the client's curtains and door.

_____ 20. Wash hands.

_____ 21. Enter the medication application in the MAR or area in the medical record as designated by the agency.

B. Administering a solid medication bucally or sublingually:

_____ 1. Assess the client and determine the nursing diagnosis.

_____ 2. Plan the expected outcomes of the medication administration.

_____ 3. Prepare to administer the drug.

_____ 4. Identify the client by comparing the information on the MAR, medication Kardex, or card with the information on the client's identification band.

_____ 5. Explain the procedure to the client.

_____ 6. Wash hands.

_____ 7. Instruct the client to place the medication between his cheek and gum (buccal administration) or under the tongue (sublingual administration). Tell the client to keep the medication in place until it is completely dissolved.

_____ 8. Open the medication packet (if the drug is packaged as a unit dose) and give the medication to the client to place. Observe him as he places the tablet in his mouth.
OR
Instruct the client to open his mouth and place the tablet yourself.

_____ 9. Explain to the client what effects to expect when the medication is absorbed. Ask him to notify you if he experiences local irritation or swelling.

_____ 10. Wash hands.

_____ 11. Enter the medication application in the MAR or area in the medical record designated by the agency.

Name ______________________________ Date ______________

Observed by ____________

SKILL 42.3 Instilling Medications

A. Instilling liquid medication into the eye:

_____ 1. Assess the client and determine the nursing diagnosis.

_____ 2. Plan the expected outcomes and gather the necessary equipment.

_____ 3. Prepare to administer the medication. Make sure the label specifically indicates that the medicine is for ophthalmic use.

_____ 4. Identify the client by comparing the information on the MAR, medication Kardex, or card with the information on the client's identification band.

_____ 5. Explain the procedure to the client.

_____ 6. Bring medication and equipment to the client's bedside.

_____ 7. Wash hands.

_____ 8. Place the client in a sitting position with his head tilted back or in a supine position with neck extended back over a pillow. Ask him to look up. Give him tissues to hold.

_____ 9. If the client has crusts or exudates around the eye, moisten a cotton ball with sterile saline and remove them.

_____ 10. Open the medication container. Fill the dropper with the correct amount of medication. Hold the dropper pointing down.

_____ 11. Pull gently downward on the skin below the client's lower eyelid.

_____ 12. Drop the correct amount of medication directly into the conjunctival sac.

_____ 13. Instruct the client to close and roll his eyes from side to side. Instruct him to remove excess medication and tears with the tissue.

_____ 14. Replace the cap on the medication container and clean the dropper if necessary.

_____ 15. Wash hands.

_____ 16. Record medication administration according to agency policy.

B. Applying ointment to the client's eye:

_____ 1. Assess the client and determine the nursing diagnosis.

_____ 2. Plan the expected outcomes and gather the necessary equipment.

_____ 3. Prepare to administer the medication. Make sure the medicine is for ophthalmic use.

_____ 4. Identify the client by comparing the information on the MAR, medication Kardex, or card with the information on the client's identification band.

_____ 5. Explain the procedure to the client.

_____ 6. Bring medication and equipment to the client's bedside.

_____ 7. Wash hands.

_____ 8. Place the client in a sitting position with his head tilted back or in a supine position with his neck extended back over a pillow. Ask him to look up. Give him tissues to hold.

_____ 9. If the client has crusts or exudates around the eye, moisten a cotton ball with sterile saline and remove them.

_____ 10. Open the tube of ointment. Carefully squeeze a very small amount of ointment onto a tissue and discard it.

_____ 11. Pull gently downward on the skin below the lower eyelid.

_____ 12. Place ointment over the entire conjunctival sac by squeezing the tube gently.

_____ 13. Instruct the client to close and roll his eyes from side to side. Instruct him to remove excess medication and tears with the tissue.

_____ 14. Replace the cap on the tube.

_____ 15. Wash hands.

_____ 16. Record medication administration according to agency policy.

C. Instilling medication into the nose:

Follow steps 1–7, substituting "otic solution" for "ophthalmic solution."

_____ 8. Place the client in a sitting position with his head tilted back or place him supine with his head hyperextended over a pillow.

_____ 9. Open the medication container. Fill the medication dropper with the correct amount of medication. Hold the dropper pointing down.

_____ 10. Place the tip of the dropper just inside the client's nares and instill the correct number of drops. Repeat in the other nares if ordered.

_____ 11. Instruct the client to hold his head tilted backward for about five minutes. Tell him to pinch the nostrils together if he feels like he might sneeze.

_____ 12. Instruct client to remove excess secretions or medication from his nose when the five minutes have passed.

_____ 13. Replace cap on the medication container and clean the dropper as necessary.

_____ 14. Wash hands.

_____ 15. Record the medication administration according to agency policy.

D. Instilling medication into the client's ear:

_____ 1. Assess the client and determine the nursing diagnosis.

_____ 2. Plan the expected outcomes and gather the necessary equipment.

_____ 3. Prepare to administer the medication.

_____ 4. Identify the client by comparing the information on the MAR, medication Kardex, or card with the information on the client's identification band.

Name ______________________________ Date ______________________________

Observed by ______________

_____ 5. Explain the procedure to the client.

_____ 6. Bring medication and equipment to the client's bedside.

_____ 7. Wash hands.

_____ 8. Position the client laterally with the ear to be medicated uppermost.

_____ 9. Fill the medication dropper with the correct amount of solution.

For an infant:

_____ 10. Pull the auricle of the ear downward and backward.

For an adult:

_____ 10. Pull the auricle of the ear upward and backward.

_____ 11. Insert the medication dropper and instill the correct amount of medication in the ear.

_____ 12. Instruct the client to remain on his side for five minutes.

_____ 13. Place a small amount of cotton into the auditory canal.

_____ 14. Replace cap of medication container and clean the dropper as necessary.

_____ 15. Wash hands.

_____ 16. Record the medication administration according to agency policy.

E. Instilling medication into the vagina:

_____ 1. Assess the client and determine the nursing diagnosis.

_____ 2. Plan the expected outcomes and gather the necessary equipment.

_____ 3. Prepare to administer the medication.

_____ 4. Identify the client by comparing the information on the MAR, medication Kardex, or card with the information on the client's identification band.

_____ 5. Explain the procedure to the client.

_____ 6. Bring medication and equipment to the client's bedside.

_____ 7. Close the door to the room and draw the curtains around the client's bed.

_____ 8. Wash hands.

_____ 9. Lower the top bedcovers and place the client supine with her knees and hips flexed and legs abducted.

_____ 10. Open the suppository package and set it within reach. Or prepare the vaginal applicator with medication. Lubricate tip with a water-soluble lubricant.

_____ 11. Don sterile gloves and spread the labia.

_____ 12. Clean the labia and orifice of the vagina with moist cotton balls held with forceps if the area is contaminated with vaginal or anal secretions. Discard the balls.

_____ 13. Insert the suppository gently into the vagina along the posterior wall using a forefinger. Or insert the applicator down and back toward the rectum about 2 inches. Depress the plunger and remove the applicator.

_____ 14. Remove and discard gloves.

_____ 15. Place a small flat pillow or folded bath blanket under the client's hips and replace top covers.

_____ 16. Instruct the client to remain in position for 15–20 minutes until the medication is dissolved and absorbed.

_____ 17. Provide a perineal pad or dressing for the client to wear when she sits or stands.

_____ 18. Wash hands.

_____ 19. Record the medication administration according to agency policy.

F. Instilling medication into the rectum:

_____ 1. Assess the client and determine the nursing diagnosis.

_____ 2. Plan the expected outcomes and gather the necessary equipment.

_____ 3. Prepare to administer the medication.

_____ 4. Identify the client by comparing the information on the MAR, medication Kardex, or card with the information on the client's identification band.

_____ 5. Explain the procedure to the client.

_____ 6. Bring medication and equipment to the client's bedside.

_____ 7. Close the door to the room and draw the curtains around the client's bed.

_____ 8. Wash hands.

_____ 9. Lower the bedcovers and position the client on his left side with right hip and knee flexed forward.

_____ 10. Open the suppository package and lubricate the suppository tip with a water-soluble jelly.

_____ 11. Don sterile gloves.

_____ 12. Separate the client's buttocks with nondominant hand to see the anus.

_____ 13. Instruct the client to take a deep breath. Insert the suppository, narrow end first, using the forefinger to direct it against the rectal wall. Insert it as far as the finger will push it in.

_____ 14. Instruct the client to squeeze the buttocks and avoid expelling the suppository.

_____ 15. Remove the gloves and discard them.

_____ 16. Replace the client's bedcovers.

_____ 17. Wash hands.

_____ 18. Record the medication administration according to agency policy.

Name ______________________ Date ______________

Observed by ____________

SKILL 42.4 Administering Parenteral Injections

A. Preparing an injection from an ampule:

_____ 1. Wash hands.

_____ 2. Prepare to administer the drug.

_____ 3. Select the correct needle and syringe for the type of administration.

_____ 4. Attach the hub of the needle to the tip of the syringe.

_____ 5. Select the correct ampule.

_____ 6. Place all the fluid in the base of the ampule by a) flicking a fingertip against the tip of the ampule or b) tightly grasping the base of the ampule and rapidly shaking downward once.

_____ 7. Hold an antiseptic swab at the top of the ampule with one hand and hold the base of the ampule with the other.

_____ 8. Break open the ampule by bending the neck away from you.

_____ 9. Remove the cap from the needle.

_____ 10. Insert the needle into the ampule so that the bevel is in the fluid.

_____ 11. Pull back on the plunger and withdraw the correct volume of solution.

_____ 12. Examine the barrel of the syringe to determine if any air bubbles are present. Gently expel the bubbles and withdraw any further solution needed to correct the volume.

_____ 13. Examine the barrel of the syringe to confirm that the correct volume is present. Correct as necessary.

_____ 14. Replace the cap on the needle.

B. Preparing an injection from a vial:

_____ 1. Wash hands.

_____ 2. Prepare for the administration of the drug.

_____ 3. Select the correct needle and syringe for the type of administration.

_____ 4. Attach the hub of the needle to the tip of the syringe.

_____ 5. Select the correct vial of medication.

_____ 6. Determine the volume of solution that contains the required dose of medication.

_____ 7. Remove the protective cap from the vial.

_____ 8. Clean the rubber stopper of the vial with the antiseptic swab.

_____ 9. Remove the protective cap from the needle.

_____ 10. Pull the plunger on the syringe back to the same volume as the required dose of medication.

_____ 11. Insert the needle through the rubber stopper.

_____ 12. Inject the air from the syringe into the vial.

_____ 13. Place the bevel of the needle under the fluid level in the vial.

_____ 14. Withdraw the exact amount of solution into the syringe.

_____ 15. Withdraw the needle from the vial.

_____ 16. Examine the barrel of the syringe to determine if any air bubbles are present. Gently expel all bubbles, repeat steps 11–15, and withdraw further solution necessary to correct the volume.

_____ 17. Examine the barrel of the syringe to confirm that the correct volume is present. Correct as necessary.

_____ 18. Replace the cap on the needle.

C. Preparing medications in a single syringe from two vials:

_____ 1. Wash hands.

_____ 2. Prepare to administer the drug.

_____ 3. Select the correct needle and syringe for the type of administration.

_____ 4. Attach the hub of the needle to the tip of the syringe.

_____ 5. Select the correct vials of medication.

_____ 6. Determine the volume of solution that contains the required dose of medication for each vial.

_____ 7. Remove the protective cap from each vial.

_____ 8. Clean the rubber stopper of each vial with the antiseptic swab.

_____ 9. Remove the protective cap from the needle.

_____ 10. Pull the plunger on the syringe back to the same volume as the total required dose of medication from each vial.

_____ 11. Determine the total volume of solution by adding the volume amount to be withdrawn from each vial.

_____ 12. Insert into vial 1 a quantity of air matching the quantity of medication desired and withdraw the syringe.

_____ 13. Insert into vial 2 a quantity of air matching the quantity of the medication desired.

_____ 14. Withdraw the correct dose of medication from vial 2.

_____ 15. Examine the syringe for accurate volume and for presence of bubbles, and adjust as necessary.

_____ 16. Insert the needle into vial 1 and withdraw the second correct dose of medication.

_____ 17. Examine the syringe for accurate total volume amount and for bubbles, and adjust as necessary.

_____ 18. Replace the cap on the needle.

D. Preparing two medications in a single syringe from a vial and an ampule:

_____ 1. Wash hands.

_____ 2. Prepare for the administration of the drug.

Name ________________________________ Date ________________

Observed by ____________

_____ 3. Select the correct needle and syringe for the type of administration.

_____ 4. Attach the hub of the needle to the tip of the syringe.

_____ 5. Select the correct vial and ampule of medication.

_____ 6. Determine the correct amount of total volume desired by adding the volume amount to be withdrawn from the vial and the volume amount to be withdrawn from the ampule.

_____ 7. Prepare the vial for removal of solution as above.

_____ 8. Inject the desired amount of air into the vial, withdraw the correct dose.

_____ 9. Open the ampule and withdraw the desired amount of solution into the syringe, as above.

_____ 10. Inspect for accurate volume amount and for bubbles; expel the bubbles and adjust the volume if necessary.

_____ 11. Replace the cap on the needle.

E. Administering an injection:

_____ 1. Assess the client to determine the nursing diagnosis.

_____ 2. Plan the expected outcomes of the medication administration.

_____ 3. Check the client's record to determine where he last received an injection, if this is a repeat.

_____ 4. Assemble the equipment and prepare the medication.

_____ 5. Take the prepared syringe to the client's bedside. Correctly identify the client by examining his identification bracelet. Explain to him that he is to receive an injection.

_____ 6. Close the door to the client's room or draw the curtains around his bed.

_____ 7. Make any assessments necessary to provide information for later evaluation of the effects of the medication.

_____ 8. Ask the client if he has a preference as to the injection site. With him, select a possible site.

_____ 9. Place the prepared injection and antiseptic swab in a location convenient to the client's bedside and injection site.

_____ 10. Assist the client to a position of comfort for receiving the injection.

_____ 11. Expose the injection site while draping the remainder of the client's body. Assess the site for suitability.

_____ 12. Clean the site with an antiseptic swab by applying swab at the center of the site and gently rotating outward in a circular fashion.

_____ 13. Hold the swab between the fingers of the nondominant hand.

_____ 14. Remove the cap from the needle and set within reach.

_____ 15. Grasp the syringe between the forefinger and thumb of the dominant hand. If the angle of insertion is 15° or 45°, rotate the needle so that the bevel is facing upward.

_____ 16. For a 15° angle insertion, stretch the skin taut between the thumb and forefinger of the nondominant hand.
For a 45° angle insertion, pinch the skin site between the thumb and forefinger of the nondominant hand.
For a 90° angle insertion, stretch the skin taut between the thumb and forefinger of the nondominant hand.

_____ 17. For subcutaneous or I.M. injection, inject the needle firmly and swiftly into the center of the prepared site until all but a small upper part of the needle shaft is inserted.

For the intradermal, inject the needle slowly and gently just under the skin surface, with the bevel facing upward.

_____ 18. Grasp the syringe with the nondominant hand. Move the finger and thumb of the dominant hand to the plunger.

_____ 19. Pull back gently on the plunger to aspirate the medication. (*Note:* Heparin is not aspirated.) If blood appears, withdraw and discard the entire syringe. Prepare a new dose of the medication and begin again.

_____ 20. If no blood appears, inject the medication slowly and evenly.

_____ 21. Hold the antiseptic swab just above the insertion site. Withdraw the needle and syringe quickly and evenly, taking care not to change the angle of insertion.

_____ 22. Move the antiseptic swab over the puncture site and massage gently. (Do not massage injected heparin.)

_____ 23. Lay the syringe aside without recapping.

_____ 24. Reposition the client and rearrange his clothing and bedcovers as necessary.

_____ 25. Open the curtains or door to his room.

_____ 26. Discard the syringe and needle in the designated receptacles.

_____ 27. Wash hands.

_____ 28. Record the injection administration according to agency policy.

F. Administering the injection via the intramuscular Z-track route:

_____ 1. Assess the client to determine the nursing diagnosis.

_____ 2. Plan the expected outcomes of the medication administration.

_____ 3. Check the client's record to determine where he last received an injection, if this is a repeat.

_____ 4. Assemble the equipment and prepare the medication.

_____ 5. Take the prepared syringe to the client's bedside. Correctly identify the client by examining his identification bracelet. Explain to him that he is to receive an injection.

_____ 6. Close the door to the client's room or draw the curtains around his bed.

_____ 7. Make any assessments necessary to provide information for later evaluation of the effects of the medication.

Name ______________________ Date ______________________

Observed by ____________

_____ 8. Ask the client if he has a preference as to injection site. With him, select a site.

_____ 9. Place the prepared injection and antiseptic swab in a location convenient to the client's bedside and injection site.

_____ 10. Assist the client to a position of comfort for receiving the injection.

_____ 11. Expose the injection site while draping the remainder of the client's body. Assess the site for suitability.

_____ 12. Clean the site by applying an antiseptic swab at the center of the site and rotating outward.

_____ 13. Hold the swab between the fingers of the nondominant hand.

_____ 14. Remove the cap from the needle and set it within reach.

_____ 15. Place the nondominant hand on the tissue just adjacent to the proposed injection site.

_____ 16. Firmly pull the superficial tissues to one side and hold them in place.

_____ 17. Inject the needle firmly and swiftly into the center of the prepared site.

_____ 18. Push the plunger and slowly inject all of the medication. Aspirate the medication by pulling back on the plunger.

_____ 19. Wait 10 seconds with the needle still in place and the superficial tissues pulled aside.

_____ 20. Simultaneously remove the needle shaft and let go of the displaced tissue. Continue as above.

G. Teaching the client how to administer his own injections:

_____ 1. Determine what the client needs to know to administer his injection safely and independently.

_____ 2. Determine what the client and his caregivers know about administering injections by interviewing them.

_____ 3. Identify learning objectives (with the client and his caregivers when appropriate and when they are able to participate).

_____ 4. Explain what is being done and why while giving the injection.

_____ 5. Encourage the client to observe and ask questions.

_____ 6. Encourage the client to participate in any way that he seems able or interested in.

_____ 7. Observe the client's emotional responses and acceptance of giving his injections.

_____ 8. Increase the amount of the client's participation as he gains comfort and skill. Begin with preparing the ampule or vial; add preparing the needle and syringe when that is mastered; next have the client draw medication into the syringe; finally, have the client do the injection himself.

_____ 9. Reinforce new information and skills as the client learns.

_____ 10. Observe as the client does his own injection. Correct him *only* when he does something that is harmful. Allow him to develop his own technique within limits of safety and accuracy.

_____ 11. Make suggestions for changes in technique when client has completed his tasks.

_____ 12. Empathize and demonstrate acceptance and caring throughout the teaching sessions.

Name ______________________________ Date ______________

Observed by ____________

CHAPTER 43 ADMINISTERING INTRAVENOUS MEDICATIONS

SKILL 43.1 Administering Intravenous Medications

A. Inserting an intermittent venous access device:

_____ 1. Explain to the client what will be done; confirm his identity by checking his name band.

_____ 2. Wash hands with antiseptic soap.

_____ 3. Attach the injection cap to the distal end of the extension tubing; maintain the sterility of the connectors.

_____ 4. Inject heparin or saline into the tubing or the intravenous access device.

_____ 5. Perform venipuncture with the intravenous access device.
OR
Perform venipuncture with the desired needle or catheter.

_____ 6. Attach primed extension set with cap to the needle or catheter.

_____ 7. Clean the injection cap with alcohol.

_____ 8. Insert syringe with heparin or saline into the cap; aspirate to ensure blood return.

_____ 9. Inject heparin or saline very slowly. Monitor for evidence of infiltration.

_____ 10. Secure access device or catheter with tape.

_____ 11. Apply a droplet of iodine ointment to venipuncture site.

_____ 12. Loop the end of the access device or tubing and secure with tape.

_____ 13. Cover the venipuncture site and taped tubing with a transparent occlusive dressing (if this is agency policy).

_____ 14. Attach a label with date and time of insertion.

_____ 15. Wash hands.

B. Irrigating or flushing a venous access device:

_____ 1. Identify the times the device is scheduled for irrigation.

_____ 2. Prepare the heparin or saline syringe; take to the client's bedside.

_____ 3. Explain to the client what will be done; confirm his identity.

_____ 4. Wash hands.

_____ 5. Inspect the injection site for evidence of inflammation.

_____ 6. Clean the cap with an alcohol swab.

_____ 7. Insert the needle of the syringe and slowly inject heparin or saline.

_____ 8. Discard the syringe.

_____ 9. Wash hands.

C. Adding medication to a primary infusion container:

_____ 1. Check the physician's orders for the right drug, dose, method, and interval of administration.

_____ 2. Wash hands.

_____ 3. Prepare additive following the instructions on the medication label.

_____ 4. Draw medication into the correct size syringe with needle.

To add to unused, new container:

_____ 5. Locate medication injection port or site on the solution container.

_____ 6. Remove protective cover (if present) and place upside down on the work surface.

_____ 7. Clean port or site with an antiseptic swab.

_____ 8. Uncap the syringe and insert the needle through the port; inject medication.

_____ 9. Replace protective cover.

_____ 10. Hold the container at each end and gently rotate from end to end.

_____ 11. Wash hands.

_____ 12. Write name and room number of client, name and dose of the additive, time and date of preparation on label; attach initials.

_____ 13. Attach label upside down on the solution container.

_____ 14. Begin administration of infusion or store until later use.

To add medication to a primary infusion while in use:

_____ 5. Check client's identity; determine the volume of solution remaining in container; document.

_____ 6. Close the tubing clamp.

_____ 7. Locate and clean injection port or site with antiseptic swab.

_____ 8. Uncap the syringe and insert needle through the port; inject the medication.

_____ 9. Remove container from IV pole.

_____ 10. Hold the container at each end and gently rotate from end to end.

_____ 11. Replace container on the standard; unclamp tubing and adjust flow rate.

_____ 12. Monitor infusion to ensure correct flow rate.

_____ 13. Wash hands.

_____ 14. Write the name and room number of client, name and dose of the additive, and time and date of the preparation on the label. Initial it.

_____ 15. Attach the label upside down on the solution container.

_____ 16. Monitor client for evidence of drug response at periodic intervals.

Name ______________________________ Date ______________________

Observed by ____________

D. Using a volume control set attached to a primary infusion:

_____ 1. Check physician's orders for the right client, drug, dose, route, and interval of administration.

_____ 2. Wash hands.

_____ 3. Prepare medication following the instructions on the medication label. Draw into a syringe.

_____ 4. Open the volume control set; close clamps above and below volume chamber.

_____ 5. Open air vent on volume chamber.

_____ 6. Insert the volume control set into the primary IV container; invert and hang on a standard.

_____ 7. Open the clamp between the IV container and the chamber; squeeze the chamber to fill one-third full with solution.

_____ 8. Prime the volume control set tubing and close the clamp.

_____ 9. Clean the chamber injection site or port with an antiseptic swab.

_____ 10. Insert the syringe with prepared medication through port; inject medication; withdraw the syringe.

_____ 11. Agitate the chamber gently.

_____ 12. Open the clamp between chamber and container; add more fluid to the chamber if desired. Close.

_____ 13. Attach a label to the chamber identifying the medication.

_____ 14. Confirm the client's identity.

_____ 15. Attach infusion tubing to the client's needle or catheter at venipuncture site.

_____ 16. Open the clamp on the tubing and adjust the drip rate to permit infusion during the desired time span.

_____ 17. Wash hands.

E. Using a secondary administration set (piggy-back set-up):

_____ 1. Check physician's orders for correct client, drug, dose, method, and interval of administration.

_____ 2. Wash hands.

_____ 3. Prepare medication by
 a. preparing bag according to instructions
 b. mixing and adding to small volume infusion container

_____ 4. Attach secondary administration set to prepared infusion container; this is now the secondary infusion.

_____ 5. Attach an intravenous needle to the distal end of the secondary tubing; maintain sterility of the tips.

_____ 6. Confirm the client's identity.

_____ 7. Hang the secondary infusion on the IV pole at or above the fluid level of the primary infusion.

_____ 8. Clean the injection port of the primary tubing with an antiseptic swab.

_____ 9. Remove the needle cover and insert the needle through injection port; secure it with tape.

_____ 10. Regulate the flow rate to ensure administration of secondary infusion within 30–60 minutes (check medication instructions for recommended infusion rate).

_____ 11. Wash hands.

_____ 12. Monitor infusion; clamp the secondary line after the medication solution is infused.

_____ 13. Adjust the flow rate of the primary line if necessary.

_____ 14. Remove secondary line and discard container, tubing, and needle.

_____ 15. Monitor primary infusion.

F. Administering IV medication directly through primary line (giving a drug bolus):

_____ 1. Check physician's orders for the right client, drug, dose, method, and interval of administration.

_____ 2. Wash hands.

_____ 3. Prepare medication in a syringe using sterile technique.

_____ 4. Explain to the client what will be done. Confirm his identity.

_____ 5. Clean the injection cap of the venous access device with an antiseptic swab.

_____ 6. Insert the syringe needle through the injection cap.

_____ 7. Inject medication very slowly over several minutes. Check medication instructions for the recommended time span of infusion.

_____ 8. Monitor the client for signs of any untoward responses to the injected medication.

_____ 9. Withdraw the syringe when all medication has been injected.

_____ 10. Dispose of equipment.

_____ 11. Wash hands.

Name ______________________ Date ______________

Observed by ____________

CHAPTER 44 MANAGING WOUNDS

SKILL 44.1 Applying Dressings

A. Preparing to apply a dressing:

_____ 1. Explain to the client what will be done and why.

_____ 2. Assess the client's level of pain and administer pain relief measures as necessary.

_____ 3. Bring equipment and supplies into the client's room. Instruct the client not to touch sterile supplies during the procedure.

_____ 4. Provide privacy.

_____ 5. Position the client so he is comfortable and the wound is accessible; drape him with a sheet or bath blanket.

_____ 6. Wash hands.

_____ 7. Place a waterproof bag within easy reach as a waste receptacle; fold the top of the bag back on itself to create a cuff.

B. Removing dressing, cleaning the wound, and reapplying a dry sterile dressing:

_____ 1. Prepare for the procedure.

_____ 2. Remove dressing binder or untie straps.

_____ 3. Loosen tape (if used) by holding the skin and peeling back the edges of the tape.

_____ 4. Remove tape by pulling parallel with the dressing.

_____ 5. Don disposable gloves.

_____ 6. Grasp a corner of the dressing at an edge away from the client's face and roll it back to remove it.

_____ 7. Observe the amount and character of any drainage on the dressing.

_____ 8. Fold the dressing inward on itself and dispose in the waste bag.

_____ 9. Remove gloves and discard in bag.

_____ 10. Wash hands.

_____ 11. Open sterile dressing tray on the overbed table and add supplies.
OR
Prepare a sterile field and add supplies.

_____ 12. Fill the basin with cleansing solution, if desired; place sterile gauze pads or cotton balls in the solution.

_____ 13. Use sterile forceps and remove any contact dressing. Discard in bag.
OR
Don't sterile gloves and remove contact dressing; discard in bag.

_____ 14. If the dressing adheres to the wound, moisten it with a small amount of solution by pouring directly from the solution container.

_____ 15. Note color, consistency, odor, and amount of any drainage. Inspect the wound for signs of dehiscence or healing.

_____ 16. Discard forceps or remove gloves and discard in bag.

_____ 17. Don sterile gloves.

_____ 18. Pick up cotton balls or gauze with forceps, keeping the tips pointing downward at all times.

_____ 19. Clean the wound:

- Using cotton balls or gauze, firmly stroke from proximal to distal, first over the incision, then moving outward. Discard used gauze; pick up fresh gauze.
- Firmly stroke an irregular wound from the center working outward with circular motions. Change cotton balls or gauze after each circular movement.

_____ 20. Dry the wound or incision in the same manner using dry cotton balls or gauze.

_____ 21. Discard forceps.

_____ 22. Apply ointments or solution to the wound as ordered by the physician, using sterile technique.

_____ 23. Apply sterile gauze directly over the wound in sufficient amounts to absorb drainage.

_____ 24. Remove and discard gloves in the waste bag.

_____ 25. Apply abdominal pads or composite pads if necessary; touch only the outside of the pad.

_____ 26. Secure dressing with tape, straps, or binders.

_____ 27. Discard remaining materials and supplies.

_____ 28. Remove the drape and position the client comfortably.

_____ 29. Wash hands.

C. Applying a wet-to-dry sterile dressing:

_____ 1. Prepare for the procedure.

_____ 2. Remove the dressing binder or untie straps.

_____ 3. Loosen tape (if used) by holding the skin and peeling back the edges of the tape.

_____ 4. Remove tape by pulling it parallel with the dressing.

_____ 5. Don sterile gloves.

_____ 6. Grasp a corner of the dressing at the edge away from the client's face and roll it back to remove it.

_____ 7. Observe the amount and character of any drainage on the dressing.

Name ______________________ Date ______________________

Observed by ______________

_____ 8. Fold the dressing inward on itself and dispose in the bag.

_____ 9. Remove gloves and discard in bag.

_____ 10. Wash hands.

_____ 11. Open a sterile dressing tray on the overbed table and add supplies.
OR
Prepare a sterile field and add supplies.

_____ 12. Pour solution for dressing in basin; pour solution for cleansing, if different, into a second basin.

_____ 13. Don sterile gloves.

_____ 14. Remove contact dressing carefully. If it adheres to the wound, inform the client that he may feel discomfort as it is peeled away.

_____ 15. Discard dressings in the bag.

_____ 16. Inspect the wound for necrotic tissue, drainage, intact sutures, and condition of the drains, if present.

_____ 17. Don the second pair of sterile gloves.

_____ 18. Saturate fine mesh gauze 4 × 4 pads in solution and wring until damp but not dripping excessively.

_____ 19. Pack wound with a moistened 4 × 4 gauze pad until all surfaces and edges are covered. Tuck edges of 4 × 4 gauze into any cavity or under skin surfaces, as necessary.

_____ 20. Remove and discard gloves in the bag.

_____ 21. Apply abdominal pads or composite pads if necessary; touch only the outside of the pad.

_____ 22. Secure dressing with tape, straps, or binders.

_____ 23. Discard remaining materials and supplies.

_____ 24. Remove drape and position the client comfortably.

_____ 25. Wash hands.

D. Applying a transparent dressing:

_____ 1. Prepare for the procedure.

_____ 2. Don clean disposable gloves.

_____ 3. Apply water or mineral oil to edges of the old transparent dressing and peel back from edges.
OR
Use an alcohol swab to loosen edges and peel back dressing.

_____ 4. Discard dressing and gloves in bag.

_____ 5. Open a sterile dressing set.

_____ 6. Pour solution into the basin; saturate 4 × 4 gauze pads in basin.

_____ 7. Don sterile gloves.

_____ 8. Clean the wound; remove exudate as necessary.

_____ 9. Clean the skin around the wound with soap and water.

_____ 10. Shave the skin up to 2 inches around the wound if excessive hair is present.

_____ 11. Discard gloves and don a second sterile pair.

_____ 12. Wipe alcohol or acetone swabs around the wound area.

_____ 13. Inspect wound for color, odor, drainage, and approximation.

_____ 14. Remove and discard gloves.

_____ 15. Begin to remove paper backing from the transparent dressing. (Use the manufacturer's recommended procedure.)

_____ 16. Place the dressing edge about 1 inch on the side of the wound distal from the nurse.

_____ 17. Lay the remaining portion of the dressing against the skin while simultaneously peeling away the paper backing.

_____ 18. Pat down and smooth the dressing as it touches the skin.

_____ 19. Rub the edges of the dressing in position until they are adhered.

_____ 20. Discard the remaining materials and supplies.

_____ 21. Remove the drape and position the client comfortably.

_____ 22. Wash hands.

E. Applying a pressure dressing:

_____ 1. Identify the body part or wound that requires pressure to prevent or stop bleeding.

_____ 2. Explain to the client what will be done and why.

_____ 3. Enlist the support and assistance of a second nurse or other health care provider if the client has bleeding.

_____ 4. Bring supplies and equipment to the bedside.

Action of the first nurse when the client is bleeding:

_____ 5. Direct pressure firmly against the bleeding site.

Action of the second nurse or when the client is not bleeding:

_____ 6. Cover the area of actual or potential bleeding with several thicknesses of gauze.

_____ 7. Apply adhesive tape with pressure on either side of the fingers of the nurse applying direct pressure; work as close to the bleeding center as possible.

_____ 8. Apply tape over the bleeding center.

_____ 9. Apply tape continually from side to side, applying firm pressure.

_____ 10. Inspect dressing for signs of further bleeding.

Name ______________________ Date ______________

Observed by __________

_____ 11. Apply elastic bandages around the site if the dressing is on an extremity.

_____ 12. Monitor distal pulses, skin color, and temperature.

_____ 13. Monitor the client's vital signs.

If the client is bleeding:

_____ 14. Remain with the client until signs indicate bleeding has stopped:

- no further blood on dressing
- vital signs within normal limits

Name ________________________________ Date ________________

Observed by ____________

SKILL 44.2 Irrigating and Suctioning Wounds

A. Irrigating the client's incision or wound:

_____ 1. Explain to the client what will be done and why.

_____ 2. Assess the client's level of pain; give analgesics 30–40 minutes before starting the irrigation.

_____ 3. Bring the equipment to the client's bedside.

_____ 4. Provide privacy.

_____ 5. Position the client so that the wound is accessible and will drain by gravity flow; ensure the client's comfort.

_____ 6. Position plastic bag for collecting soiled dressing and discarded supplies.

_____ 7. Wash hands.

_____ 8. Remove the client's clothing to expose the wound.

_____ 9. Place a waterproof pad under the wound area.

_____ 10. Place clean basin at the drainage outlet of the wound.

_____ 11. Wash hands.

_____ 12. Prepare a sterile field with irrigating syringe, catheter, dressing materials, and basin.

_____ 13. Fill the sterile basin with the prescribed solution in the amount ordered at 90°F.

_____ 14. Don clean gloves and remove the soiled dressing; discard into bag.

_____ 15. Inspect wound for evidence of healing, dehiscence, and inflammation.

_____ 16. Inspect wound for the character, amount, color, and odor of the drainage.

_____ 17. Inspect the skin surrounding the wound for excoriation, redness, or inflammation.

_____ 18. Don sterile gloves.

To irrigate an open wound:

_____ 19. Fill a syringe with solution.

_____ 20. Flush the wound gently beginning at the upper surface.

_____ 21. Repeat until all the solution is used or the solution drains clear into the basin.

To irrigate a deep wound:

_____ 22. Attach the soft catheter to the irrigating syringe.

_____ 23. Fill the syringe and lubricate the catheter tip with the solution.

_____ 24. Insert the catheter tip gently into the deepest portion of the wound and flush gently until you feel resistance; pull back 0.5–1 inch.

_____ 25. Repeat until all of the solution is used or the returning solution is clear.

_____ 26. Dry the wound edges and skin with dry sterile gauze.

_____ 27. Apply a sterile dressing.

_____ 28. Remove and dispose of gloves.

_____ 29. Secure dressing with tape, binder, or bandage.

_____ 30. Remove drainage basin; empty.

_____ 31. Remove the waterproof pad.

_____ 32. Reposition the client comfortably.

_____ 33. Dispose of equipment.

_____ 34. Wash hands.

B. Emptying a wound suction reservoir:

_____ 1. Explain to the client what will be done and why.

_____ 2. Bring the equipment to the room.

_____ 3. Provide privacy.

_____ 4. Wash hands.

_____ 5. Position the client, if necessary.

_____ 6. Locate the empty port on the reservoir.

_____ 7. Place a sterile container next to the reservoir.

_____ 8. Open the port.

_____ 9. Tilt the reservoir so that drainage escapes through the port.

_____ 10. Squeeze the reservoir flat until all drainage is removed.

_____ 11. Cover the sterile collection container.

_____ 12. Reestablish suction by squeezing the reservoir flat.

_____ 13. Wipe the outside edge of the port with an alcohol sponge; secure the plug.

_____ 14. Reposition the reservoir below the level of the wound.

_____ 15. Monitor the collecting apparatus for sufficient vacuum, patency of the tubing, and absence of tension against the wound.

_____ 16. Note color, amount, and consistency of the drainage.

_____ 17. Proceed with dressing change if necessary.

_____ 18. Reposition the client comfortably if necessary.

_____ 19. Wash hands.

_____ 20. Label collection container with correct information.

Name ______________________________ Date ______________________

Observed by ____________

SKILL 44.3 Removing Sutures or Staples

____ 1. Explain to the client what will be done and why.

____ 2. Bring equipment to the room.

____ 3. Provide privacy.

____ 4. Wash hands.

____ 5. Position the client so that the dressing or incision is exposed.

____ 6. Make a cuff on the opening of the waterproof bag; place within reach.

____ 7. Open sterile suture removal tray or prepare a sterile field and place supplies on it.

____ 8. Saturate 4 × 4 gauze pads with antiseptic solution. Or prepare antiseptic swabs.

____ 9. Don clean gloves.

____ 10. Remove and discard any dressing covering the wound.

____ 11. Inspect the wound for signs of dehiscence or infection.

____ 12. Discard gloves and don sterile gloves.

____ 13. Cleanse sutures or staples with antiseptic swabs, moving from proximal to distal. Discard swab after using each surface.

To remove staples:

____ 14. Place lower jaw of surgical staple remover under the first proximal staple.

____ 15. Close staple remover so that the upper jaw depresses the center of the staple.

____ 16. Lift the staple remover and staple from the skin when both ends of the staple are visible.

____ 17. Discard staple in bag.

____ 18. Repeat steps 14–17 on every other staple. If no evidence of wound separation is present, remove the remaining staples if ordered.

To remove intermittent sutures:

____ 19. Place a dry sterile gauze pad near the wound.

____ 20. Grasp the scissors with your dominant hand and hold the forceps in the other.

____ 21. Pick up the knot of the suture with the forceps and draw away from the skin surface.

____ 22. Slip the curved end of the scissors under the distal end of the suture and cut it at the skin surface.

_____ 23. Pull the suture gently out of the skin with the forceps; place it on the gauze pad.

_____ 24. Repeat steps 19–23 on every other suture. If no evidence of wound separation is present, remove the remaining sutures if ordered.

To remove continuous sutures:

_____ 25. Place a dry sterile gauze pad near the wound.

_____ 26. Grasp the scissors with your dominant hand and hold the forceps in the other.

_____ 27. Pick up the knot of the suture with the forceps and draw away from the skin surface.

_____ 28. Slip the curved end of the scissors under the distal end of the suture and cut the first suture distal to the knot.

_____ 29. Cut the second suture on the same side.

_____ 30. Pull the knot gently from the skin and place it on the gauze pad.

_____ 31. Repeat steps 27–31 until all spiral sutures have been removed.

When all sutures or staples are removed:

_____ 32. Cleanse entire suture line from proximal to distal with antiseptic swab.

_____ 33. Allow the incision and skin to dry.

_____ 34. Place butterfly strips or reinforced tape strips perpendicularly across the incision, every inch.

_____ 35. Place light dressing over the incision, if ordered.

_____ 36. Reposition the client.

_____ 37. Dispose of materials.

_____ 38. Wash hands.

Name ____________________ Date ____________________

Observed by ____________

SKILL 44.4 Applying Bandages

_____ 1. Explain the procedure and its purpose to the client.

_____ 2. Collect the elastic bandage(s) and fasteners.

_____ 3. Wash hands.

_____ 4. Close door or draw bedside curtains to give the client privacy.

_____ 5. Assist the client to assume a comfortable position, maintaining a position of normal function for his body.

_____ 6. Place padding over bony prominences and separate skin surfaces.

_____ 7. Start the bandage from distal area (stand facing the client) and wrap toward the proximal area.

_____ 8. Hold the bandage in the dominant hand with the roll up.

To make a circular turn:

_____ 9. Unroll 3–4 inches of the bandage.

_____ 10. Hold the end of the bandage in place on top of the distal body part using the fingers of your nondominant hand.

_____ 11. Leave a portion of the distal body part exposed, such as the toes or fingers.

_____ 12. Bring the bandage down and around the body part, unrolling and stretching slightly if it is elastic.

_____ 13. Wrap the bandage directly over the held end and fasten it with safety pins, clips, or tape.

To make a spiral turn:

_____ 14. Start the application and make a circular turn. Continue to wrap the bandage around the extremity using a 30° upward angle each turn, overlapping preceding bandage width by approximately one-half to two-thirds.

_____ 15. Proceed with wrapping until you reach the proximal border.

_____ 16. Complete the bandage with two circular turns and fasten with clip, tape, or safety pin.

To make a spiral-reverse turn:

_____ 14. Start the application and make a circular turn. Place the thumb of your nondominant hand on the upper center edge of the anchored bandage.

_____ 15. Fold the bandage over the thumb and back on the bandage itself halfway through each turn.

_____ 16. Slide the thumb from under the next bandage and hold for the next turn.

_____ 17. Advance bandage around limb overlapping one-half to two-thirds of the previous turn, making turns at the same point of the limb.

_____ 18. Continue to wrap to the distal boundary. Fasten with two circular turns, and clips, tape, or safety pin.

OR

Wrap at least 2 inches beyond underlying dressing and fasten.

To make figure-8 turns:

_____ 14. Start the application and make a circular turn. Anchor the bandage below the joint.

_____ 15. Bring the bandage obliquely above and behind joint, around and down obliquely below the joint.

_____ 16. Cover one-half to two-thirds of the width of the previous bandage turn.

_____ 17. End the bandage above the joint with two circular turns.

_____ 18. Fasten with tape, safety pins, or clips.

To make a recurrent turn:

_____ 14. Start the application and make a circular turn. Anchor bandage at the proximal end of body part with two circular turns.

_____ 15. Turn the roll perpendicular to the circular turns and place the bandage centrally over the distal end.

_____ 16. Bring the bandage roll back over the end to the right of center, holding the bandage in place.

_____ 17. Overlap one-half to two-thirds width of bandage with each turn.

_____ 18. Bring the bandage back over to the left of center.

_____ 19. Continue in this manner until the area is covered.

_____ 20. End the bandage with two circular turns over the initial circular turns.

_____ 21. Fasten with clips, safety pins, or tape.

To wrap a spica bandage:

_____ 14. Start the application and make a circular turn. Anchor with two circular turns.

_____ 15. Bring the bandage up and around the body part.

_____ 16. Wrap the bandage down and around the other body part, forming a figure-8.

_____ 17. Continue in this pattern until the area is covered. Leave the tips of fingers and toes exposed.

_____ 18. End with two circular turns.

_____ 19. Fasten with tape, safety pins, or clips.

For all bandage types:

_____ 20. Inspect the bandage at frequent intervals for intactness and uniform tension; make a neurovascular assessment of the distal extremity.

Name ______________________ Date ______________________

Observed by ____________

SKILL 44.5 Applying a Binder

A. Preparing for applying a binder:

_____ 1. Explain the procedure to the client.

_____ 2. Take supplies to the bedside.

_____ 3. Wash hands.

_____ 4. Close the door or draw bedside curtains.

B. Applying an abdominal binder (straight):

_____ 1. Prepare for the procedure.

_____ 2. Position client in supine position, head slightly elevated, knees slightly flexed.

_____ 3. Fanfold the binder to its midline.

_____ 4. Assist or ask the client to roll to his side, facing away from you. If he has an incision, instruct him to support it with his hands.

_____ 5. Place fanfolded binder under the client, with its upper border at the waist and lower border at the gluteal folds.

_____ 6. Assist the client to roll toward you over the fanfolded binder.

_____ 7. Reach over the client and straighten the fanfolded binder until it is smooth and wrinkle-free.

_____ 8. Instruct the client to roll back to a supine position.

_____ 9. Pad bony prominences.

_____ 10. Check the dressing, if present, to ensure that it covers wound edges. Reinforce dressing if necessary.

_____ 11. Bring the furthest portion of the binder firmly over the client's abdomen.

_____ 12. Place the nearest binder end over the center of the abdomen, while holding tension on the other binder.

_____ 13. Secure by placing safety pins horizontally or secure the Velcro closure from the distal to proximal edges. Rub the Velcro surfaces firmly together to ensure full contact.

_____ 14. Place darts or tucks as needed to provide a snug fit. Allow room for breathing.

C. Applying a scultetus binder:

_____ 1. Prepare for the procedure.

_____ 2. Position the client in supine position, head slightly elevated, knees slightly flexed.

_____ 3. Fanfold the binder to its midline.

_____ 4. Assist or ask the client to roll to his side, facing away from you. If he has an incision, instruct him to support it with his hands.

_____ 5. Place the fanfolded binder under the client, with its upper border at the waist and lower border at the gluteal folds.

_____ 6. Assist the client to roll toward you over the fanfolded binder.

_____ 7. Reach over the client and straighten the fanfolded binder until it is smooth and wrinkle-free.

_____ 8. Instruct the client to roll back to a supine position.

_____ 9. Pad bony prominences.

_____ 10. Check the dressing, if present, to ensure that it covers wound edges. Reinforce dressing if necessary.

_____ 11. Bring the distal tail on the side opposite you across the client's abdomen and hold it firm against the abdomen; if it is longer than the abdomen, fold it back on itself.

_____ 12. Bring the opposite tail across the abdomen while maintaining tension on the first tail.

_____ 13. Fasten tail with safety pin or Velcro.

OR

Repeat steps 11 and 12, smoothing away wrinkles, until all tails are in place.

_____ 14. Sculpture tails to accommodate body shape.

_____ 15. Fasten visible tail ends with safety pins or Velcro straps.

D. Applying a single or double T-binder:

_____ 1. Prepare for the procedure.

_____ 2. Assist the client to a dorsal recumbent position.

_____ 3. Have the client raise his hips.

_____ 4. Check or change the perineal rectal dressing.

_____ 5. Assist the client to turn away from you.

_____ 6. Place the horizontal band (waistband) around the waist above the iliac crest.

_____ 7. Bring the remaining strap (perineal strap) down the midback and through the perineal area to the lower abdomen.

_____ 8. Attach perineal strap to the waistband by overlapping and securing with a horizontal safety pin.

If a double-T binder:

_____ 9. Apply in the same manner but place the perineal straps on either side of the genitalia.

_____ 10. Observe the client for comfort as he lies, sits, or stands.

_____ 11. Adjust dressings and binder as needed for comfort and to reduce pressure and rubbing.

_____ 12. Instruct the client to remove and reapply binders as necessary.

Name ____________________ Date ____________________

Observed by ____________

E. **Applying a breast binder:**

_____ 1. Prepare for the procedure.

_____ 2. Assist the client to place her arms through the armholes of vest.

OR

Place the binder on bed, with the straps open at top, and assist client to a supine position on top of binder.

_____ 3. Place cotton padding under the breasts.

_____ 4. Secure binder securely at the nipple level with vertical safety pins or Velcro closures.

_____ 5. Continue securing below the center closure, then above.

_____ 6. Secure the last bottom closure with closure with a horizontal safety pin.

_____ 7. Monitor the client's comfort and ability to breathe. Adjust the binder as needed.

_____ 8. Fasten straps with safety pins if required.

F. **Applying a triangular bandage (sling):**

_____ 1. Explain the procedure to the client.

_____ 2. Bring the triangular bandage to the bedside.

_____ 3. Wash hands.

_____ 4. Close door or draw bedside curtains.

_____ 5. Place the client in a sitting position with fingers higher than hand, hand higher than the arm and elbow flexed 90°, in correct alignment.

_____ 6. Place open end of bandage on the uninjured shoulder.

_____ 7. Place open bandage under the affected arm with the longest edge at the elbow.

_____ 8. Bring bandage's other point up over the arm, across the affected shoulder, and around the neck.

_____ 9. Adjust the arm for the correct angle and alignment.

_____ 10. Tie a square knot with the points at the shoulder level on the unaffected side.

_____ 11. Support the wrist and hand of the affected arm by manipulating the edge of the bandage.

_____ 12. Fold the apex smoothly around the elbow and fasten it with a safety pin.

_____ 13. Apply padding to areas where the bandage presses against the soft tissues. (This may happen around the neck, the axilla, and between the wrist and a cast, if present.)

_____ 14. Inspect the bandage for proper support of the arm, alignment of the arm, and pressure of the knot against the shoulders; assess the neurovascular condition of the skin and arms.

_____ 15. Instruct the client or his caregiver to apply the sling using these same steps.

Name ______________________ Date ______________

Observed by ____________

CHAPTER 45 APPLYING HEAT OR COLD

SKILL 45.1 Applying Heat

A. Preparing the client:

_____ 1. Explain to the client what will be done.

_____ 2. Bring equipment into the room.

_____ 3. Provide privacy.

_____ 4. Wash hands.

_____ 5. Assist the client to assume a comfortable position with the area to be treated exposed.

B. Applying a hot water bottle:

_____ 1. Prepare the client.

_____ 2. Fill the bottle two-thirds full of 115°F (45°C) water.

_____ 3. Expel excess air from the bottle by squeezing or pushing with the flat of the hand.

_____ 4. Secure the stopper tightly. Hold the bottle upside down to check for leaks.

_____ 5. Dry the bottle and wrap it with a towel or place it in a bottle cover.

_____ 6. Test the temperature of the bottle by placing it against the inner aspect of your forearm.

_____ 7. Inspect the client's skin while placing the hot water bottle on the prescribed area.

_____ 8. Observe for signs of burning and ask the client if the bottle feels too hot.

_____ 9. Position the hot water bottle against the site. Support with a pillow as necessary.

_____ 10. Continue to observe the application site for five minutes.

_____ 11. Remove the hot water bottle if signs of burning occur: excessive pain or redness of the skin surface.

_____ 12. Remove the bottle after the prescribed length of time.

_____ 13. Question the client about his comfort level; inspect his skin.

_____ 14. Wash hands.

C. Applying an aquathermia pad or heating pad:

_____ 1. Prepare the client.

_____ 2. Connect the unit to an energy source.

_____ 3. Cover the pad with a bath towel or enclosing case. Secure with tape or ties. DO NOT USE SAFETY PINS.

_____ 4. Ensure that the skin is dry.

_____ 5. Test the temperature of the pad by placing against the inner aspect of your forearm.

_____ 6. Inspect the client's skin while placing the pad on the application site.

_____ 7. Continually monitor the temperature settings of the pad.

_____ 8. Monitor the client for five minutes for burning: inspect the skin for redness or excessive heat; ask the client if he feels any pain or discomfort.

_____ 9. Remove the pad after the prescribed time. (Usually this is 15–20 minutes.)

_____ 10. Observe the skin; ask the client if he feels more comfortable now.

_____ 11. Assist the client to a comfortable position.

_____ 12. Wash hands.

D. Applying dry heat indirectly with a heat lamp:

_____ 1. Explain what will be done to the client.

_____ 2. Bring the equipment to the room.

_____ 3. Provide privacy.

_____ 4. Wash hands.

_____ 5. Help the client to assume a comfortable position.

_____ 6. Drape the client so that the treatment site is exposed.

_____ 7. Dry the skin treatment area with a towel.

_____ 8. Check the heat lamp bulb to determine the correct distance of the lamp from the treatment area.

_____ 9. Turn on the lamp and direct it at the treatment area.

_____ 10. Instruct the client not to touch the bulb or bring unaffected sites near the bulb.

_____ 11. Leave the lamp in position for 10–20 minutes.

_____ 12. Assess the client's skin every five minutes. Question the client to make sure he is comfortable.

_____ 13. Remove the lamp. Note condition of skin at the treatment site.

_____ 14. Return the client to position of comfort.

_____ 15. Wash hands.

E. Applying a heat cradle:

_____ 1. Explain what will be done to the client.

_____ 2. Bring equipment to the room.

_____ 3. Provide privacy.

_____ 4. Wash hands.

_____ 5. Assist the client to assume a comfortable position.

Name ______________________________ Date ______________________

Observed by ____________

_____ 6. Drape the client so that the treatment site is exposed.

_____ 7. Dry the skin treatment area with a towel.

_____ 8. Check the wattage of the heat cradle's bulb; use a 25-watt bulb at a distance of 16–18 inches.

_____ 9. Fanfold covers to the end of the bed.

_____ 10. Position the heat cradle over the area to be treated and secure.

_____ 11. Turn the cradle light on; check the distance of the bulb from the skin area.

_____ 12. Make a tent by placing a bath blanket or sheet over the top of the cradle; do not allow the sheet to touch the bulb.

_____ 13. Instruct the client not to touch the bulb or bring unaffected sites near the bulb.

_____ 14. Leave the lamp in position for 10–20 minutes.

_____ 15. Assess the client's skin every five minutes. Question the client to make sure he is comfortable.

_____ 16. Remove the lamp. Note condition of skin at the treatment site.

_____ 17. Return the client to position of comfort.

_____ 18. Wash hands.

F. Applying hot moist compresses:

_____ 1. Explain to the client what will be done and why.

_____ 2. Bring the equipment to the client's room.

_____ 3. Provide privacy.

_____ 4. Wash hands.

_____ 5. Assist the client to assume a comfortable position with the application site accessible.

_____ 6. Place a waterproof pad under the client at the application site.

_____ 7. Drape the client with a bath blanket to expose the application site.

_____ 8. Place a towel with plastic under the application site.

_____ 9. Wash hands.

_____ 10. Turn on the Aquathermia pad.

_____ 11. Open a sterile pack and pour warm solution into the sterile basin.

_____ 12. Place sterile gauze compresses into the solution. (Place commercially prepared compresses in the designated heat source.)

_____ 13. Don clean gloves.

_____ 14. Remove the existing dressing and discard.

_____ 15. Remove and discard gloves.

_____ 16. Assess the condition of the wound or skin.

_____ 17. Don sterile gloves.

_____ 18. Apply a thin layer of petroleum jelly around the periphery of the wound with sterile swabs.

_____ 19. Check temperature of solution with a thermometer.

_____ 20. Wring out a gauze compress and place it directly over wound.

_____ 21. Observe client for his response; ask him if he feels comfortable.

_____ 22. Apply another moist gauze snugly to the remainder of wound if no redness or discomfort is noted.

_____ 23. Wrap plastic and towel over the compress and secure with safety pins or tape.

24. Place heating pad over the area.

_____ 25. Monitor site and client's responses for 10 minutes to make sure the heat is not burning the skin.

_____ 26. Discard gloves and wash hands.

_____ 27. Remove heat source, towel, and plastic after 20–30 minutes.

_____ 28. Don disposable gloves.

_____ 29. Remove the compress and discard it.

_____ 30. Assess the condition of the skin or wound.

_____ 31. Reapply sterile dressing as ordered.

_____ 32. Assist the client to position of comfort.

_____ 33. Dispose of used equipment.

_____ 34. Wash hands.

G. Providing a warm soak or sitz bath:

_____ 1. Explain to the client what will be done and why.

_____ 2. Prepare the equipment.

_____ 3. Wash hands.

_____ 4. Transport the client to the tub or area where the treatment occurs.

_____ 5. Provide privacy.

_____ 6. Fill the basin, tub, or sitz bath with water or a solution of 98–105°F (37–41°C) using a bath thermometer to confirm water temperature.

_____ 7. Pad the edges of basin or tub with washcloths or towels.

_____ 8. Assist the client to undress and immerse his body part into the basin or sitz bath. Drape his exposed body with a bath blanket.

_____ 9. Ask the client if he feels comfortable; adjust water temperature if necessary.

Name ______________________ Date ______________________

Observed by ____________

_____ 10. Maintain water temperature at a constant level if temperature controls are present.

_____ 11. Remove the body part from the basin midway through the soak; empty the solution and refill the basin with warmed solution; put the body part back into the basin.

_____ 12. Assess client continually for comfort and response to the procedure.

_____ 13. Remove body part from soak or bath after 15–20 minutes or as instructed by the physician.

_____ 14. Dry the body part with a towel; use a sterile towel if the skin integrity is impaired.

_____ 15. Inspect the body part; reapply dressings if necessary.

_____ 16. Wash hands.

_____ 17. Help the client dress and return to his room.

Name ______________________________ Date ______________________________

Observed by ____________

SKILL 45.2 Applying Cold

A. Applying a cold moist compress:

_____ 1. Explain to the client what will be done and why.

_____ 2. Bring supplies and equipment to the room.

_____ 3. Provide privacy.

_____ 4. Wash hands.

_____ 5. Assist the client to a position of comfort.

_____ 6. Place towel or waterproof pad under the application site.

_____ 7. Drape the client so the application site is accessible.

_____ 8. Place ice solution in basin and check the temperature.

_____ 9. Wash hands and don sterile or clean gloves.

_____ 10. Place gauze or cloth into the solution.

_____ 11. Wring out excessive solution.

_____ 12. Apply the compress to the site; mold to the body contours.

_____ 13. Inspect the condition of the site while applying the compress.

_____ 14. Observe the application site for five minutes and question the client regarding his comfort.

_____ 15. Remove and discard gloves.

_____ 16. Leave the compress in position for 15–20 minutes or as ordered.

_____ 17. Don gloves and remove compress; dry skin area.

_____ 18. Inspect the condition of the application site.

_____ 19. Assist the client to a comfortable position.

_____ 20. Discard equipment.

_____ 21. Wash hands.

B. Applying an ice bag, collar, or pack:

_____ 1. Explain to the client what will be done and why.

_____ 2. Bring supplies and equipment into the room.

_____ 3. Provide privacy.

_____ 4. Wash hands.

_____ 5. Assist the client to a comfortable position; support immobilized body as necessary.

_____ 6. Fill ice bag, collar, or pack two-thirds full of ice. (Prepare commercial packs as directed.)

_____ 7. Remove excess air and seal tightly.

_____ 8. Wipe dry.

_____ 9. Place the ice container in a pillowcase or wrap it in a towel; secure the wrapping.

_____ 10. Inspect the application site.

_____ 11. Apply the ice container to body part; secure it with pillows, elastic bandages, bath blankets, etc.

_____ 12. Inspect skin after five minutes.

_____ 13. Remove ice container after the designated time.

_____ 14. Observe the application site for condition.

_____ 15. Assist client to resume comfortable position.

_____ 16. Wash hands.

C. Giving a cooling sponge bath:

_____ 1. Explain to the client what will be done and why.

_____ 2. Bring the equipment to the room.

_____ 3. Provide privacy.

_____ 4. Wash hands.

_____ 5. Close windows and doors.

_____ 6. Assess the client's vital signs.

_____ 7. Remove the top bedding; place a bath blanket over the client and remove clothing.

_____ 8. Place water in basin and check the temperature (90°F, or 32°C). (If client is a child, place 2 inches of water in a bathtub.)

_____ 9. Immerse washcloths in cool water.

_____ 10. Wring cloths until they are no longer dripping wet but moist.

_____ 11. Place wet cloths to axillae and groin. (Sit the child in the tub, providing appropriate body support, for 20–30 minutes.)

_____ 12. Place wet cloths over the arms and legs; avoid sponging chest or abdomen.

_____ 13. Monitor the client's responses; assess vital signs every 10 minutes and record.

_____ 14. Replace cloths as they warm, usually every five minutes.

_____ 15. Place cloths on back and buttocks for 3–5 minutes.

_____ 16. Change water as needed.

_____ 17. Discontinue applying cloths when the body temperature is slightly above normal.

Name ______________________________ Date ______________

Observed by ____________

_____ 18. Pat the moist body surfaces dry with a towel.

_____ 19. Replace the client's clothing and cover him with a sheet.

_____ 20. Assess the client's vital signs and responses.

_____ 21. Remove supplies and equipment.

_____ 22. Wash hands.

Name ______________________________ Date ______________

Observed by __________

CHAPTER 46 MANAGING DECUBITUS ULCERS

SKILL 46.1 Managing the Decubitus Ulcer

A. Managing the client with a Stage I decubitus ulcer:

_____ a. Place the client on a protective mattress surface (an air mattress, alternating pressure mattress, eggcrate or foam mattress, or sheepskin).

_____ b. Apply foam or sheepskin heel or elbow protectors.

_____ c. Turn and position the client every two hours or less.

_____ d. Inspect the skin frequently for evidence of further damage.

_____ e. Avoid positioning the client on the involved area until signs and symptoms disappear.

_____ f. Place a trapeze on an overhead bar so the client can move himself if he is able.

_____ g. Keep skin meticulously dry and free of secretions or excretions.

_____ h. Avoid use of soaps, perfumed lotions, powders, or other lubricants with an alcohol base.

_____ i. Encourage well-balanced nutritional intake with emphasis on high-protein foods.

_____ j. Encourage sufficient fluid intake daily to greater-than-average amounts for the client's age and weight.

_____ k. Avoid massaging identified areas of ischemia but massage other vulnerable areas frequently.

_____ l. Cushion the bony prominences if the client sits in a chair or wheelchair.

B. Managing the client with a Stage II decubitus ulcer:

_____ a. Continue the same measures initiated under Stage I.

_____ b. Clean the ulcer using sterile technique with one of these agents or as the physician prescribes:

- half-strength hydrogen peroxide
- or quarter- to half-strength povidone-iodine

_____ c. Rinse the cleansed ulcer with normal saline.

_____ d. Avoid puncturing or injuring blisters.

_____ e. Apply topical medications as prescribed by the physician.

For the dry treatment:

_____ f. Dry the ulcer after cleaning it and expose it under a heat lamp for 20 minutes at 18–20 inches (45–50 cm).

_____ g. Check skin every five minutes for signs of thermal injury while exposed to heat.

_____ h. Apply a sterile light dressing (4 × 4 gauze pads) over the broken skin area and approximately 2 inches peripheral to it. Secure with paper tape.

OR

Leave the ulcer undressed.

For the wet treatment:

_____ i. Clean the wound as instructed above and dry thoroughly.

_____ j. Apply a transparent dressing over the ulcer and approximately 2 inches peripheral to it. Leave the dressing in place until it falls off.

C. Managing the client with a Stage III decubitus ulcer:

_____ a. Continue the measures initiated in Stages I and II.

_____ b. Take an aerobic culture and an anerobic culture of the wound exudate and send them both to the laboratory correctly identified.

_____ c. Consult with the physician regarding medications or specific treatment measures.

_____ d. Order dietary changes that increases the amount of protein and vitamin C.

_____ e. Increase the fluid intake to greater than normal amounts for the client's age and body weight.

_____ f. Clean the wound as described in Stage II.

_____ g. Irrigate the ulcer with half-strength hydrogen peroxide or povidone-iodine (or as the physician prescribes) using sterile technique.

_____ h. Debride the necrotic tissue and eschar by vigorous irrigation and cleansing with saturated sterile 4 × 4 gauze pads.

_____ i. Apply sterile wet-to-dry dressings for continued debridement.

_____ j. Apply topical medications as prescribed by the physician using sterile technique.

D. Managing the client with a Stage IV decubitus ulcer:

_____ a. Continue the measures initiated in Stages I, II, and III.

_____ b. Consult with the physician regarding pharmacotherapy or surgical intervention.

Name ______________________________ Date ______________________

Observed by ______________

CHAPTER 47 PREPARING THE CLIENT FOR SURGERY

SKILL 47.1 Preparing the Client for Surgery

A. Teaching the client about his surgical procedure:

_____ 1. Schedule with the client a mutually acceptable time for teaching.

_____ 2. Invite the client's family members or significant others to be present.

_____ 3. Gather appropriate teaching aids, such as diagrams, charts, pamphlets, or videotape presentations.

_____ 4. Arrive promptly at the appointed time and setting for the teaching episode.

_____ 5. Ensure the client's comfort.

_____ 6. Outline the educational goals in terms understandable to the client.

_____ 7. Present the material in the manner that seems most conducive to the client's learning.

_____ 8. Describe the environment of the operating room and recovery room; explain what types of equipment or machinery will be present, if any, following surgery.

_____ 9. Explain general types of nursing interventions that will be performed after surgery.

_____ 10. Assure the client that a nurse will be present and available to assist the client however necessary.

_____ 11. Explain the behaviors or activities expected of the client.

_____ 12. Teach the client the following techniques:

- deep breathing
- coughing
- use of the incentive spirometer
- leg exercises
- use of any equipment to be employed after surgery

_____ 13. Provide time for questions.

_____ 14. Answer questions as honestly and completely as possible but avoid vivid, frightening information or scenarios.

_____ 15. Observe the client's responses carefully, looking for cues of comprehension, confusion, or anxiety.

_____ 16. Reinforce positively the client's learning responses.

_____ 17. Use the simplest possible method of evaluating learning objectives.

_____ 18. Provide constructive criticism in situations where the client's skills or knowledge require improvement.

B. Preparing the client for surgery on the night before the scheduled event:

_____ 1. Consult the physician's orders for preoperative instructions.

_____ 2. Arrange to do all physical preparations at the designated time, or at a time convenient for the client.

_____ 3. Suggest that the client spend time with his significant others.

_____ 4. Perform ordered physical preparations after client has had time with his significant others.

- bowel preparation (enema)
- skin shaving

_____ 5. Encourage the client to talk about his impending surgery.

_____ 6. Reinforce the client's learning regarding his surgery.

_____ 7. Ask if the client has any further questions or concerns; answer all questions as completely as possible.

_____ 8. Demonstrate empathy and acceptance of any anxiety or fear expressed by the client.

_____ 9. Direct or assist the client to take a shower with antiseptic soap.

_____ 10. Offer to provide back massage when the client is in bed.

_____ 11. Remain vigilant to client's anxiety or fear of impending surgery.

_____ 12. Administer ordered medications at the designated time.

_____ 13. Secure an "NPO" sign on the client's bed or unit or door.

_____ 14. Create a soothing environment in the client's room; meet his desires for temperature, quiet, light or dark, and privacy.

C. Preparing the operative skin site:

_____ 1. Consult the physician's orders to determine how much of the body area to shave.

_____ 2. Explain to the client how the skin is to be prepared for surgery.

_____ 3. Provide privacy.

_____ 4. Wash hands.

_____ 5. Position the client so that the body area is exposed.

_____ 6. Place a protective pad under the client.

_____ 7. Adjust the lighting.

_____ 8. Saturate cleansing gauze sponges with antiseptic solution.

_____ 9. Don sterile gloves.

_____ 10. Cleanse the skin with sponges beginning at the center of the surgical site and moving in a circular fashion outward.

_____ 11. Discard sponges after each complete circle.

_____ 12. Stretch the skin taut with your free hand and, using a disposable razor, shave the skin beginning at the center of the site and moving outward using firm, steady strokes. Follow hair growth patterns.

_____ 13. Discard the razor when it becomes dull and use a fresh one as often as necessary.

Name ______________________________ Date ______________________

Observed by ______________

When all skin area has been shaved:

_____ 14. Repeat steps 10 and 11 until the site is rescrubbed.

_____ 15. Rinse the site with fresh, warm water and blot dry with sterile gauze sponges.

_____ 16. Remove gloves and discard sponges, razors, and other equipment.

_____ 17. Remove the protective pad from bed.

_____ 18. Help the client don a clean hospital gown.

_____ 19. Wash hands.

D. Preparing the client just prior to surgery:

_____ 1. Consult the physician's orders for preoperative instructions.

_____ 2. Examine the client's health record to confirm that all essential information is included.

_____ 3. Confirm the presence of the informed consent form.

_____ 4. Use the agency's preoperative checklist.

_____ 5. Check the client's identification.

_____ 6. Record the client's vital signs.

_____ 7. Assist the client to shower with antiseptic soap.

_____ 8. Instruct the female client to remove all makeup and nail polish.

_____ 9. Provide the client with a clean gown to don after the shower.

_____ 10. Ask the client to remove all jewelry or other valuables. Ask the significant others to hold them; or place them in a locked, secure place.

_____ 11. Remain alert to the client's anxiety or questions. Respond as necessary.

_____ 12. Perform ordered interventions at the required time:

- intravenous solutions and medications
- urinary catheterization
- nasogastric intubation

Before giving the preoperative medications:

_____ 13. Instruct the client to empty his bladder.

_____ 14. Remove all prostheses from the client:

- dentures
- eyeglasses or contact lenses
- artificial limbs
- hearing aids

_____ 15. Store prostheses in a secure place.

_____ 16. Administer the preoperative medications.

_____ 17. Explain to the client that he may become sleepy and feel cotton-mouthed.

_____ 18. Raise the client's siderails and place the bed in the lowest position.

_____ 19. Secure the call signal within the client's reach.

_____ 20. Encourage his significant others to remain with the client until time for him to leave for the operating room.

E. Transporting the client to the operating room:

_____ 1. Review the agency's preoperative checklist.

_____ 2. Inform client and his significant others that it is time to leave.

_____ 3. Transfer the client to the transport cart using safety precautions.

_____ 4. Direct the family to the appropriate waiting area.

Name ______________________________ Date ______________________

Observed by ____________

CHAPTER 48 MANAGING THE POSTOPERATIVE CLIENT

SKILL 48.1 Managing the Postoperative Client

A. Assessing the client upon return from the recovery room:

_____ 1. Note the client's general appearance, observing facial expression, body posture, and presence of diaphoresis, pallor, or other abnormal conditions.

_____ 2. Assess the client's alertness and awareness.

_____ 3. Take the client's pulse and blood pressure; compare to previous readings.

_____ 4. Take the client's temperature; compare to previous readings.

_____ 5. Assess the client's rate, depth, and quality of respirations; compare to previous assessments.

_____ 6. Auscultate the client's lung sounds throughout the thorax.

_____ 7. Inspect the intravenous infusion for solution type, amount in bottle, additives, drip rate, or infusion pump controls. Inspect the venipuncture site for redness, swelling, and intactness.

_____ 8. Inspect the client's wound, if it is not dressed. Note the approximation of the wound edges and condition of the sutures; the amount, color, and consistency of drainage, if present.

_____ 9. Inspect the client's dressing. Note amount, color, and consistency of drainage, if present. Look to see if drainage has pooled under the body.

_____ 10. Check to determine that all drainage tubes are patent; inspect drainage for amount, color, and consistency:

- tubes in the wound
- urinary catheter
- nasogastric tube
- chest tubes
- T-tube

_____ 11. Check to see if other therapeutic aids (oxygen cannula, ventilators, monitoring equipment) are functional.

_____ 12. Examine the client's skin color and palpate the skin for temperature and moisture on the trunk and extremities.

_____ 13. Assess for peripheral pulses if surgery warrants it.

_____ 14. Determine the client's level of pain and his present management of it.

B. Implementing postoperative measures:

_____ 1. Regulate the intravenous infusion as necessary.

_____ 2. Attach drains to collection bags or suction supply if necessary.

_____ 3. Attach therapeutic aids as necessary.

_____ 4. Reinforce the wound as necessary.

_____ 5. Instruct the client to take deep breaths and cough. Splint the incision with a folded bath blanket to minimize discomfort.

_____ 6. Encourage the client to void if he does not have an indwelling catheter and has not recently urinated in the recovery room.

_____ 7. Determine what position is safe for the client according to his condition. If he is alert and aware and his surgery does not contraindicate it, place him in a position of comfort.

_____ 8. Raise the siderails and attach the call signal within the client's reach.

_____ 9. Medicate for pain if the client expresses discomfort and has not received analgesia recently.

_____ 10. Notify his significant others that the client has returned to his unit; invite them to visit if the client's condition and interest permit.

_____ 11. Leave client to rest.

C. Managing the postoperative course:

_____ 1. Assess the client's level of awareness and alertness according to the postoperative assessment schedule.

_____ 2. Assess the client's cardiovascular function and tissue perfusion according to the postoperative assessment schedule.

- Assess vital signs.
- Inspect skin color; palpate skin temperature.
- Assess for peripheral pulses.

_____ 3. Assess the client's temperature.

_____ 4. Assess the client's respiratory function according to postoperative assessment schedule.

- Assess respiratory rate and quality.
- Auscultate lung sounds.

_____ 5. Maintain adequate respiratory function.

- Position oxygen cannula and maintain the ordered flow.
- Turn the client every two hours from side to side while he is in bed.
- Position the client in Fowler's position or dangling and direct him to cough and deep breathe every two hours during the first 48 hours after surgery and every four to eight hours thereafter. Splint the incision when he coughs.
- Direct the client to use the incentive spirometer every two hours for 48 hours if ordered.

_____ 6. Assess fluid and electrolyte balance and renal function.

- Monitor fluid intake and output.
- Examine the client for signs of fluid or electrolyte imbalance.
- Monitor blood electrolyte levels for adequacy.

Name ______________________________ Date ______________

Observed by ______________

_____ 7. Maintain adequate fluid balance.

- Manage the intravenous fluids replacement as ordered.
- Encourage intake of sufficient fluids after the client is taking oral fluids.

_____ 8. Maintain adequate urinary function.

If client has a catheter:

- Position catheter tubing to facilitate gravity drainage.
- Empty drainage bag when it is full or every eight hours.

If client is voiding naturally:

- Encourage the client to void every two hours.

_____ 9. Assess gastrointestinal function.

- Monitor fluid intake and output.
- Monitor patency of and amount, color, and consistency of drainage if nasogastric tube is present.
- Begin auscultating the abdomen for presence of bowel sounds during the first eight hours after surgery and continue regular auscultation until the client has sounds present in all four quadrants or is passing flatus or feces.
- Monitor the amount of and reaction to food intake.

_____ 10. Maintain adequate gastrointestinal function.

- Withhold fluids or food according to the physician's orders or until the client is without nausea and bowel sounds are present in all four abdominal quadrants.
- Increase the client's dietary intake from clear liquids to a regular diet only as he tolerates it or according to physician's orders.
- Encourage the client to eat a diet balanced with nutrients that will promote healing.

_____ 11. Assess the surgical wound for healing on the postoperative assessment schedule.

- Inspect the wound dressing to make sure it is dry and intact.
- Inspect the wound for drainage; identify the amount, color, and consistency of drainage.
- Inspect the wound drains for amount, consistency, and color of drainage.
- Monitor for signs of wound infection.

_____ 12. Provide wound care.

- Change the wound dressing when it becomes soiled with drainage or loose. If necessary, reinforce the dressing.
- Irrigate the wound if ordered.
- Empty, advance, or change the drains as necessary.

_____ 13. Manage the client's postoperative pain.

- Assess the quality and nature of pain regularly.
- Provide comfort measures such as position change as needed.
- Administer analgesia on a regular basis during the first two or three days after surgery. Schedule analgesic administration approximately 30 minutes to one hour prior to physically taxing activities.

_____ 14. Return client to full mobility.

- Instruct client to flex his legs and hips or to move them from side to side every two hours while he is in bed.
- Measure for, order, and apply antiembolic stockings.
- Begin ambulation as early as possible.
- Encourage the client to walk at least three to four times daily beginning the second day, gradually increasing the frequency and duration of his activity.

_____ 15. Provide sufficient rest and sleep.

- Group scheduled activities and allow lengthy periods of uninterrupted rest or sleep.
- Provide analgesia on a regular basis.
- Limit visitors if the client appears tired by them.

_____ 16. Manage the client's postoperative anxiety or mood changes.

- Monitor for signs of anxiety.
- Provide therapeutic interactions.

_____ 17. Prevent postoperative infections.

- Provide aseptic wound care.
- Provide pulmonary physiotherapy.
- Maintain adequate fluid intake.
- Ensure sufficient rest.

_____ 18. Monitor for signs of thrombophlebitis formation.

- Instruct the client to dorsiflex and plantar flex both legs and feet. Monitor for evidence of pain with these maneuvers.
- Watch the client move or ambulate; observe for signs of leg pain upon exercise.
- Inspect the lower extremities for redness, swelling; palpate for tender areas.

D. Teaching the client and his caregivers these strategies if he returns home after day surgery:

_____ 1. Monitor the temperature and pulse.

_____ 2. Encourage deep breathing and coughing at regular intervals.

_____ 3. Monitor the client's dressing for drainage. Draw a line around the drainage line with a pen; if the drainage increases each hour, contact the agency.

_____ 4. Monitor drainage tubes for evidence of abnormal or excessive drainage.

_____ 5. Monitor the client's urinary output.

Name ______________________ Date ______________________

Observed by ____________

____ 6. Increase the client's food and fluid intake gradually. Signs and symptoms of readiness are taught as well as signs and symptoms of potential gastrointestinal blocks.

____ 7. Monitor for the return of normal bowel elimination habits.

____ 8. Ambulate the client gradually but effectively.

____ 9. Change the dressing and monitor wound healing.

____ 10. Help the client to return to independent self-care in all his activities of daily living.

Name ______________________ Date ______________

Observed by ____________

CHAPTER 49 SUPPORTING THE DYING CLIENT AND THE FAMILY

SKILL 49.1 Supporting the Dying Client

A. Physically caring for the dying client:

_____ 1. Manage the client's pain through available pain relief measures.

_____ 2. Position the client upright if he is having difficulty breathing.

_____ 3. Encourage movement and activity as the client is able. Place a trapeze over his bed for him to use to move.

_____ 4. Perform passive range-of-motion exercises to all extremities if this does not increase the client's pain.

_____ 5. Position and turn the bed-bound client every hour or two.

_____ 6. Use pillows or other supportive devices to maintain body alignment.

_____ 7. Place a supportive mattress surface under the immobile client.

_____ 8. Assist with or provide personal hygiene: bathing, hair, and nail care.

_____ 9. Assist with or apply makeup to the female client if she desires.

_____ 10. Massage skin areas over pressure points.

_____ 11. Lubricate dry skin with the client's preferred lotions or creams.

_____ 12. Change dressings frequently.

_____ 13. Offer, assist with, or provide mouth care: provide mouthwashes or cleanse the mouth with antimicrobial solutions.

_____ 14. Lubricate dry oral mucous membranes frequently.

_____ 15. Offer additional bedclothing or covers if the client complains of cold.

_____ 16. Provide appealing food or drink as the client desires. If the client is unable to eat unassisted, offer small sips or bites of food frequently.

_____ 17. Monitor urinary output for volume, character, and frequency.

_____ 18. Consider insertion of indwelling catheter if the client has urinary retention.

_____ 19. Monitor bowel elimination for frequency and character of stools.

_____ 20. Cleanse the perineal area and change the client's bedclothing immediately after incontinence. Use absorbent undergarments for the woman client; apply an external catheter for the urinary incontinent man.

_____ 21. Use room deodorizers if the client's wounds or incontinence create odors.

_____ 22. Encourage rest. Give tranquilizers or sedatives when needed.

_____ 23. Provide safety measures as needed: siderails on bed, restraints, etc.

B. Providing emotional care of the dying:

_____ 1. Make yourself available for conversation, listening, or simply touching as often as possible.

_____ 2. Answer the client's questions honestly and openly.

_____ 3. Arrange the client's personal belongings attractively within his reach or vision.

_____ 4. Position the client near a window or room door, if possible.

_____ 5. Encourage visits by the client's significant others.

_____ 6. Encourage his significant others to touch and talk with the unconscious client.

_____ 7. Provide music through a radio or tape recorder if desired by the client.

_____ 8. Arrange for pastoral visits if desired by the client.

_____ 9. Support religious or spiritual practices of the client.

_____ 10. Read to the client from his favorite books if he requests; if he is unconscious, ask the family what he might find meaningful.

_____ 11. Permit the presence of pets in the client's home.

_____ 12. Arrange for the client to sign a donor card if he wishes.

Name ______________________ Date ______________________

Observed by ____________

SKILL 49.2 Supporting Grieving

A. Aiding the mourners immediately following the client's death:

_____ 1. Guide the mourners to a room or area that provides privacy.

_____ 2. Remain with the solitary mourner until other support persons arrive. However, leave if the mourner requests it and he appears safe to be alone.

_____ 3. Contact a clergyman and ask for his presence if the mourner requests this or is receptive to the notion.

_____ 4. Encourage the mourner to express his feelings through talk or behaviors such as crying.

_____ 5. Listen carefully to the mourner as he talks for cues about his feelings and desires. Attend to his wishes if possible.

_____ 6. Answer questions honestly and directly if the mourners ask about the death process or the disposition of the body.

_____ 7. Avoid rationalization or reassuring statements that block effective communication.

_____ 8. Offer to make phone calls or contact support persons on behalf of the mourner.

_____ 9. Accept statements of denial or disbelief. Do not attempt to force reality on the mourner if he is not ready.

_____ 10. Accept without judgment whatever grieving behaviors are present.

_____ 11. Offer coffee, tea, juice, or solid nourishment to family members.

_____ 12. Avoid trite comments such as, "He is at peace now," or "You'll feel better later."

_____ 13. Offer hugs or hold the mourner's hands or touch him if he is receptive.

B. Supporting bereavement in the days or weeks following the death:

_____ 1. Attend the funeral, if possible.

_____ 2. Make a follow-up visit to the client's home, after the funeral, to express concern and caring.

_____ 3. Contact the family by phone or letter if a personal visit is not possible. Express caring and concern for their situation.

_____ 4. Offer comments such as, "Tell me about your mother . . . ", to the mourner who is unable to express grieving.

Name ______________________________ Date ______________________

Observed by ____________

CHAPTER 50 PROVIDING POSTMORTEM CARE

SKILL 50.1 Providing Postmortem Care

_____ 1. Ask other clients, family members, or visitors to leave the room before initiating procedures.

_____ 2. Explain to any remaining clients what is being done and why. Be honest but respectful of their feelings.

_____ 3. Close the door to the room or draw the curtains around the bed.

_____ 4. Don disposable gloves.

_____ 5. Check the identification on the body.

_____ 6. Close the eyelids if they are open; place a gauze pad or cotton ball over each eye to secure the lids down if they won't remain shut.

_____ 7. Place the body in straight alignment with arms and legs extended.

_____ 8. Place a pillow under the head and shoulders or raise the head of the bed about 15°.

_____ 9. Position the arms with palms downward on the abdomen. Do not place one hand on top of the other; the lower hand will become discolored.

_____ 10. Place the client's dentures in the mouth if agency policy permits. If not possible, place them in a labeled storage container.

_____ 11. Close the mouth. If the jaw drops, roll a small towel or washcloth and prop it under the chin.

_____ 12. Detach all equipment: intravenous bottles, drainage bags, suction apparatus, oxygen tubes.

_____ 13. Remove soiled dressings or any tape from the skin by gently peeling back. Take care not to lacerate the skin. If wounds are present, cover with a light gauze dressing and secure with paper tape.

_____ 14. Place absorbent pads between the buttocks near the anus or urethra.

_____ 15. Remove tubing from body cavities as the agency policy requires.

_____ 16. Remove jewelry or body prosthesis, other than dentures, and label it.

_____ 17. Wash soiled body areas with plain water and pat dry very gently.

_____ 18. Place the body in a clean gown.

_____ 19. Comb or brush the hair neatly.

_____ 20. Gather, identify, and list all the client's belongings. Place them in the bag for safekeeping.

If the mourners wish to view the body:

_____ 21. Draw clean bed linens over the body to shoulder level.

_____ 22. Call the mourners to the bedside; leave them alone with the body or stay with them as they desire.

_____ 23. Transfer the bag with the client's belongings to the family. If agency policy dictates, have the family sign a receipt.

When the mourners no longer wish to view the body:

_____ 24. Attach identification tags to the designated body parts. Usually the agency identification is left in place and an ID tag is placed on the ankle. If the wrist band is absent, attach a second ID tag to the wrist.

_____ 25. Tie the ankles together with gauze if this is agency policy.

_____ 26. Roll the body to one side and slip the shroud or sheet directly under the body; roll the body back to a supine position.

_____ 27. Drape the shroud according to agency policy or the instructions on the package.

_____ 28. Secure the drape with masking tape or ties according to the shroud package instructions.

_____ 29. Attach another identification tag to the outside of the shroud.

_____ 30. Arrange for removal to the agency morgue by following policy.

_____ 31. Use care when transferring the body to a gurney; ensure proper alignment and avoid unnecessary pressure against the tissues.

_____ 32. Transport the body as inconspicuously as possible.

_____ 33. Remove gloves and wash hands.

_____ 34. Arrange for stripping and cleaning the bed unit according to agency policy.

Name ________________________________ Date ________________

Observed by __________

CHAPTER 51 COLLECTING AND TESTING SPECIMENS

SKILL 51.1 Collecting Cultures from the Nose or Throat

A. Culturing the pharynx:

_____ 1. Explain the exact procedure to the client. Inform him that he will feel a tickling sensation in his throat and may even gag as his throat is swabbed.

_____ 2. Wash hands.

_____ 3. Instruct the client to sit upright or help him into the position.

_____ 4. Place tissues and emesis basin within the client's reach.

_____ 5. Ready the swab by loosening it from the culture tube; set it within reach.

_____ 6. Instruct the client to tilt his head back and open his mouth.

_____ 7. Depress the tongue with the tongue depressor while illuminating the pharynx with the penlight.

_____ 8. Inspect the pharynx for reddened or inflamed areas or patches of exudate.

_____ 9. Set the penlight aside and grasp the swab.

_____ 10. Insert the swab through the mouth, carefully avoiding the tongue, teeth, or cheeks.

_____ 11. Rub the swab quickly but firmly over the area of inflammation or patchy exudate.

_____ 12. Withdraw the swab quickly without touching the oral tissues.

_____ 13. Replace the swab in the culture tube.

_____ 14. Crush ampule of culture media at the bottom of the tube; insert swab tip into the media.

_____ 15. Secure the top of the culture tube.

_____ 16. Discard tongue blade in trash collector.

_____ 17. Provide comfort measures for the client as necessary.

_____ 18. Wash hands.

_____ 19. Secure labels to the culture tube.

_____ 20. Send the culture tube to the laboratory according to agency guidelines.

B. Culturing the nasal mucosa:

_____ 1. Explain the exact procedure to the client. Tell him that he will feel itching and discomfort as the swab passes through the nose.

_____ 2. Wash hands.

_____ 3. Instruct the client to sit upright or help him into the position.

_____ 4. Place tissues within the client's reach.

_____ 5. Ready the swab by loosening it from the culture tube; set it within reach.

_____ 6. Instruct the client to blow his nose.

_____ 7. Instruct the client to tilt his head backward.

_____ 8. Inspect the nostrils to determine patency, using the penlight for illumination.

_____ 9. Insert the wire swab gently through the most patent nostril, avoiding touching the nasal tissue.

_____ 10. Force the swab through the resistance met when it enters the turbinates.

_____ 11. Place the tip of the swab against the turbinate tissue and rotate.

_____ 12. Withdraw the swab quickly without touching the sides of the nares.

_____ 13. Replace the swab in the culture tube.

_____ 14. Crush an ampule of culture medium at the bottom of the tube; insert swab tip into the medium.

_____ 15. Secure the top of the culture tube.

_____ 16. Discard tongue blade in trash collector.

_____ 17. Provide comfort measures for the client as necessary.

_____ 18. Wash hands.

_____ 19. Secure labels to the culture tube.

_____ 20. Send the culture tube to the laboratory according to agency guidelines.

Name ______________________________ Date ______________________

Observed by ____________

SKILL 51.2 Collecting Sputum Specimens

A. Collecting a sputum specimen expectorated by the client:

_____ 1. Explain to the client what will be done. Instruct him in whatever way is necessary.

_____ 2. Wash hands.

_____ 3. Draw the bedside curtains or close the door to the room if the client desires privacy.

_____ 4. Position the client so that he is upright. This can be in high Fowler's, dangling, or standing position.

_____ 5. Give the specimen container to the client with the cover removed. Warn him not to touch the inside of the container.

_____ 6. Encourage the client to take several deep breaths with full expiration.

_____ 7. Instruct the client to cough deeply, raising secretions from the deep airways.

_____ 8. Instruct the client to expectorate directly into the container.

_____ 9. Direct the client to repeat the deep breathing and coughing sequence until approximately 3 ml of sputum is in the container.

_____ 10. Place the cover securely on the container; attach an identifying label.

_____ 11. Provide comfort measures for the client as necessary.

_____ 12. Wash hands.

_____ 13. Send the specimen container to the laboratory according to agency guidelines.

B. Collecting a sputum specimen by suctioning:

_____ 1. Explain to the client what will be done. Instruct him in whatever way is necessary.

_____ 2. Wash hands.

_____ 3. Draw the bedside curtains or close the door to the room if the client desires privacy.

_____ 4. Position client in high Fowler's position.

_____ 5. Connect the tubing from the suction device to the collection trap.

_____ 6. Open the sterile saline bottle; place the cap inside up next to the bottle.

_____ 7. Open the sterile suction kit using sterile technique.

_____ 8. Don a sterile glove on the dominant hand.

_____ 9. Prepare the cup with gloved hand.

_____ 10. Pour saline into the cup with ungloved hand. Replace cap.

_____ 11. Hold the end of the collection trap in ungloved hand.

_____ 12. Pick up the suction catheter with gloved hand and connect it to collection trap.

_____ 13. Wrap the catheter around the gloved hand.

_____ 14. Turn on the suction source with the ungloved hand.

_____ 15. Dip the end of the catheter into the saline.

_____ 16. Insert the tip of the catheter through the nares, endotracheal tube, or tracheostomy; gently advance the catheter into the trachea.

_____ 17. Encourage the client to cough.

_____ 18. Apply suction for 5–10 seconds during the cough by placing gloved thumb over the valve. Stop suction by removing thumb.

_____ 19. Wait at least one full minute and repeat steps 15–18 until 5 ml of sputum is collected in the trap. Observe the client for dyspnea, color changes, restlessness, or irritability.

_____ 20. Withdraw the catheter gently; turn off suction.

_____ 21. Offer the client tissues.

_____ 22. Disconnect catheter from collection trap; gather in gloved hand; remove glove inside out around the catheter and discard.

_____ 23. Disconnect sputum trap from suction tubing.

_____ 24. Connect tubing on sputum trap to the adapter on the trap.

_____ 25. Provide comfort measures for the client as necessary.

_____ 26. Wash hands.

_____ 27. Attach label to sputum trap and send to the laboratory according to agency guidelines.

Name ____________________ Date ____________________

Observed by ____________

SKILL 51.3 Collecting and Testing Gastric Secretions

_____ 1. Explain to the client what will be done.

_____ 2. Wash hands.

_____ 3. Provide privacy.

_____ 4. Place the client in high Fowler's position. Place towel or waterproof pad around his shoulders.

_____ 5. Insert nasogastric tube, if one is not present.

_____ 6. Detach nasogastric tube from suction source and unclamp.

_____ 7. Insert bulb syringe into distal end of nasogastric tube and aspirate approximately 5–10 cc. Inspect aspirated specimen for character and color.

_____ 8. Set syringe aside if doing the testing yourself; insert contents of syringe into a clean specimen container if being sent to a laboratory.

_____ 9. Reattach nasogastric tube to suction source (or remove if inserted for specimen collection).

_____ 10. Reposition the client comfortably.

_____ 11. Label the specimen container properly and send to the laboratory according to agency guidelines.

_____ 12. Wash hands.

If nurse is testing specimen:

_____ 13. Follow the instructions on the package for testing secretions for pH or occult blood.

_____ 14. Dispose of remaining specimen and materials.

_____ 15. Wash hands.

_____ 16. Inform the client of the results.

Name ______________________________ Date ______________________

Observed by ____________

SKILL 51.4 Drawing and Testing Blood Specimens

A. Collecting and testing capillary blood for glucose:

____ 1. Explain to the client what will be done. Check his identification bracelet.

____ 2. Instruct the adult client to wash his hands thoroughly. Cleanse the infant's foot.

____ 3. Wash hands and don gloves.

____ 4. Assist the client to a comfortable position.

____ 5. Prepare the reagent strip according to the manufacturer's instructions.

____ 6. Examine the client's hands (or the infant client's heel) to select a puncture site.

____ 7. Lower the client's hand (or foot) and massage the selected site with a finger.

____ 8. Clean the site with an antiseptic swab. Allow to air dry.

____ 9. Remove protective cap from the lancet or needle. Insert in puncture device, if used.

____ 10. Grasp lancet or needle with hand and quickly prick the prepared site.

OR

Place puncture device against the prepared site and push the release mechanism.

____ 11. Remove first drop of blood with gauze pad and discard.

____ 12. Milk or squeeze the finger or heel proximal to the puncture site.

____ 13. Place the reagent strip next to the site and gently cover strip with blood, according to manufacturer's instructions.

____ 14. Remove strip and begin timing mechanism.

____ 15. Place gauze pad over the site; apply pressure for one to two minutes or until bleeding stops.

____ 16. Follow the manufacturer's instructions for the remainder of the glucose test.

____ 17. Assist the client to a comfortable position. Tell him the test results.

____ 18. Discard used supplies and equipment.

____ 19. Remove gloves and wash hands.

B. Drawing blood from a vein:

____ 1. Explain to the client what will be done. Check his identification bracelet.

____ 2. Wash hands and don gloves.

____ 3. Attach needle to syringe or attach vacuum container needle to the needle holder and insert a vacuum tube. Place extra vacuum container tubes next to venipuncture site.

_____ 4. Position client so that his arm is extended with palm up on a table or pillow.

_____ 5. Inspect the client's antecubital fossa for visible veins.

_____ 6. Secure the tourniquet approximately 5 to 6 inches above the site; check for presence of distal pulse.

_____ 7. Instruct the client to open and clench fist several times.

_____ 8. Select a vein that is visible and firm on palpation.

_____ 9. Clean the site with antiseptic swab.

_____ 10. Place thumb of hand on the vein distal to the puncture site; press down lightly until skin over the vein is taut.

_____ 11. Insert needle, with bevel up, at a 30° angle approximately $\frac{1}{2}$ inch distal to the puncture site. Note a slight "give" sensation as the needle pierces the vein.

If using a syringe and needle:

_____ 12. Draw very gently on the syringe plunger and watch for blood return.

_____ 13. Advance needle carefully if blood return is slow. Hold steady; slowly and deliberately withdraw plunger and draw blood into syringe.

_____ 14. Withdraw needle quickly when desired volume of blood fills the syringe.

If using a vacuum container:

_____ 15. Hold vacuum container securely and push tube into the needle of the holder; avoid pushing needle into vein.

_____ 16. Watch for blood flow into the tube.

_____ 17. Hold vacuum container securely and remove tube when desired volume of blood is present; insert next tube if desired.

_____ 18. Remove vacuum container and needle quickly when all the tubes are filled.

For both syringe and vacuum container:

_____ 19. Release tourniquet with free hand.

_____ 20. Place gauze pad against puncture site and apply pressure for one to two minutes or until bleeding stops.

_____ 21. Transfer blood drawn by syringe to specimen tubes. Gently rotate tubes if additives present.

_____ 22. Label the specimen tubes correctly.

_____ 23. Inspect puncture site for bleeding. Attach bandage if client desires.

_____ 24. Assist client to comfortable position.

_____ 25. Discard used syringes and needles according to agency guidelines.

_____ 26. Remove gloves and wash hands.

_____ 27. Send specimens to laboratory according to agency guidelines.

Name ______________________________ Date ______________

Observed by ______________

C. Drawing blood from an arterial puncture for blood gas analysis:

_____ 1. Explain to the client what will be done. Check his identification bracelet.

_____ 2. Wash hands.

_____ 3. Prepare syringe: aspirate 0.5 ml of heparin 1:1,000 units/ml from vial; pull plunger the entire length of the syringe barrel; eject remaining heparin from syringe.

_____ 4. Position client comfortably with arm extended.

_____ 5. Don gloves.

_____ 6. Palpate radial or brachial arteries with fingertips. Locate maximal pulsation site.

_____ 7. Stabilize radial artery by hyperextending the wrist; stabilize brachial artery by hyperextending elbow.

_____ 8. Clean the puncture site over area of maximum pulsation with antiseptic swab.

_____ 9. Hold swab in fingertips and palpate pulsation again. Keep fingertips proximal to site.

_____ 10. Grasp syringe and insert needle, bevel up, at 45° angle directly into the artery.

_____ 11. Watch the syringe barrel for a pulsating return of blood. Stop advancing the needle when this is seen.

_____ 12. Draw 2–3 ml of blood into the syringe.

_____ 13. Hold antiseptic swab over puncture site and withdraw needle; apply pressure immediately.

_____ 14. Maintain continuous pressure over site for 5 minutes (or 10 minutes if the client is receiving anticoagulants).

_____ 15. Clean the site for any blood that oozed out of puncture site.

_____ 16. Monitor site for bleeding by inspection and palpation.

_____ 17. Apply pressure dressing if bleeding continues.

To prepare the blood for laboratory analysis:

_____ 18. Expel extra air from barrel of syringe and replace the needle cap.

_____ 19. Place identification label on the syringe.

_____ 20. Place syringe in container of crushed ice.

_____ 21. Remove gloves and wash hands.

_____ 22. Document required information on the requisition form.

_____ 23. Send to the laboratory immediately.

Name ______________________ Date ______________

Observed by ____________

SKILL 51.5 Collecting Wound Drainage Specimens

_____ 1. Explain to the client what will be done.

_____ 2. Administer analgesics approximately 45–60 minutes before procedure if appropriate.

_____ 3. Provide privacy.

_____ 4. Wash hands.

_____ 5. Assist the client to move so that his position permits access to the wound.

_____ 6. Drape the client so that the wound is exposed.

_____ 7. Don disposable gloves.

_____ 8. Remove the wound dressing and discard in receptacle.

_____ 9. Inspect wound; identify areas of exudate.

_____ 10. Discard gloves and wash hands.

_____ 11. Prepare sterile dressing supplies and culture tube.

_____ 12. Don sterile gloves.

To collect an aerobic specimen:

_____ 13. Remove cotton-tipped applicator from culture tube.

_____ 14. Insert tip of applicator in area of drainage; rotate so that the entire cotton swab is covered.

_____ 15. Replace applicator in the culture tube; ensure its placement in the culture medium.

To collect an anaerobic specimen:

_____ 16. Remove cotton-tipped applicator from anaerobic culture tube.

_____ 17. Insert tip of applicator into the wound cavity; rotate so that the entire cotton swab is covered.

_____ 18. Replace applicator in the culture tube; ensure its placement in the culture medium.

For each type of specimen:

_____ 19. Set specimen tube aside.

_____ 20. Continue wound care as ordered.

_____ 21. Remove gloves and wash hands.

_____ 22. Ensure the client's comfort.

_____ 23. Attach label to the specimen tube and send with requisition to the laboratory.

Name ____________________ Date ____________________

Observed by ____________

SKILL 51.6 Collecting and Testing Urine Specimens

A. Collecting a clean urine specimen for urinalysis:

_____ 1. Explain the need for a urine specimen and how it is to be collected. Assess the client's understanding and ability to void and produce a urine specimen.

_____ 2. Provide a collecting receptacle for the client to use.

If nurse is to obtain specimen:

_____ 3. Wash hands and don clean gloves; place a urinal or bedpan in position; instruct the client to void.

_____ 4. Remove urinal or bedpan after client voids; empty urine into specimen collecting container.

_____ 5. Discard gloves and wash hands.

_____ 6. Place the urine specimen in the designated specimen container.

_____ 7. Label the specimen container with the client's name, room, and bed number, and the hour and date of collection.

_____ 8. Send the collected specimen for diagnostic procedures.

B. Instructions for the client collecting midstream urine specimen:

_____ 1. Wash hands thoroughly.

_____ 2. Cleanse perineal area around urinary meatus using supplied disposable washcloth.

_____ 3. Wash hands again.

_____ 4. Soak the cotton balls with antiseptic soap.

_____ 5. Using a cotton ball, cleanse around external meatus with a single stroke.

_____ 6. Discard cotton ball after one use.

_____ 7. Continue action of cleansing, discarding all balls used.

_____ 8. Void small amount; hold the urine stream.

_____ 9. Void urine into the sterile specimen container, holding container only on the outside.

_____ 10. Stop voiding when container is about three-quarters full; void remaining urine in toilet, bedpan, or urinal.

_____ 11. Wash hands.

C. Collecting a midstream urine specimen from a client:

_____ 1. Wash hands and don clean gloves.

_____ 2. Soak the cotton balls with disinfectant.

_____ 3. Place the female client on a bedpan; position a urinal near the male client's penis.

_____ 4. Wash the perineal area or penis with a disposable washcloth; discard the washcloth.

_____ 5. Wash hands and don clean gloves.

_____ 6. Cleanse area around meatus with cotton ball using one stroke if the client is male.

OR

Cleanse from pubis to anus with a cotton ball using one stroke if the client is a female.

_____ 7. Discard cotton balls after each stroke.

_____ 8. Instruct the client to void small amount in the bedpan or urinal and then hold the urine stream.

_____ 9. Place the specimen collecting receptacle near the urinary meatus and instruct the client to void again.

_____ 10. Instruct the client to hold the urine stream again, after the receptacle is three-quarters full.

_____ 11. Remove the receptacle, and instruct the client to finish voiding into the bedpan or urinal.

_____ 12. Place a sterile cap on the specimen receptacle.

_____ 13. Remove bedpan or urinal; leave the client comfortable.

_____ 14. Discard gloves and wash hands.

_____ 15. Label the specimen receptacle with information on the client's name, room number, and date and time specimen was given; send specimen for testing.

D. Collecting a urine specimen from a closed urinary drainage system:

_____ 1. Explain to the client what will be done.

_____ 2. Wash hands.

_____ 3. Provide privacy.

_____ 4. Inspect the urinary drainage tubing for amount of urine in the tubing.

_____ 5. Clamp the tubing (if it contains little urine) by using a U clamp or folding the tubing and securing a rubber band around the fold.

_____ 6. Leave the clamp in place for 10–15 minutes.

_____ 7. Locate the specimen port on catheter or drainage equipment.

_____ 8. Clean the port with an antiseptic swab.

_____ 9. Don clean gloves and insert needle of the 10 cc syringe through the port.

_____ 10. Withdraw 10 cc of urine from the tubing.

_____ 11. Expel the urine into the sterile collection container; close it.

_____ 12. Remove the clamp from the drainage system; ensure proper position.

_____ 13. Assist the client to a comfortable position.

Name ______________________ Date ______________

Observed by ______________

_____ 14. Discard gloves and wash hands.

_____ 15. Label the container and send to the laboratory.

E. Collecting a 24-hour urine specimen:

_____ 1. Explain the procedure to the client.

_____ 2. Obtain the designated large size collection container from the laboratory.

_____ 3. Label the container with the client's name and test.

_____ 4. Place the container in a larger container filled with ice; place in the client's bathroom or nearby storage area.

_____ 5. Instruct the client to void and discard the specimen.

_____ 6. Record the time and date of discarded specimen on the collection container. This is the starting time of the collection.

_____ 7. Ensure that all voided urine is placed in the container during the next 24 hours.

_____ 8. Instruct the client to void exactly 24 hours after the discarded specimen; this is the ending time of the collection.

_____ 9. Add the final voided urine to the collection bottle.

_____ 10. Record the time and date of the final voided urine on the container.

_____ 11. Send the container and requisition to the laboratory.

F. Collecting a urine specimen from an infant or toddler:

_____ 1. Explain the procedure to the child's parents, if they are present.

_____ 2. Bring supplies to the child's crib.

_____ 3. Wash hands.

_____ 4. Remove child's diaper.

_____ 5. On a boy, wash the area around base of the penis.

_____ 6. On a girl, wash the labia majora.

_____ 7. Dry carefully.

_____ 8. Remove paper backing from adhesive on collector.

_____ 9. On a girl, apply the adhesive part of collector to the labia so that the opening is around urinary meatus.

_____ 10. On a boy, apply adhesive portion of the collector to perineum so that the opening is around the penis and scrotum.

_____ 11. Apply pressure so that the adhesive fits snugly against the perineum and there are no leaks.

_____ 12. Place a diaper on the child.

_____ 13. Position the child comfortably.

_____ 14. Wash hands.

_____ 15. Check the collector every 10–15 minutes to determine if urine is present.

_____ 16. When urine is present, carefully peel adhesive around opening of collector, taking care not to spill urine contents.

_____ 17. Remove collector.

_____ 18. Transfer urine to specimen container.

_____ 19. Wash hands.

_____ 20. Replace diaper and clothing on the child.

_____ 21. Label and send container to laboratory.

G. Test urine for contents:

_____ 1. Explain to the client what will be done.

_____ 2. Read instructions on the testing kit to determine how much urine is needed.

_____ 3. Wash hands and don clean gloves.

_____ 4. Collect urine specimen.

_____ 5. Take specimen to a work area.

_____ 6. Follow instructions on the test package exactly.

_____ 7. Discard urine and testing materials when test is completed.

_____ 8. Discard gloves and wash hands.

_____ 9. Inform the client of the results.

Name ______________________ Date ______________

Observed by __________

SKILL 51.7 Collecting and Testing Stools

A. Collecting a stool specimen:

_____ 1. Explain the purpose of the test to the client.

_____ 2. Describe how the specimen is to be collected.

_____ 3. Instruct the client to void before defecating; discard the urine; then save his stools in a bedpan or urine collecting hat; discard toilet paper separately.

If the client is unable to collect specimen:

_____ 4. Don disposable gloves.

_____ 5. Remove bedpan (or commode pan) with stool after the client evacuates it.

_____ 6. Take bedpan to bathroom or dirty work area.

_____ 7. Use tongue blades to transfer stool from bedpan to specimen container. Transfer as much as is required for the test.

_____ 8. Discard tongue blades and excess stool; wash bedpan.

_____ 9. Discard gloves and wash hands.

_____ 10. Label specimen container with appropriate identification and send to laboratory.

B. Testing a stool specimen for occult blood:

_____ 1. Explain to the client what will be done.

_____ 2. Read the instructions on the test packet to determine how much stool is required and how the stool is tested.

_____ 3. Don disposable gloves.

_____ 4. Collect specimen and remove to bathroom or storage area.

_____ 5. Use tongue blade to transfer a small amount of stool to testing paper.

_____ 6. Implement test procedure as instructed by packet. Record results.

_____ 7. Dispose of excess stool; clean bedpan or container; discard test materials.

_____ 8. Wash hands.

_____ 9. Report test results to the client.

Name ______________________________ Date ______________

Observed by ____________

CHAPTER 52 ASSISTING WITH DIAGNOSTIC EXAMINATIONS OR PROCEDURES

SKILL 52.1 Preparing for and Assisting with the Pelvic Examination

A. Preparing the client for a pelvic examination:

_____ 1. Explain the purpose and process of the exam to the client.

_____ 2. Instruct the client to void.

_____ 3. Instruct or assist the client to undress and don a hospital gown.

_____ 4. Wash hands.

_____ 5. Place the client in a lithotomy position on the examination table or in bed. If stirrups are available, place her feet in the stirrups.

_____ 6. Place a drape over the client's lower body extending from the waist to her feet.

_____ 7. Prepare speculum for use by rinsing under warm water.

_____ 8. Place gloves, lubricant, slides, scraper, and cotton-tipped applicators on the work area.

_____ 9. Check the examination light for function; place at the distal end of the examination table.

_____ 10. Notify the physician that the client is ready.

_____ 11. Wash hands.

B. Assisting the physician with the pelvic examination:

_____ 1. Arrange the client's drape so that the perineum is exposed.

_____ 2. Direct the examination light on the perineum.

_____ 3. Stand at the client's shoulders throughout the exam.

_____ 4. Hand the physician the instruments he requests.

_____ 5. Instruct the client to take deep breaths and relax the pelvic muscles during the exam.

_____ 6. Assist the client with perineal care at the completion of the exam.

_____ 7. Assist the client to dress if necessary.

_____ 8. Wash hands.

_____ 9. Label the cytology container and send to the laboratory.

_____ 10. Clean or dispose of equipment as necessary.

Name ________________________________ Date ________________

Observed by ____________

SKILL 52.2 Preparing the Client for Electrophysiologic Tests

A. Preparing the client for an electrocardiogram:

_____ 1. Explain the purpose and the process of the EKG to the client.

_____ 2. Answer any questions or concerns.

B. Preparing the client for an electroencephalogram or evoked potentials:

_____ 1. Explain the purpose and the process of the EEG to the client.

_____ 2. Answer any questions or concerns.

_____ 3. Instruct or assist the client to shampoo his hair.

_____ 4. Administer any sedative or hypnotics as ordered.

After the test:

_____ 5. Instruct or assist the client to shampoo his hair.

C. Preparing the client for an electromyelogram:

_____ 1. Explain the purpose and the process of the EMG.

_____ 2. Answer any questions or concerns.

After the test:

_____ 3. Monitor the electrode insertion site for hemorrhage or hematoma formation.

Name ______________________________ Date ______________

Observed by ____________

SKILL 52.3 Preparing and Managing the Client Having Radiologic Studies

A. Preparing the client for a flat-plate x-ray, CAT scan without contrast media, or an MRI scan:

____ 1. Explain to the client what will be done and why.

____ 2. Instruct or assist the client to don a hospital gown and pajama bottoms.

____ 3. Instruct the client to remove any metallic objects from the body area to be x-rayed.

____ 4. Administer any medications that are ordered.

B. Preparing the client for a dye injection study:

____ 1. Determine if the informed consent is signed.

____ 2. Ask the client if he knows what will be done and why.

____ 3. Provide further explanations as necessary.

____ 4. Institute food and fluid restrictions as required for the examination. Administer intravenous fluids if ordered.

____ 5. Provide empathy and caring as needed.

____ 6. Obtain vital signs and document in the medical record.

In the hour before the study:

____ 7. Instruct or assist the client to don a hospital gown and pajama bottoms.

____ 8. Instruct the client to remove jewelry or prostheses.

____ 9. Instruct the client to void.

____ 10. Give preparation medications at the time ordered.

____ 11. Assist or transfer the client to a wheelchair or stretcher for transportation to radiology.

When the client returns from radiology:

____ 12. Assist the client to assume required position or encourage activity if no restrictions are ordered.

____ 13. Obtain the vital signs; compare with data recorded before.

____ 14. Assess the dye injection site, if present.

____ 15. Provide food or fluids if allowed. Force fluids after a myelogram.

____ 16. Monitor for signs of dye reactions such as nausea, vomiting, low urine output, and altered sensory or motor function.

____ 17. Monitor for signs of vascular compromise (after angiography) such as absent peripheral pulses, cool skin, numbness, tingling, or paralysis of a part.

____ 18. Give pain medications if warranted.

C. Preparing the client for a barium contrast study:

_____ 1. Determine if the informed consent is signed.

_____ 2. Ask the client if he knows what will be done and why.

_____ 3. Provide further explanations as necessary.

_____ 4. Institute food and fluid restrictions as required for the examination. Administer intravenous fluids if ordered.

_____ 5. Give cathartics or perform enema as ordered.

_____ 6. Instruct client not to smoke prior to the exam if upper gastrointestinal (GI) series is being done.

_____ 7. Provide empathy and caring as needed.

When the client returns:

_____ 8. Encourage client to resume prior activity levels.

_____ 9. Resume previous diet intake. Force fluids if not contraindicated.

_____ 10. Administer laxatives and enemas as ordered.

_____ 11. Monitor the results of laxatives and enemas.

Name ______________________________ Date ______________

Observed by ____________

SKILL 52.4 Assisting with a Tissue or Fluid Biopsy

A. Preparing the adult client and assisting during a lumbar puncture:

_____ 1. Explain the purpose and process of the procedure to the client.

_____ 2. Instruct the client to void prior to the procedure.

_____ 3. Provide privacy where the procedure is done.

_____ 4. Wash hands.

_____ 5. Assess the client's vital signs.

_____ 6. Instruct the client to remove his clothing and lie on the examination table or bed. Assist him if necessary. Cover him with a drape.

_____ 7. Position the client laterally with his back at the edge of the table or bed.

_____ 8. Draw the client's knees up to his abdomen and flex his chin toward his chest.

_____ 9. Reposition the drape so that the back is exposed.

_____ 10. Place all equipment on a table within the physician's reach.

During the lumbar puncture:

_____ 11. Provide reassurance and comfort to the client as needed; coach him to take deep breaths and relax.

_____ 12. Explain each step of the procedure as the physician implements it.

_____ 13. Hold the client's arms and legs in position if necessary.

_____ 14. Hand supplies or equipment to the physician as requested.

_____ 15. Note the "opening pressure" of the fluid when stated by the physician; assess the color and clarity of the spinal fluid.

_____ 16. Monitor the client for untoward responses.

_____ 17. Collect specimen containers from the physician and label as indicated.

_____ 18. Wash hands when the procedure is completed.

Following the procedure:

_____ 19. Cover the client and assist to a flat, supine position. Encourage him to remain in this position for 12 hours or as the physician recommends.

_____ 20. Assess the vital signs; compare with values recorded before the procedure.

_____ 21. Assess the client for changes in his level of consciousness.

_____ 22. Encourage the client to force fluids if not contraindicated by other conditions.

_____ 23. Don gloves and discard used equipment according to agency policy.

B. Prepare the infant or toddler and assisting during a lumbar puncture:

_____ 1. Explain the purpose and process of the procedure to the infant's parents. Ask them to remain outside of the examining room.

_____ 2. Wash hands.

_____ 3. Place all the equipment on a table near the examination table.

_____ 4. Place the infant on the examination table and undress him.

_____ 5. Position the infant on his side facing the nurse.

_____ 6. Grasp the infant's knees with one hand and draw his legs up to his abdomen.

_____ 7. Grasp the infant's neck with the other hand and pull his head toward his chest. (The infant will be curled in a fetal position facing the nurse.)

During the procedure:

_____ 8. Maintain the infant in the position.

_____ 9. Monitor the infant's breathing patterns.

_____ 10. Have a second nurse assist the physician with the procedure.

Following the procedure:

_____ 11. Release the infant from his position and cuddle him. Monitor his breathing patterns.

_____ 12. Permit his parents to hold and cuddle the infant as soon as possible.

_____ 13. Wash hands.

_____ 14. Don gloves and discard used equipment according to agency policy.

C. Preparing the client and assisting with a liver biopsy:

_____ 1. Explain the purpose and process of the procedure to the client.

_____ 2. Administer sedatives (if ordered) at the correct time.

_____ 3. Instruct the client to void prior to the procedure.

_____ 4. Provide privacy where the procedure is done.

_____ 5. Wash hands.

_____ 6. Place the equipment on a table adjacent to the examination table.

_____ 7. Assess the client's vital signs.

_____ 8. Assist or instruct the client to remove his clothing and lie on the examination table or bed. Cover him with a drape.

_____ 9. Place the client in a supine position toward the edge of the examination table.

_____ 10. Raise the client's right arm above his head; position his hand behind his neck; turn his head to the left.

_____ 11. Reposition the drape to expose the right chest and upper abdomen.

During the procedure:

_____ 12. Instruct the client to remain motionless.

_____ 13. Instruct the client to take a deep breath and hold it as the physician inserts the needle for the biopsy.

Name ______________________ Date ______________________

Observed by ____________

_____ 14. Instruct the client to breathe normally after the needle is withdrawn.

_____ 15. Label specimens as instructed.

After the biopsy:

_____ 16. Apply dressing to puncture site.

_____ 17. Place the client on his right side with a folded bath blanket or sand bag next to the puncture site for one hour.

_____ 18. Assess the client's vital signs; compare with values recorded before the procedure.

_____ 19. Instruct the client to remain in bed for 24 hours.

_____ 20. Assess the puncture site and vital signs for evidence of hemorrhage every 15 minutes for one hour; every hour for 12 hours and every four hours for 24 hours after that, or as the physician orders.

_____ 21. Don gloves and discard used equipment according to agency policy.

D. Preparing the client and assisting with a bone marrow biopsy:

_____ 1. Explain the purpose and process of the procedure to the client.

_____ 2. Administer sedatives (if ordered) at the correct time.

_____ 3. Instruct the client to void prior to the procedure.

_____ 4. Provide privacy where the procedure is done.

_____ 5. Wash hands.

_____ 6. Arrange equipment on a table adjacent to the examination table.

_____ 7. Assess the client's vital signs.

_____ 8. Assist the client to remove his clothing and lie on the examination table or bed; cover with a drape.

_____ 9. Place the client in the proper position: supine if the sternum or anterior iliac crest site is used; prone if posterior iliac crest site is used.

_____ 10. Reposition the drape so that the site is exposed.

During the procedure:

_____ 11. Instruct the client to remain motionless.

_____ 12. Assist the physician as requested.

_____ 13. Provide emotional comfort as the biopsy needle is inserted.

_____ 14. Label the specimens as instructed.

_____ 15. Don gloves and discard used equipment according to agency policy.

After the procedure:

_____ 16. Apply pressure to the puncture site for 5–10 minutes.

_____ **17.** Apply dressing to puncture site.

_____ **18.** Assess the client's vital signs and compare with values recorded before the procedure.

_____ **19.** Assist the client to a position of comfort.

_____ **20.** Wash hands.

_____ **21.** Monitor the puncture site for bleeding for 24 hours.

Name ______________________________ Date ______________________

Observed by ____________

SKILL 52.5 Assisting with Centesis

A. Preparing the client and assisting with a thoracentesis:

_____ 1. Explain to the client what will be done and why. Instruct him not to cough during the procedure.

_____ 2. Ensure that the consent form is signed.

_____ 3. Administer cough suppressant medication, if ordered, at least one hour prior to the procedure.

_____ 4. Provide privacy.

_____ 5. Wash hands.

_____ 6. Assess the client's vital signs.

_____ 7. Assist the client to dangling position at his bedside or on an examination table.

_____ 8. Position an overbed table in front of the client; place pillows or padding on the table.

_____ 9. Assist the client to lean forward with arms draped over the overbed table. Drape as necessary.

If client is unable to sit upright:

_____ 8. Position laterally in bed or on the examination table.

_____ 9. Place affected side of chest uppermost. Drape as necessary.

_____ 10. Place the thoracentesis tray and supplies adjacent to the client.

_____ 11. Notify the physician.

To assist the physician during the thoracentesis:

_____ 12. Open sterile supplies as directed by the physician.

_____ 13. Clean the rubber stopper of the anesthetic vial and hold it upside down when directed by the physician. (The physician inserts the sterile syringe and needle in the vial to withdraw the correct amount of anesthetic.)

_____ 14. Note the exact location of the puncture and the time of needle insertion.

_____ 15. Note characteristics of the aspirated fluid: color, volume, clarity, and viscosity.

_____ 16. Assist with the placement of a dressing over the puncture site.

_____ 17. Collect specimens and label as directed by the physician.

To monitor and assist the client during the thoracentesis:

_____ 18. Assist the client to maintain the desired position throughout the procedure.

_____ 19. Monitor the client's respirations for dyspnea, cough, or expectorated blood.

_____ 20. Monitor skin and nail bed color for evidence of hypoxia.

_____ 21. Monitor the client's pulse rate for changes.

To monitor and assist the client after the thoracentesis:

_____ 22. Assist the client to a high Fowler's position when the procedure is completed.

_____ 23. Auscultate the client's breath sounds.

_____ 24. Monitor the client's vital signs q 15 minutes × 4 and then q 1 hour × 4 or as the physician orders.

_____ 25. Observe the dressing for hemorrhage or fluid drainage.

_____ 26. Don gloves and discard used equipment according to agency policy.

_____ 27. Wash hands.

_____ 28. Obtain chest x-ray and send specimens as ordered.

B. Preparing the client and assisting with a paracentesis:

_____ 1. Explain to the client what will be done and why. Explain to him that he must remain still during the procedure.

_____ 2. Ensure that a consent form is signed.

_____ 3. Provide privacy.

_____ 4. Wash hands.

_____ 5. Shave the puncture site if ordered.

_____ 6. Instruct or assist the client to void.

_____ 7. Assist the client to a sitting position on a chair.
OR
Position in high Fowler's in bed.

_____ 8. Assess the vital signs.

_____ 9. Measure the abdomen girth at the umbilical level; record.

_____ 10. Place paracentesis tray and other equipment at the bedside.

_____ 11. Notify the physician.

To assist the physician:

_____ 12. Open sterile supplies as directed by the physician.

_____ 13. Clean the rubber stopper of the anesthetic vial and hold it upside down when directed by the physician. (The physician inserts the sterile syringe and needle in the vial to withdraw the correct amount of anesthetic.)

_____ 14. Note the exact location of the puncture and the time of needle insertion.

_____ 15. Note characteristics of the aspirated fluid: color, volume, clarity, and viscosity.

_____ 16. Assist with the placement of a dressing over the puncture site.

_____ 17. Collect specimens and label as directed by the physician.

Name ____________________ Date ____________________

Observed by ____________

To monitor and assist the client during the paracentesis:

_____ 18. Assist the client to maintain the desired position throughout the procedure.

_____ 19. Monitor the client's vital signs every 15 minutes throughout the procedure.

_____ 20. Assess for lightheadedness, vertigo, diaphoresis, pallor, tachycardia, dyspnea, or hypotension. Report these signs to physician immediately.

To monitor and assist the client after the paracentesis:

_____ 21. Assist the client to a comfortable position.

_____ 22. Remeasure the abdominal girth at the umbilicus; compare with preprocedure measurement.

_____ 23. Monitor the client's vital signs q 15 minutes × 4 and then q 1 hour 4 or as the physician orders.

_____ 24. Observe the dressing for hemorrhage or fluid drainage.

_____ 25. Don gloves and discard used equipment according to agency policy.

_____ 26. Wash hands.

_____ 27. Send specimens to laboratory as ordered.

Name ______________________________ Date ______________

Observed by ____________

SKILL 52.6 Assisting with Direct Visualization Procedures

A. Preparing the client and assisting with a bronchoscopy or endoscopy:

_____ 1. Explain to the client what will be done and why.

_____ 2. Ensure that a consent form is signed.

_____ 3. Keep the client NPO for 8–10 hours if ordered.

_____ 4. Wash hands.

_____ 5. Administer sedatives at least one hour prior to the procedure or as ordered.

_____ 6. Assess vital signs.

_____ 7. Remove the client's dentures or eyeglasses and store in a safe place.

For bronchoscopy:

_____ 8. Place the client in a supine position with his neck extended and arms at his sides. (This is the position when a flexible fiberoptic scope is used. Usually the client is in the operating room when a rigid scope is used.)

For endoscopy:

_____ 9. Place client in left lateral position. Attach suction catheter to source; check for proper function.

_____ 10. Notify physician that the client is ready.

To assist the client and physician during the bronchoscopy or endoscopy:

_____ 11. Assist the physician to don sterile gown.

_____ 12. Open sterile supplies or equipment as directed by the physician.

_____ 13. Dim illumination in the examination area.

_____ 14. Assist physician as directed.

_____ 15. Collect specimens and label as directed by the physician.

To monitor the client during and following the bronchoscopy or endoscopy:

_____ 16. Encourage the client to relax and breathe through his nose (if scope is passed through mouth) or mouth (if scope is passed through nares).

_____ 17. Assess vital signs, particularly breathing patterns. Assess skin color.

_____ 18. Remove excess lubricant from client's nares or mouth if necessary following removal of the scope.

_____ 19. Don gloves and clean equipment; dispose of supplies.

_____ 20. Wash hands.

B. Preparing the client and assisting with a proctoscopy or colonoscopy:

_____ 1. Explain to the client what will be done and why.

_____ 2. Ensure that a consent form is signed.

_____ 3. Administer enema or laxatives as ordered. Assess character of expelled stool.

_____ 4. Wash hands.

_____ 5. Place client in knee-chest position on examination table or bed; or place client supine on examination table with hips flexed and feet in stirrups.

_____ 6. Drape the client so that perineal area is exposed.

_____ 7. Position lamp so that it will illuminate the perineal area.

_____ 8. Place equipment next to the examination area.

_____ 9. Attach proctoscope to suction source.

_____ 10. Notify physician that client is ready.

To assist the client and the physician during the procedure:

_____ 11. Hand equipment or supplies to the physician as requested.

_____ 12. Assist the client to maintain his position.

_____ 13. Provide emotional support to the client as needed.

At the completion of the procedure:

_____ 14. Assist the client with perineal care as necessary.

_____ 15. Assist client to assume a position of comfort.

_____ 16. Don gloves and clean equipment as necessary; dispose of used supplies.

_____ 17. Wash hands.

ANSWERS TO SELF-TESTS AND CASE STUDIES

CHAPTER 1 SELF-TEST

1. acute care, home care, community
2. B, A, D, C
3. 1) define nursing practice; 2) regulate licensure; 3) regulate nursing education
4. Negligence is failure to do something a reasonable person would do; malpractice is negligence by a professional person through misconduct or lack of expected skills or knowledge.
5. The Patient's Bill of Rights is a set of statements that explain basic rights such as dignity, privacy, confidentiality, and informed consent. Most states require the health care agency to prepare the Bill.
6. Professional liability means nurses accept legal responsibility for their knowledge and actions. Confidential communication means nurses do not divulge client information to people outside of the immediate health care team. Informed consent means nurses do not permit invasive procedures to be performed on the client without written permission from the client.
7. C, A, D, E, B
8. a. implementation. b. planning. c. assessment. d. evaluation. e. making a nursing diagnosis.

CHAPTER 2 SELF-TEST

1. home visit, caregiver
2. Socioeconomic trends are changes in the financial support of health care, advances of medical technology resulting in an aging population, changes in the composition and function of the family, growing health awareness, and consumerism.
3. Health maintenance provides basic services such as assisting with personal hygiene under the supervision of a nurse who visits periodically. Intermediate services provide direct nursing supervision with rehabilitation or health management. Intensive services provide continuous, skilled nursing management.
4. A home care nurse may be a direct care provider, coordinator, teacher, casefinder, counselor, and resource locator.

CHAPTER 3 SELF-TEST

1. In a therapeutic interaction, one of the parties has an obligation to remain present and available for the other party. There is no obligation in a social conversation.
2. sender, medium for transmitting message, receiver
3. inability to speak, difficulty speaking or verbalizing, inability or refusal to speak, a stutter or slurred speech, difficulty forming words or sentences, difficulty ex-

pressing thoughts verbally, disorientation, dyspnea, difficult cultural background, physical or anatomic barrier, decreased circulation to the brain, psychological barrier, developmental disability, defects in neurotransmission or psychosis

4. broad opening: indicates the nurse wishes the client to select the topic of conversation
   general lead: encourages the client to continue
   silence: indicates the nurse expects the client to begin the conversation
   focusing: encourages the client to examine a specific point; accentuates its importance
   seeking clarification: ensures that the nurse has accurately interpreted the client's communication
   sharing observations: the nurse helps the client become aware of what is happening; provides an opportunity for the client to talk about it
   offering self: communicates interest, caring, and understanding
   suggesting collaboration: gives the client control over care and responsibility for meeting his own needs
   giving information: contributes to the client's information
5. reassurance: discounts the client's feelings
   giving approval: may limit client's expression in the future if they are different than those approved
   introducing an unrelated topic: prevents the client from continuing to discuss the topic at hand
   interpreting: may be perceived as an invasion of privacy and be threatening to the client
   agreeing: may prevent the client from changing his mind
   rejecting: causes the client to feel that his feelings are not important
   disapproving: belittles or judges the client's thoughts or feelings
   disagreeing: communicates lack of acceptance
   advising: discourages client from autonomous, independent thoughts or actions
   defending: suggests that the client cannot criticize or express feelings and thoughts of that which is defended
6. The interview is goal-oriented and purposeful; the therapeutic interaction has purpose but usually does not have a well-defined goal.
7. The medical history focuses on the client's physical and emotional clinical manifestations that suggest a medical problem that is treatable by the physician; the nursing history focuses on the client's perceptions, expectations of health care, and clinical characteristics that suggest a nursing problem that is treatable by the nurse.
8. A, C, B, B, A, C

CHAPTER 4 SELF-TEST

1. affective domain: the part of the intellect that relates to attitudes and feelings
   cognitive domain: the part of the intellect that relates to information
   psychomotor domain: the part of the intellect that relates to physical skills of manipulation
2. inability to explain information or demonstrate a skill
3. knowledge of the information, alternative, readiness
4. suitable environment, acceptance of the learner, positive reinforcement of learning, and constructive criticism

CHAPTER 5 SELF-TEST

1. It is a verbal and graphic documentation of current health status, health history, and events of his present health problems as identified, monitored, and treated by the health care team of the agency.
2. communication, research, education, statistical documentation, review of services and legal evidence of health care and status
3. The client owns the information regarding himself; the agency owns the actual document.
4. All entries into a source-oriented record are made according to source; all entries into a problem-oriented record are made according to the problem.
5. G, H, D, A, E, B, F, C
6. Centrally records pertinent information necessary for the nurse to manage the client.
7. S, O, S, S, O, O, O

CHAPTER 6 SELF-TEST

1. Gives intent and direction to client care; communicates to other nurses; used as basis for client–nurse assignments; establishes mechanism for evaluation of nursing actions; educates the student.
2. A standardized care plan is a set of identified problems with prepared outcomes and nursing orders that may be applied to a number of clients; the individualized care plan is created solely on the basis of one client's problems.
3. a. blue around the mouth and unable to breathe
   b. cough that leaves him exhausted
   c. inability to concentrate right now
   d. itchy skin under the cast
4. NO, YES, YES, NO
5. "three times a day," "before he leaves the hospital," "each morning"

UNIT I CASE STUDY

1. This is an open-ended question that is effective because the client answered with information that was important to her.
2. verbalizing the implied
3. This is a direct question that proved effective because the client gave a specific answer.
4. This is clarification; it effectively encouraged the client to confirm that something does bother her, fatigue.
5. This is an open-ended question and a general lead; it encouraged the client to talk about her perceptions of her fatigue.
6. verbalizing the implied
7. This is an open-ended question; it elicited information effectively.
8. This is selective reflection; it effectively encourages the client to talk about breast-feeding.
9. This is a direct question that focuses (a communication skill) on the client's feelings.
10. This is a communication block; specifically, the nurse changed the subject. It

blocked further discussion of the breast-feeding problem. A more appropriate response might be, "You are troubled by your husband's reaction," which makes an observation. Another appropriate response is to repeat, "Isn't right . . . ?" which is selective reflection. Both responses encourage the client to talk further about her feelings.

11. This is a communication block; specifically because the nurse cannot accurately predict what will happen to the baby. It discouraged further communication because the client felt she had to agree with the nurse. A more appropriate response might be, "This is a difficult time for you, with a tiny baby and two young children to care for." This statement is making an observation as well as demonstrating empathy, thus encouraging further sharing of feelings.

CHAPTER 7 SELF-TEST

1. fire: Limit smoking; post "danger" signs when oxygen is in use; store flammable materials properly; know fire reporting and managing policies.
   falls: Keep beds in low position; use siderails appropriately; clear pathways; assist with walking; lock wheels on furniture, wheelchairs, and gurneys; provide adequate lighting; remove spilled or slippery objects from the floor; use restraints.
   accidental poisoning: Clearly label and store medications and chemicals properly.
2. a. in use. b. in use. c. in use.
3. Cross out ability to eat by self and body temperature.
4. a. wrist restraint. b. belt or jacket restraint. c. elbow or mitt restraint.
5. infectious agent, reservoir, portal of exit, method of transmission, portal of entry, susceptible host
6. A, B, A, A, B
7. T, F, T, F, F, F
8. E, A, D, C, B

CHAPTER 8 SELF-TEST

1. The nurse assesses for characteristics of level of consciousness, weakness, fatigue, shortness of breath, and immobility.
2. right, left
3. a. 1. b. 3. c. 7. d. 2. e. 6. f. 5. g. 4.
4. Elastic stockings exert pressure against the muscles and superficial veins that force venous blood into the deeper veins and enhance return blood flow to the heart and prevents stasis.

CHAPTER 9 SELF-TEST

1. protection, regulation of body temperature, excretion of body wastes, sensory perception, vitamin D production
2. C, A, B, D, E
3. Wrinkling, sagging, and color changes due to loss of collagen, elastin, changes in pigmentation and vasculature, and inability to hold moisture.
4. Potential impairment of skin integrity.
5. The primary purpose of AM care is to assist the client with his morning activities

of daily living: toileting, washing face and hands, and preparing for breakfast. The primary purpose of PM care is to assist the client to prepare for sleep.

6. inability to wash body or body parts by himself; unable to prepare bath water or regulate the water temperature
7. Skin assessment; assessment of other body systems, such as musculoskeletal or cardiovascular; client education regarding hygiene or skin care; establishment of a therapeutic relationship.
8. Limits potential transfer of microorganisms from the anus toward the urethra.
9. Self-care deficit; Alteration in comfort; Pain; Impairment of skin integrity; Sleep-pattern disturbance.
10. effleurage, petrissage, friction, tapotement

CHAPTER 10 SELF-TEST

1. mucosa: epithelial tissue that forms the protective coating on some body surfaces
   mucus: fluid secreted by mucosa
   saliva: fluid composed of mucus and a digestive enzyme
   papillae: cellular projections located on the tongue
   dentin: the enamel tissue of teeth
   plaque: gummy mass of food particles and microorganisms that accumulates on the gums and teeth
   caries: tooth decay
   gingiva: the gums
2. ineffective oral hygiene, malnourishment, dehydration, no intake of oral fluids or food, mouth breathing, exposure to harmful chemical or mechanical irritants that have damaged mucous membranes, oral trauma or infection
3. laterally with the face pointing downward
4. Grasp the denture firmly and slip one fingertip under the edge to break the suction; gently remove the denture.
5. sclera: protects inner eye structures
   iris: controls the opening of the pupil
   pupil: controls the amount of light entering the eye
   lacrimal apparatus: manufactures, circulates, and drains tears
6. blink reflex; inner, outer; suction, special or saline
7. Terminal hair is coarse, pigmented, located only on some body parts; vellus is soft, fine, and almost transparent and located on all body surfaces except the palms of the hands and soles of the feet.
8. The shampoo board is used to collect rinse water when shampooing the client in bed.
9. Loosen the hair with fingers, divide it into workable sections, and use a wide-tooth comb or pick to free the tangles by working from the ends toward the scalp.
10. T, T, F, F, T, T

UNIT II CASE STUDY

1. Potential for injury related to weakness and paralysis
2. The client is without bodily injury or harm during his hospitalization.
3. Keep siderails up while the client is in bed.
   Place call signal within reach of his functional hand.

Keep frequently used possessions within reach of his functional hand.
Use a restraint when the client is sitting in a chair.
Frequently monitor to check on his safety.

4. Partial self-care deficit: grooming and dressing related to weakness and paralysis
5. These are possible:
   The client reports that he has experienced minimal discomfort during the removal and replacement of his clothing.
   The client's clothing is clean and neatly positioned.
   The client demonstrates how to put on or remove various pieces of clothing that he is presently unable to put on or remove.
6. Potential impaired skin integrity related to immobility
7. The client's skin remains intact and without discomfort to the client.
8. Frequently turn and reposition the client.
   Gently massage the skin area at regular intervals.
   Keep the affected skin area clean and dry.
   Continue to monitor and note any changes in color or sensation.

CHAPTER 11 SELF-TEST

1. functional special senses, examine with deliberation and calm, ability to recognize and differentiate between normal and abnormal findings, ability to concentrate or focus on technique used, accurate technique, use objectivity, accurately communicate findings
2. inspection: all aspects of appearance: size, shape, color, location
   palpation: temperature, texture, shapes, placement or location of lesions or organs
   percussion: tissue density and location
   auscultation: characteristics of sounds
3. a. inspection, palpation. b. auscultation. c. inspection, palpation. d. inspection, percussion, palpation, and auscultation. e. auscultation. f. percussion and palpation. g. inspection, palpation. h. inspection, palpation.

CHAPTER 12 SELF-TEST

1. C, D, B, A
2. The circadian cycle causes slight body temperature fluctuation during a 24-hour period of time.
3. pyrexia, infection
4. On the Fahrenheit thermometer, normal is 98.6°; on the Centigrade thermometer, normal is 37°.
5. oral: 3–11 minutes
   rectal: 2–4 minutes
   axillary: 10 minutes
6. exercise: increases pulse rate although cardiovascular conditioning lowers resting pulse rate
   emotions: may slow or increase pulse rate
   body temperature: higher than normal temperature increases pulse rate and lower than normal temperature lowers the rate
   pathology: depends on pathology, but infection increases rate; heart failure increases the rate; changes in blood volume increase rate, and increased intracranial pressure may cause rate fluctuations

7. tachypnea: fast, even respiratory rate
   bradypnea: slow, even respiratory rate
   hyperpnea: deep, even respiratory rate
   apnea: absence of respiration
   dyspnea: subjective sensation of shortness of breath
   orthopnea: difficulty breathing unless in an upright position
8. systole, contracts, diastole, relaxes
9. circulating blood volume: More volume increases blood pressure; less volume lowers it.
   peripheral vascular resistance: Greater resistance increases blood pressure; lesser resistance lowers it.
   blood viscosity: More viscous blood increases blood pressure.
   vascular tone: Loss of tone may lower diastolic pressure.
10. The auscultatory gap is a temporary disappearance of Korotkoff's sounds when monitoring blood pressure. It occurs in some cardiovascular abnormalities. Clinically, the examiner must apply sufficient external pressure to the arteries to detect a gap.

CHAPTER 13 SELF-TEST

1. age: Body water is highest at birth and gradually decreases with age.
   sex: After puberty, males have a higher percentage of muscle weight than females; females have a higher percentage of fat tissue than males.
   morphology: Physical shape and size affects proportion of tissues; for example, thicker, heavier bones increase tissue weight.
   nutrition: Adequate balance of nutrients is essential for development of tissues; imbalances, such as greater proportion of fat and carbohydrates in the diet, may result in disproportionate amount of fat tissue.
2. age: Growth rate of the body height is constant from birth until maturity; height is constant until later adulthood when it begins to decline.
   sex: Males are generally taller than females after puberty.
   race: May affect stature; for example, Caucasians are generally taller than Orientals.
   heredity: Height is genetically influenced.
   nutrition: Body height is directly affected by sound nutrition; the better the nutrition, the greater the body height.

CHAPTER 14 SELF-TEST

1. introduction of nurse to the client: begins the therapeutic relationship
   orientation of the client to his room and facilities: acquaints the client with his surroundings, which helps relieve anxiety regarding the unknown
   orientation of the client to the agency: same as above
   information regarding Patient's Bill of Rights: gives information to the client that contributes to his sense of power or control over his own life
   admission interview: identifies those health factors that will impact on his agency relationship.
   assessment of vital signs: provides baseline data for later comparisons.
2. a. Knowledge deficit related to delivery process
   b. Health management deficit related to aging
   c. Anxiety related to impending surgery

3. The referral communicates client information to the receiving agency so that appropriate health management continues with minimal interruption. Some of the information communicated is client's health history, recent illness events, current therapies and medications, current condition, and future plans.
4. The nurse may identify the Nichols' specific concerns; evaluate their home situation, identify who is available to support them at home, provide health teaching regarding the medication administration and physical therapy to compensate for losses and refer them to a home health agency for continuing care.

UNIT III CASE STUDY

1. **Objective**
   age 79 years
   lives by self
   does own cooking
   pulse 100 and irregular
   respirations 24 and even
   temperature 38.2°C
   blood pressure 142/70
   skin warm
   swollen ankles
   weight gain of 12 pounds in 7 days

   Subjective
   failing vision
   short of breath
   difficulty breathing lying down
   sensation of palpitations in chest
   dizzy
   feels hot
   sweaty
   feels sick
2. breathing rate assessed by observation or inspection
   breath sounds assessed by auscultation
   skin color assessed by inspection
   skin temperature assessed by palpation
   heart rate assessed by palpation (peripheral pulse) or auscultation (apical pulse)
   blood pressure assessed by auscultation (or palpation)
3. difficulty breathing: dyspnea
   discomfort in breathing except in an upright position: orthopnea
   rapid breathing: tachypnea
   slow breathing: bradypnea
   high blood pressure: hypertension
   low blood pressure: hypotension
   rapid heart beat: tachycardia
   slow heart beat: bradycardia
   swelling of the soft tissues: edema
4. Pulse is not normal; it is rapid. This is called tachycardia. Its irregular rhythm is called dysrhythmia.
5. Respirations are not normal but are rapid. This is called tachypnea.
6. Temperature is not normal, it is elevated. Elevated temperature is pyrexia. He is febrile.
7. Systolic is 142; diastolic is 70.

CHAPTER 15 SELF-TEST

1. C, D, B, E, A
2. bone, skeleton, periosteum, marrow, ligaments, cartilage, tendons
3. appearance, posture, gait, muscular strength

4. Activities of daily living are those universally performed, routine, daily events such as bathing, dressing, grooming, eating, and toileting.
5. bedrest: client remains in bed except for toileting or brief walks.
   up ad lib: client is out of bed as much as he wishes.
6. A. Total self-care deficit. B. Partial self-care deficit: bathing and dressing. C. Impaired physical mobility.

CHAPTER 16 SELF-TEST

1. gravity, base of support, center of gravity, line of gravity
2. G, I, H, B, D, J, E, C, F, A
3. standing: 1) Head is erect; 2) shoulders at same level directly over hips; 3) arms fall at the same with elbows slightly flexed; 4) fingers slightly flexed; 5) hips at the same level and directly over the legs and feet; 6) abdomen does not protrude; 7) knees slightly flexed; 8) ankles in functional position; 9) toes point forward and slightly lateral.
   sitting: 1) Head is erect with eyes forward, chin tucked in; 2) spine retains natural curves and rests on hips and buttocks; 3) shoulders are level; 4) arms are flexed and rest on lap or chair armrests; 5) thighs are horizontal to the floor and rest on chair seat; 6) knees are flexed at 90°; 7) feet rest on floor with ankles in functional position.
   lying: 1) Neck muscles are not stretched or twisted; 2) face is centered between the shoulders; 3) shoulders are level and in natural relationship to the head; 4) arms are flexed and positioned without compression under the body; 5) body trunk is not twisted, and shoulders and hips are level and equally distant from each other; 6) hips and knees are slightly flexed or comfortably flexed and positioned so that neither leg is compressed under the body; 7) legs are positioned approximately parallel to each other; 8) ankles are in functional position from the lower leg.
4. a. Roll, push, or pull a person or object rather than lift it.
   b. Position feet and legs farther apart when using force to push or pull another object or person.
   c. Use a smooth surface to push or pull an object rather than a rough or uneven surface.
   d. Lower the head of the bed when moving the client up in bed.
5. supine: lying flat on the back
   dorsal recumbent: lying flat on the back with head and shoulders resting on a pillow
   prone: lying flat on the abdomen
   lateral: lying on the side
   Fowler's: sitting upright
   Sims': side-lying position with the face and body trunk turned toward the bed surface
   dangling: sitting on the side of the bed
6. Trendelenberg: Thoracic cavity must be lower than the abdomen.
   reverse Trendelenberg: Keeps the abdominal contents below the diaphragm in a hiatus hernia.
   lithotomy: Used during examination or surgery on the perineum or pelvis.
   knee-chest: Used during examination of the rectum.
7. 1) client safety; 2) maintenance of client's posture and body alignment; 3) nurse's safety through use of proper body mechanics
8. 1) amount of purposeful movement; 2) amount of joint movement; 3) amount of muscular strength; 4) mechanical restrictions on joint or body movements; 5)

client reports of fatigue or weakness; 6) client's shortness of breath; 7) presence of risk factors for skin breakdown
9. Partial self-care deficit related to hemiplegia

CHAPTER 17 SELF-TEST

1. unoccupied bed: Linens are changed when client is out of bed.
   occupied bed: Linens are changed when the client is in bed.
   open bed: Top linens are fanfolded on the foot of the bed, ready to be drawn over the client when he gets in bed.
   closed bed: Top linens are drawn to the head of the bed.
   anesthesia bed: Top linens are fanfolded to one side of the bed, ready to be drawn over the client as he is transferred from a gurney to the bed.
2. 1) ability of the client to get out of bed or tolerate the activity of bedmaking if he remains in bed; 2) appearance of bed linens; 3) soiling of bed linens; 4) which linens must be changed; 5) when is the most convenient time to change linens
3. The drawsheet is placed over the midsection of the mattress, on top of the bottom sheet, to protect the bottom sheet from soiling or perspiration. If the drawsheet is soiled, it is readily changed.
4. 1) limit handling or shaking linens; 2) avoid touching soiled or used linens with clean linens; 3) avoid placing clean linens on soiled surfaces; 4) discard used linens in laundry hamper or chute immediately; 5) wash hands before and after linen change; 6) wear clean gloves during linen change; 7) hold bundled soiled linens away from uniform
5. 1) raise bed to a comfortable height; 2) work on one side of the bed at a time; 3) use proper body mechanics throughout the activity

CHAPTER 18 SELF-TEST

1. functional, action, flexor, extensor, extensor, flexor, joint range of motion, ankylosis, contracture, atrophy
2. E, G, F, H, J, B, D, C, I, A
3. Passive range of motion is the movement of the joint through its range without using its attached muscles. Energy is supplied by another means.
4. positive effects of active ROM: maintains joint action, improves muscle tone through contraction and relaxation, and uses body stores of energy
   negative effects of active motion: may deplete energy stores in debilitated person, may cause further damage or pain if joint or muscle injury is present
   positive effects of passive ROM: maintains joint action without using body's energy stores, if person is weak or debilitated
   negative effects: does not maintain muscle tone
5. 1) amount of purposeful joint movement possible; 2) limits of activity; 3) any joint limitations; 4) presence of joint pain, stiffness, swelling, or inflammation; 5) risk factors for contracture development
6. Strengthens and conditions muscles even though joints may be immobilized.
7. Gait is style of walking; pace is the number of steps taken during a given period of time.
8. progressive ambulation: gradually increasing the amount of activity

assisted ambulation: walking with the help of a mechanical aid or another person
independent ambulation: walking without any help

9. Impaired physical mobility; Potential for injury related to weakness, fatigue, impairments; Potential or actual activity intolerance.
10. 1) client's physical disability; 2) client's level of awareness of surroundings; 3) ability to balance and use correct body alignment; 4) presence of weakness, paralysis; 5) weight-bearing ability; 6) use of upper extremities

CHAPTER 19 SELF-TEST

1. cardiovascular: 1) increased cardiac workload; 2) orthostatic hypotension; 3) venous stasis
   respiratory: 1) decreased lung expansion; 2) pooled pulmonary secretions
   musculoskeletal: 1) loss of physical endurance; 2) loss of muscular tone and mass; 3) joint stiffening
   urinary: 1) urinary stasis; 2) development of urinary stones
   integumentary: 1) impaired circulation; 2) development of pressure ulcers
2. age, presence of pathology, length of immobility, extent of immobility and overall general health
3. cardiovascular: 1) exercise; 2) increased fluid intake; 3) application of antiembolic stockings or devices
   respiratory: 1) proper positioning; 2) pulmonary physiotherapy
   musculoskeletal: 1) active or passive exercise; 2) ambulation; 3) supportive devices
   urinary: 1) increased fluid intake; 2) exercise; 3) sufficient opportunity for voiding
   integumentary: 1) basic hygiene; 2) skin stimulation; 3) turning and repositioning; 4) protective mattress surfaces
4. pressure points are those skin areas that are vulnerable to breakdown and are located over bony prominences in most instances.
5. immobility, presence of shearing forces, friction or pressure, reddened bony prominences, reduced tactile sensation
6. turning frame: maintains strict body alignment while being rotated from supine to prone (and back) laterally
   CircOlectric bed: maintains strict body alignment while being rotated from supine to prone (and back) vertically
   Clinitron bed: reduces pressure against skin surface

CHAPTER 20 SELF-TEST

1. strain: muscle or tendon damage because of overuse
   sprain: damage to ligament fibers caused by overstretching muscles
   laceration: break or tear in muscle or other soft tissue
   dislocation: change in the normal relationship of the articulating bones in a joint
   fracture: interruption of the continuity of the bone
   fracture: interruption of the continuity of the bone
2. C, B, D, A, E
3. splint: external device that maintains joint in its functional position after injury

brace: external device that provides stability for a body part while permitting joint movement

cast: external device that immobilizes joints proximal and distal to a fracture or surgical site

4. Neurovascular assessments include color, sensation, and movement:
   1) Note skin color for evidence of erythema and pallor; blanch the skin by pressing against it with the fingers for 5 seconds and note how long until color returns (normal is approximately 3 seconds); feel skin for changes in temperature.
   2) Test sensation by pinching or scratching the surface of the extremity and asking the client to identify the sensation.
   3) Assess movement by asking the client to wiggle his fingers or toes.
5. Plaster of Paris casts take longer to dry (24 hours), may crumble if moistened, permit some air and moisture to penetrate, and have slight movement. Synthetic casts dry in 30 minutes, are impermeable to water or air, and are so hard they may break if subjected to slight movement.
6. 1) Check the fingers frequently for skin color and temperature and have Johnny wiggle his fingers to check movement.
   2) Inspect the skin around the edges of the cast each day for any damage; check more often if Johnny feels irritation or pain.
   3) Do not stick any object into the cast to scratch the skin; if itching occurs, blow cold air from a hair dryer toward the itchy area.
   4) Remove any small objects that are loose in the cast with a vacuum cleaner.
   5) Call the clinic or physician immediately if Johnny has fever, more pain than usual, or any unusual discomfort.
7. Skin traction is applied externally; skeletal traction is applied to a pin or bar that is attached to the bone.
8. 1) skin condition at the point of attachment, whether skin or skeletal; 2) circulatory status distal to the injury; 3) neuromuscular status distal to the injury; 4) skin condition on any pressure points; 5) any evidence suggesting a complication of immobility

UNIT IV CASE STUDY

1.

Subjective Data	**Objective Data**
likes the "hotel"	age 87
pain and stiffness in joints	slender
	white hair
	friendly, talkative
	wears bifocals and hearing aid
	osteoarthritis
	joint stiffness
	cannot grasp small objects
	immobilized in Buck's extension
	able to lift upper body from bed

2. Impaired physical mobility related to immobilization in traction
3. The client is without the musculoskeletal complications of immobility as evidenced by joint flexibility, normal muscle tone, and verbal reports of comfort.
4. Change the client's position every two hours (these are possible: raise or lower head of the bed; flex or extend nonaffected leg).

   Place a footboard against the nonaffected foot to maintain its functional position.

Perform passive range-of-motion exercises to all nonaffected joints every four hours. Encourage client to exercise independently.
Monitor for joint or muscular pain and treat when necessary.

5. Potential for injury related to immobility and confusion
6. The client is without injury during hospitalization.
7. Keep siderails up at all times unless nurse is at the bedside.
   Position call signal within the client's reach.
   Place frequently used possessions within reach of the client (such as tissues, water cup, television control, or telephone).
   Monitor at regular intervals (every two hours).
8. Potential for impaired skin integrity related to immobility and age
9. The client's skin remains pink, soft, and intact during her hospitalization.
10. At the foot or ankle, observe skin color; apply pressure against the skin for a brief period and monitor return of skin color upon release; gently rub the skin with object and assess the client's perception of sensation; palpate the skin for temperature.

CHAPTER 21 SELF-TEST

1. physiologic manifestations: muscular tension, tremor, perspiration, pallor, dilated pupils, increased rate and depth of respiration, increased pulse, increased blood pressure, diarrhea, urinary frequency and urgency, decreased appetite, and dry mouth
   behavioral manifestations: attempts to control or manipulate the environment, regression to earlier patterns of behavior, suspicion, hostility, aggression, excessive complaints of dissatisfaction, overreaction to minor inconveniences
2. Mr. Carter: denial
   Ms. Gray: suppression
   John: displacement
   Peter: projection
3. describes a perceived threat; expresses feeling of apprehension, dread, nervousness or concern about a threatening event, person, or object; verbalizes expectation of danger to self; questions or seeks information; is restless; changes the pitch of the voice or has vocal tremors; increases rate of verbalization; has hand tremors; has increased muscle tension; narrows or fixes focus of attention; perspires profusely; increased heart or respiratory rates; elevated blood pressure; reacts with unprovoked anger, hostility, or suspicion
4. Move the client to a small, quiet space, if he is in a large, open area; stay with him and remain calm; ensure adequate lighting.
5. 1) Use therapeutic skills of communication; 2) communicate in short, simple questions; 3) use quiet, firm tone of voice; 4) avoid use of false reassurance; 5) accept expression of negative feelings; 6) be sensitive to the client's feelings and needs; 7) avoid negating, belittling, or discounting the client's feelings or experiences; 8) express empathy; 9) use touch.

CHAPTER 22 SELF-TEST

1. 1) mechanical, such as pressure; 2) thermal, such as intense heat that burns tissues; 3) chemical, such as the release of histamine or bradykinin that causes tissue destruction; or 4) ischemic, such as blood vessel blockage that causes tissue destruction because of lack of oxygen

2. nociceptors, noxious stimuli, afferent, fiber, gate control, block, threshold, tolerance
3. pain intensity: severity of pain
   intermittent pain: occurs on a regular or irregular schedule but does subside at times
   intractable pain: constant pain that is unresponsive to treatment
   diffuse pain: experienced over a wide area and not clearly pinpointed by the sufferer
   localized pain: confined to a body area that is identifiable to the sufferer
   radiating pain: perceived as rapidly and repeatedly moving in a wavelike fashion
   referred pain: perceived in a body area some distance from the stimuli
   phantom pain: painful sensation perceived in an absent body part, such as an amputated limb
4. rapid heart and respiratory rate, blood pressure changes, dry mouth, and dilated pupils when pain is acute with rapid onset; slowed heart and respiratory rate, constricted pupils, and moist mouth when pain is chronic. Sufferer may experience sweating, pallor, or withdrawal from noxious stimuli
5. verbalization of pain; vocalization with grunts, groans, or screams; facial expressions of grimacing, frowning, clenching the jaw, tightly closing the eyes; guarding, limping, limiting motion in a body part
6. E, C, B, H, G, F, D, A

UNIT V CASE STUDY

1. B. He is denying the inevitability of his wife's death.
2. C. Susan is rationalizing that she will be okay; she probably really feels terrified at the impending loss of her mother.
3. A. Jeff is very angry because of his mother's illness but since he can't be angry with her because that would hurt too much, he displaces his anger on his father.
4. D. Jared is fantasizing about something that is important to him; it helps him avoid feeling the pain of his mother's illness.
5. Eric is withdrawing from social interaction with the family or the nurse. This prevents him from facing the painful situation.
6. Each member of the Maynard family learns to express anxiety over Joan's illness in a healthy manner, as evidenced by their ability to plan realistically for the future.
7. Demonstrate interest and concern for each family member.
   Use active listening skills.
   Use therapeutic skills of communication to facilitate expression of feelings. Avoid blocks.
   Accept expression of negative feelings.
   Be sensitive to the client's feelings and needs.
   Use nonverbal cues, such as touch, to communicate caring.
   Promote problem solving.
8. Joan experiences a more tolerable pain level as confirmed by her nonverbal behaviors and verbal reports.
9. Remove any painful stimuli from her environment.
   Use relaxation techniques; teach family members the techniques.
   Employ distraction through more social interaction with family members.
   Use therapeutic touch; teach family members the technique.

CHAPTER 23 SELF-TEST

1. 45, 75, age, amount of body fat, intracellular, extracellular
2. perspiration, medications, vomiting, diarrhea, excess urine output
3. Actual fluid volume deficit; Actual fluid volume excess
4. 1,260 cc total
5. nutritionist: health care specialist who assesses and identifies nutritional needs, plans nutritional therapy, and teaches nutrition
   diet history: interview that identifies eating patterns and habits
   food intake study: documentation of actual amount of food and fluid ingested during a given period
   anthropometrics: measurements of body and muscle sizes
6. body height, weight, and skinfold thickness
7. hair: dull, fine or very coarse, color changes, easily plucked
   eyes: dull, fissures on eyelids
   mouth: pale or very red conjunctiva, Bitot's spots, swollen or red lips, fissures at corners of mouth, ulcerated mucosa, absent or abnormally positioned teeth, receding gum line, fragile gums that bleed easily, swollen or purplish tongue
   skin: dry, flaky, swollen or discolored areas, petechiae
   nails: spoon shaped, brittle, or ridged
   heart: tachycardia, dysrhythmias, or enlarged heart
8. Alteration in nutrition: more than body requirements
   Alteration in nutrition: less than body requirements

CHAPTER 24 SELF-TEST

1. B
2. C
3. B
4. B
5. A
6. C
7. C
8. A

CHAPTER 25 SELF-TEST

1. D, E, B, A, C
2. decompression: removing flatus, secretions, and other gastric contents
   gavage: inserting fluids and nutrients directly into the stomach
   lavage: irrigating the internal organ with a liquid solution
   compression: applying pressure against cavity walls for hemostasis
3. suction: pulls fluids or gases from area of low pressure toward area of high pressure
   force of gravity: permits drainage of fluids downward
   tube diameter: Large diameter drains more fluid than small diameter.
   viscosity: Thin fluids flow faster than thick fluids.

tube length: Longer tubes decrease flow rate because of friction created by the lumen of the tube.

4. Measure the distance from the client's earlobe to the tip of the nose to the xiphoid process and mark on the tube.
5. aspirating gastric contents; auscultating the epigastrium for a bubbling or rushing sound as air is injected into the external end of the tube; and confirming with x-ray
6. Irrigation is done to establish or maintain the patency of the tube.
7. enteral, proteins, fats, carbohydrates, the client's nutritional needs, and diarrhea
8. This determines how much food remains in the stomach. If the stomach is not emptying, gastric distress, nausea, vomiting, and aspiration may result if feedings are continued.

CHAPTER 26 SELF-TEST

1. fluid volume depletion (dehydration): less than normal intake, dilute urine, rapid and sudden weight loss, thirst, loss of skin turgor, dry mucous membranes, sunken eyeballs, hypotension, rapid pulse, depressed fontanelles in infants, and possible rise in body temperature

   fluid volume overload (overhydration): edema, sudden and rapid weight gain, restlessness and anxiety, altered mental awareness, shortness of breath, moist lung sounds, jugular vein distention and changes in the blood pressure

   fluid concentration disturbances: same as volume depletion plus lowering levels of consciousness, oliguria progressing to anuria and signs of increasing intracranial pressure

   fluid composition disturbances: muscle weakness, diminished tendon reflexes, paralytic ileus, and changes in heart conduction
2. replacement therapy: indicates fluids are given to replace those lost

   open line: intact intravenous route is available

   keep open: very small amounts of fluids are infused over long periods of time
3. replace fluids and nutrients, electrolyte, isotonic, replace blood volume, blood products, water, dextran
4. B, F, C, H, D, A, G, E
5. type of solution being given, duration of the infusion, client's age, and condition of the client's veins
6. gravity, position of limb or vein, patency of the tube, infiltration
7. 33 gtt/minute
8. 31.2 gtt/minute
9. too fast
10. 12.5 gtt/minute

CHAPTER 27 SELF-TEST

1. total parenteral nutrition: intravenous administration via a central vein of all essential nutrients in a liquid preparation

   hyperalimentation: another term for TPN

   nitrogen balance: blood indicator of the available protein for tissue repair and growth

   catabolism: breakdown of substances
2. Negative nitrogen balance occurs when body stores of protein, rather than carbohydrates or fats, are used for energy by catabolism.

3. starvation, massive injuries or burns, malignancies, or chronic gastrointestinal disorders
4. The concentration of nutrients is less irritating to the larger central vein than a peripheral vein. Thrombophlebitis is less likely to occur.
5. systemic fever, local redness, swelling, purulent exudate from the puncture site
6. pneumothorax
7. Arterial rather than venous puncture. It is treated by withdrawing the catheter and applying pressure to the puncture site for 5–10 minutes.
8. Potential for infection

UNIT VI CASE STUDY

1. **Objective**
   vomiting for three days
   weight loss of 14 pounds
   dry, sticky mucous membranes
   diminished skin turgor

   Subjective
   nausea for four days
   severe epigastric cramps
   unable to eat or drink for four days
2. Fluid volume deficit related to prolonged vomiting
3. The client's body fluid is conserved and replaced so that body weight is stabilized and skin turgor is firm.
4. I = 2,275 cc; O = 2,800 cc
5. Provides a continuous flow of air through the tube into the stomach so that the suction pressure never increases above a level that would damage the gastric tissues.
6. size 18 to 20
7. either 145 or 146 cc/hour
8. 125 cc/hour
9. apply a water soluble lubricant around the nostril.
10. approximately 119 cc/hour.
11. The tube may not be patent at all. The nasogastric tube should be irrigated to ensure patency.
12. Suggest infiltration at the venipuncture site. It may be confirmed by palpating the site for temperature; cool temperature suggests fluid in the tissues. Also lower the infusion container below the level of the site to see if blood returns; if it does not, it suggests the needle or catheter is not in the vein.

CHAPTER 28 SELF-TEST

1. blood, acid-base, kidneys, ureters, arterial blood pressure, and renin.
2. The pressure of urine against the bladder walls triggers visceral afferent impulses that signal efferent visceral impulses to contract the detrusor muscles and relax the neck of the bladder and internal sphincter. The body involuntarily opens the external sphincter and urine is eliminated.
3. C, D, B, F, A, E
4. urgency: sensation of needing to urinate immediately
   dysuria: painful or uncomfortable urination
   hesitancy: difficulty starting the urinary flow
   nocturia: desire to urinate during the night
   enuresis: inability to retain urine in the bladder during the night
   incontinence: inability to retain urine in the bladder

5. Stress incontinence
   Impairment of urinary elimination: retention

CHAPTER 29 SELF-TEST

1. A
2. A
3. C
4. A
5. B

CHAPTER 30 SELF-TEST

1. adult women: French 12, 14, 16
   adult men: French 16, 18, 20
   children? French 6, 8, 10
2. to avoid introducing microorganisms into the normal sterile urinary tract
3. 1) length of time since last voiding; 2) amount of fluid intake since last voiding; 3) distended bladder upon palpation; 4) verbal reports of bladder discomfort from the client
4. NO, YES, YES, YES, NO
5. 1) Ask the client to take a deep breath and bear down.
   2) Change the angle of the penis toward the abdomen.
6. Straight catheter is used for removing urine one time; an indwelling catheter remains in the bladder to drain it continually. Straight catheter is a long, slender, flexible tube with a single lumen; an indwelling catheter is a long, slender, flexible tube with a double lumen and a Y-branch at the distal end which contains one lumen. The second lumen of the indwelling catheter is used to inflate a balloon that rests just inside the bladder to anchor the catheter in place.
7. Alteration of urinary elimination: incontinence; Actual or potential skin integrity impairment
8. In an irrigation, a solution is inserted into the bladder via a catheter and then drained out; in an instillation, a solution is inserted into the bladder via a catheter and held in place.
9. 1) Provides hemostasis against a surgical incision.
   2) Rinses tissue debris and blood clots following bladder, prostate, or urethra surgery.
10. 375 cc

CHAPTER 31 SELF-TEST

1. chyme, peristalsis, feces, large intestine, intra-abdominal pressure, conscious, gastrocolic reflex
2. 1) age; 2) food intake; 3) fluid intake; 4) exercise; 5) medications; 6) opportunity for defecation; 7) consistent habits; 8) emotions
3. melena: black, tarry stools
   steatorrhea: stools with visible fat

impaction: large mass of hardened stool in the colon
flatus: intestinal gas
eructation: burping

4. Mr. Roberts: Alteration in bowel elimination: constipation
   Ms. Henry: Alteration in bowel elimination: diarrhea
5. Rebound tenderness is the pain or guarding that occurs *after* palpation of the abdomen. It is elicited by deep, firm pressure against the abdomen that is quickly released.

CHAPTER 32 SELF-TEST

1. 1) encouraging a response to the gastrocolic reflex; 2) proper positioning; 3) providing sufficient time and privacy; 4) increasing fluid intake; 5) encouraging intake of food that adds bulk to the stool
2. A laxative stimulates peristalsis and causes gentle elimination of stool; a cathartic has a stronger action and may cause liquid feces to evacuate.
3. cleansing enema: removes feces and flatus from the rectum
   retention enema: softens or lubricates stool
   return-flow enema: relieves flatulence
4. 1) encourage exercise; 2) have the client drink carbonated beverages or chamomile tea; 3) have the client assume a knee-chest position; 4) apply heat to the abdomen; 5) insert a rectal tube
5. Fecal impaction is suspected when the client complains of pain, anorexia, or a feeling of fullness in the abdomen. He may have diarrhea stools after an absence of any stools for several days. Upon examination, the client has a hardened, palpable mass in the left lower quadrant or a hardened mass upon digital examination of the rectum.

CHAPTER 33 SELF-TEST

1. C, E, F, A, B, D
2. sigmoid colostomy: formed stool
   colostomy in the cecum: liquid stool but may be semiformed
   ileostomy: liquid stool
   urostomy: urine
3. appliance: apparatus attached to the stoma to collect effluent
   faceplate: applied to peristomal skin to prevent leakage of effluent onto the skin surface
   skin barrier: protects skin from exposure to effluent
   skin sealant: liquid skin barrier
4. 1) reason for the procedure; 2) surgery and aftereffects; 3) actual physical changes; and 4) meaning of the procedure to the client
5. Mr. Griego: Knowledge deficit
   Ms. Larson: Body image disturbance
   Mr. Altman: Impaired skin integrity
6. Colostomies most likely to evacuate formed stool are transverse, descending, or sigmoid.
7. B, A, D, C

UNIT VII CASE STUDY

1. feeling of needing to urinate frequently: urgency
   inability to start urinary stream: hesitancy
   burning when passing urine: dysuria
2. S: Reports full feeling in bladder; feels urge to void but can't begin urinary stream; dysuria. Reports limiting fluid intake.
   O: Odor of urine emanating from clothing; clothing has moist spots.
3. C
4. The client's incontinence is managed so that the client remains dry, odor-free, and without embarrassment.
5. S: Reports abdominal pain; flatus in the past month or so; reports diarrhea × 2 weeks; formed stool rare.
   O: Hyperactive bowel sounds × 4 quadrants; large mass palpated in left lower quadrant. Hardened stool digitally palpated in rectum.
6. A
7. The client passes a soft, formed stool at least once a day.
8. 1) Digitally remove present fecal impaction.
   2) Administer a small-volume retention enema to remove fecal impaction.
   3) Increase fluid intake.
   4) Increase exercise.
   5) Add fiber or other bulk foods to diet.
   6) Consult physician for pharmacologic therapy.
9. 1) Monitor food intake to identify gas-forming foods; eliminate them from diet.
   2) Increase exercise.
   3) Suggest drinking carbonated beverages or chamomile tea for relief of flatus.

CHAPTER 34 SELF-TEST

1. Through the nostril, the nasal cavity, the oropharynx, the pharynx, the larynx, the trachea, the bifurcation of the bronchi, a bronchus, a bronchiole, the alveolar, across the alveolar-capillary membrane, and taken up by a red blood cell.
2. nasal turbinates: moistens and warms inhaled air
   nasal cilia: filters inhaled air
   epiglottis: prevents food and fluids from passing into the larynx when closed and permits air to pass into the larynx when open
   olfactory receptors: receives smell stimuli
   surfactant: decreases surface tension on the lining of the alveoli, which prevents the alveolar wall from collapsing upon itself
   alveolar-capillary membrane: permits the exchange of gases by means of diffusion
3. nasal mucosa: moist and pink
   posterior pharynx: moist, pink, without areas of swelling, redness, or patches of exudate
   posterior chest: symmetric with straight spine; scapulae are of even height and distance on either side of the spine; chest expands slightly during inspiration
   spine: straight and centered in the midline of the back
   chest expansion: symmetric and slight with inspiration
   anterior chest: symmetric, suprasternal notch in midline directly above the manubrium and sternum; clavicles at the same level; costal margins are symmetric. Chest movement is symmetric and easy.

4. Mr. Yung: Ineffective breathing pattern
   Robbie Andrews: Ineffective airway clearance
   Mrs. Stalk: Impaired gaseous exchange

CHAPTER 35 SELF-TEST

1. Pulmonary hygiene is the body's protective mechanism that prevents the accumulation of mucus, secretions, and other debris in the airways.
2. cough: protective voluntary and reflex mechanism that forces air and accumulated secretions and debris from the airway by increasing the thoracic cavity volume and increasing intrathoracic pressure
   mucociliary transport system: removes secretions and foreign particles from airways by trapping them in a viscous mucous and propelling them toward the throat with the cilia
   mucus: traps particles and moistens lining of airways
3. Sputum is a combination of mucus, dust, microbial debris, and cell fragments that accumulates and is coughed out of the airways. It is examined for consistency, color, and volume.
4. deep breathing: improves forcible exhalation
   pursed-lip breathing: increases effective exhalation and decreases the work of breathing
   abdominal breathing: uses the diaphragm to alter intrathoracic pressure and facilitate airflow in and out of the lungs
5. controlled coughing, incentive spirometry, percussion and vibration, and postural drainage

CHAPTER 36 SELF-TEST

1. G, B, E, F, D, A, C
2. The chemical stimulus for respiration is the relative concentration of oxygen and carbon dioxide in the blood; the free hydrogen ions stimulate the chemoreceptors in the carotid and aortic sinuses.
3. Oxygen-induced hypoventilation occurs when the person is without the normal chemical stimulus for breathing. Because of prolonged hypercapnea, the chemoreceptors are dulled. High concentrations of oxygen in the blood shut off the hypoxic drive and the person's breathing slows or ceases.
4. Oxygen toxicity results from breathing high concentrations of oxygen for a prolonged period of time; it causes cellular damage or destruction.
5. Impaired gas exchange
6. Be sure all electrical connections are intact; post "Danger: Oxygen in Use" and "No Smoking" signs, and be alert to any hazardous materials that may cause spontaneous combustion.
7. addition of water to oxygen to decrease mucosal drying; monitoring the placement of the cannula against the nasal skin and the area above the ears for pressure and subsequent skin ischemia
8. The mask is designed so that the client receives almost pure oxygen and little room air. If the tubing is kinked or blocked, the client will receive no oxygen.

CHAPTER 37 SELF-TEST

1. pneumothorax: Air is in the pleural space.
   open pneumothorax: Air has entered the pleural space from outside the body and interferes with lung expansion.
   closed pneumothorax: Air has entered the pleural space but cannot escape.
   spontaneous pneumothorax: Air has entered the pleural space through no apparent cause.
   tension pneumothorax: The lung collapses because of air in the chest.
   hemopneumothorax: Air and blood have entered the pleural space.
2. air, fluid, collection chamber, greater, under 2 cm water, suction
3. Client assessments: rate, depth, regularity of breathing and symmetry of chest expansion; breath sounds; monitor for crepitus at insertion site; monitor dressing around insertion site for evidence of drainage.
   Equipment assessments: monitor for air leaks; monitor collection chambers for fluctuations corresponding to respirations; make sure the unit is below chest level to allow drainage by gravity; if suction is on, gentle, continuous bubbling will occur in the water.

CHAPTER 38 SELF-TEST

1. 1) foreign object in the airway; 2) retained secretions; 3) loss of muscular control of the tongue; 4) tissue edema or enlargement
2. patent airway: an open, unobstructed pathway for air to enter and exit the respiratory system
   intubation: placing a tube in the airway
   extubation: removing a tube from the airway
   tracheostomy: artificial opening from the throat into the trachea
3. Introduction of microorganisms by way of a suction catheter may result in undesirable infections of the airway.
4. Bubbling or rattling respiratory sounds, rapid, moist respirations, cyanotic mucous membranes.
5. 3, 5, 4, 2, 1
6. outer cannula: separates soft tissues and tracheal cartilage to form stoma
   inner cannula: fits within outer cannula; removed for cleaning
   obturator: plugs the end of the tube to protect mucosa from trauma during insertion of the cannula
   cuff: when inflated, provides an airtight seal to prevent air from leaking above the tracheostomy
7. "You have a tracheostomy, which is an opening from your throat to your trachea or windpipe. This has affected the ability of your larynx or voice box to make sounds. If you want to speak, place your finger over the tip of the opening and you will be able to form sounds."

CHAPTER 39 SELF-TEST

1. blood pH: 7.35 to 7.45
   percentage of formed blood elements: 42–47 percent
   erythrocytes per cubic mm of blood: 4.5–5.5 million

leukocytes per cubic mm of blood: 5,000–10,000
thrombocytes per cubic mm of blood: 150,000–250,000

2. leukocytes: phagocytosis of microorganisms, detoxification of toxic proteins and development of immunities
   erythrocytes: gas transport
   thrombocytes: clot formation
3. vena cava, right atrium, tricuspid valve, right ventricle, pulmonic valve, pulmonary artery, pulmonary capillaries, pulmonary vein, left atrium, mitral valve, left ventricle, aortic valve, aorta
4. S_1: closure of mitral valve
   S_2: closure of aortic valve
   S_3 (ventricular gallop): opening of mitral valve for rapid ventricular filling
   S_4 (atrial gallop): atrial contraction to enhance ventricular filling
   murmur: abnormal blood flow turbulence
5. Mr. Perkins: Alteration in tissue perfusion
   Mrs. Cohen: Alteration in cardiac output: decreased
   Mr. Consoli: Impaired gas exchange

CHAPTER 40 SELF-TEST

1. The heart stops beating (absent pulses) followed by cessation of respirations within 60 seconds.
2. The lungs stop breathing followed by cessation of heart beat within one or two minutes.
3. 1) artificial respiration; 2) external cardiac compression
4. establishing and maintaining effective ventilation by intubation; establishing an intravenous route for the administration of fluids and medications; applying defibrillation to reestablish normal cardiac rhythm; and administration medications to restore normal blood pH and restore circulatory function
5. resuscitation: restoration of vital functions that have ceased
   defibrillation: external application of electrical shock to restore normal sinus rhythm
   cardiac tamponade: compression of the heart due to blood accumulation within the pericardial sac
6. A: clearing the airway
   B: initiating artificial breathing
   C: initiating cardiac compression

UNIT VIII CASE STUDY

1. The sounds in the left chest are rales; the sounds in the right upper chest are rhonchi. When sounds are not heard at all, they are described as diminished or absent.
2. S: Reports feeling very tired with little energy to walk to the bathroom. Pain on inhalation; most intense in lower right chest. Reports difficulty breathing; worse lying down.
   O: Respiration: 26, guarded, shallow. Pulse 94; blood pressure 154/88. Rales over left chest; rhonchi in right upper chest; diminished lung sounds in lower right chest. Dusky color; cyanosis of mucous membranes.

3. Ineffective airway clearance related to accumulated secretions
   Ineffective breathing pattern related to respiratory disease
   Activity intolerance related to respiratory disease
   Alteration in comfort: pain related to respiratory disease
4. Ineffective airway clearance is the most urgent problem because of the body's urgent need for oxygen to maintain cell life, particularly of the brain.
5. Outcome: The client is able to effectively remove secretions from airways as evidenced by return of normal breathing patterns, vital signs within normal limits and absence of adventitious breath sounds.

   Measures: Encourage fluid intake.
   Maintain client in position of comfort.
   Encourage deep breathing and coughing at regular intervals (perhaps every 2 hours) with rest periods between.
   Perform percussion, vibration, and postural drainage as per physician's orders.
6. The bubbler adds moisture to the oxygen mixture; this is necessary because of the drying effect on mucous membranes and respiratory secretions.
7. 1) Keep the cannula properly attached so that the nasal prongs are in the nostrils and the tubing secured around the client's head or ears.
   2) Monitor the oxygen flow meter to ensure continuous flow of oxygen at the ordered rate.
   3) Inspect nostrils every four hours and lubricate with water-soluble lubricant if the skin is dry or irritated.
8. Position the client on his left side with his shoulders lower than his waist.
9. Position yourself so that you are upright and your feet are firmly on the floor. Place a pillow flat against your abdomen. Take two or three deep breaths, expanding your chest as fully as you can. Hold a tissue in your hand. Lean forward, take another breath, hold it briefly and then tighten your abdominal muscles and cough from deep inside your chest, forcing any sputum out and into the tissue. Pause 15 seconds, breathe normally, and repeat.
10. Encourage Mr. Fettini to rest as much as possible; group activities so that he can perform several actions at the same time and rest between; provide a bedside commode; make meals small so that he doesn't tire while eating but frequent so that he can get enough calories.

CHAPTER 41 SELF-TEST

1. E, G, H, D, I, F, C, A, K, J, L, B
2. 1,000, 0.1, 1,000, 0.1, 1, 32, 0.5 or ½, 16, 8
3. 1) form and stability; 2) classification
4. Parts are date written, name of client, name of medication, dosage, route of administration, time and intervals of administration, and physician's signature.
5. standing order: continually in effect until physician terminates it
   automatic stop order: automatically discontinued if it is not renewed by a certain date
   p.r.n. order: given only as needed
   single order: given only once
   STAT order: given immediately
6. oral: by mouth
   parenteral: by injection into a body tissue
   topical: applied to the skin or mucous membranes

instillation: inserted into a body cavity
inhalation: breathed into the lungs
intravenous: injected into the blood

7. 1) right client; 2) right drug; 3) right dose; 4) right route; 5) right time
8. a. two pills
   b. 0.75 ml
   c. two pills
   d. ½ pill
   e. 10 pills
   f. 0.5 ml

CHAPTER 42 SELF-TEST

1. Oral route
   Advantages: 1) convenience; 2) cost (they are cheaper)
   Disadvantages: 1) requires conscientious and compliant client; 2) may have unpleasant taste; 3) may irritate mucosa; 4) may be destroyed by gastric acids or enzymes; 5) slower to enter general circulation
2. Parenteral route
   Advantages: 1) fast absorption; 2) bypasses enteral digestion that may destroy them; 3) may be given to the unconscious or uncooperative client
   Disadvantages: 1) causes anxiety in some people; 2) may cause pain or local irritation; 3) increases risk for infection; 4) may not be self-administered by some persons
3. topical: on the skin
   buccal: between the cheek and gum in the mouth
   sublingual: under the tongue
   instillation: in body cavities
   subcutaneous: between the skin and muscle tissues
   intramuscular: in the muscle tissue
   intradermal: between the layers of the skin
4. ampule: sealed glass container with narrowed neck. An ampule usually contains a single dose
   vial: glass bottle with rubber stopper or seal that is pierced by needle to withdraw contents
   prepared disposable injection unit: a prepackaged barrel of medication with attached needle that fits into reusable syringe; after injection, the barrel is discarded
5. ventrogluteal: anterior superior iliac spine and iliac crest
   dorsogluteal: iliac crest and gluteal fold
   deltoid: acromial process and axilla
   vastus lateralis: greater trochanter and knee
   rectus femoris: inguinal fold and knee
6. The displaced skin and subcutaneous tissues (while injecting medication into the muscle) return to normal position when the needle is removed, thus sealing the medication under the layers of skin and subcutaneous tissue, preventing irritation in the needle channel.
7. Susie: 18, 1½, or 2
   Mr. Nelson: 25 or 26, ⅝ or ½
   Mrs. Jessup: 20, 1 or 1¼, or 1½
   Tom Sanders: 26, ½, or ⅝

CHAPTER 43 SELF-TEST

1. Advantages: 1) prompt results because medications are circulated to the body tissues immediately; 2) blood levels are easy to maintain.
   Disadvantages: 1) if administered too rapidly, high blood concentrations of toxic levels may result; 2) may cause adverse local effect on vasculature; 3) creates direct route from contaminated skin to blood
2. primary intravenous administration: instillation of a medication directing through a venous catheter or needle
   secondary intravenous administration: instillation of a medication by attaching a secondary set or line to the primary line
   intermittent venous access device: needle or catheter that remains permanently inserted into the vein; its distal end is capped but pierced with a needle at intervals to insert medication or fluid
   volume control set: an intravenous chamber that is attached to the primary bottle or bag to draw a given volume of solution from the primary bottle; this volume is mixed with medication and then administered intravenously
   admixture: medication given intravenously with other drugs or solutions
   bolus: small volume of medication that is given directly through an intravenous route
3. 1) adding to a primary container before infusion is begun; 2) adding to the primary container after infusion has begun
4. The volume control set is attached to the primary solution bottle or bag by inserting a tubing into the bottle (or bag) port. A given amount of the solution is drawn into the control set chamber by opening the clamp between the chambers. Medication is inserted by a syringe into a port in the chamber and mixed with the solution. The clamps on the intravenous tubing are opened and the mixture is infused.
5. A container of medication mixed with infusion solution is hung on the IV standard at a level at or above the primary container. Its tubing is attached to the primary tubing by inserting a needle into an injection port. When both tubings are unclamped, the comingled solution flows into the vein.

UNIT IX CASE STUDY

1. All but one is complete. Incomplete order is for multiple vitamins; the route of administration is missing.
2. The schedule is

0600	cefotoxin
0700	regular and NPH insulin
0800	calcium carbonate
0900	multiple vitamins
1200	cefotoxin
1200	calcium carbonate
1300	multiple vitamins
1700	multiple vitamins
1700	calcium carbonate
1800	cefotoxin
2400	cefotoxin

3. The five rights are right client, right drug, right dose, right route, and right time.
4. Decide which drug you wish to draw first. Draw a volume of air that equals

the dose of the second drug into the syringe; insert the syringe into the second drug vial and eject the volume of air. Withdraw the syringe; draw a volume of air that equals the dose of the first drug into the syringe; insert the syringe into the first drug vial and eject the volume of air. Draw the desired volume of drug into the syringe; remove from vial. Carefully insert the needle into the second vial and withdraw the exact desired volume of drug.

5. Check the client's identification by looking at the name bracelet.
6. Use a 45° angle.
7. Check the medication administration record to determine the last time the client received the drug. If an interval equal to or greater than the ordered interval has occurred, you may administer the drug again.
8. Narcotics are kept in a locked cabinet or drawer.
9. 2 ml
10. 21, 22, or 23 gauge needles are acceptable.
11. Ventrogluteal is best; dorsogluteal is also desirable.
12. Give four unit doses.
13. Add 10,000 units of heparin.
14. 50 drops per minute
15. Knowledge deficit about prescribed medications
16. The client understands the purpose and effects of the prescribed medications as evidenced by her correct verbal explanations.
17. 7.5 ml
18. Add the 7.5 ml of reconstituted medication to a small-volume infusion container with 50 ml normal saline. Attach a secondary administration set to this container. Attach a large-bore needle to the distal end of the secondary tubing; hang the secondary set on an IV pole at the same level or higher than the primary infusion that contains heparin. After cleansing the injection port on the primary tubing, insert the secondary needle through the port; opening the flow rate on the secondary set so that the 50 ml are infused in 20 minutes.

CHAPTER 44 SELF-TEST

1. In a closed wound, the skin is not broken; in an open wound, it is.
   An intentional wound is made deliberately and an unintentional wound is made accidentally.
   A clean wound is free of pathogenic organisms and a contaminated wound contains many pathogenic organisms.
2. C, D, E, F, A, B
3. inflammatory phase: Fibrin forms a scab or eschar; vasodilation; leukocytes and macrophages migrate to the wound site; new epithelial cells grow from edge of wound to center.
   proliferative phase: Fibrin network forms fibrinoblasts and is reabsorbed; blood vessels, fibroblasts, and lymph produce granulation tissue, which forms the scar.
   maturation phase: Small blood vessels disappear; collagen fiber is replaced; scar reduces in size; scar tissue does not regain full strength for a year.
4. first intention: surgical incision
   second intention: abrasion
   third intention: surgical wound left open for drainage of exudates until healing can occur
5. abrasion, contaminated, serous, no risk factors, impaired skin integrity
6. accidental, open, purulent, yes, smoking history, impaired skin integrity
7. hemostasis: blood clotting

evisceration: separation of wound edges with the protrusion of viscera
dehiscence: separation of wound edges

8. wet-to-dry dressings: debridement of wounds
   dry sterile dressings: protection of wounds from microorganisms; absorbs drainage
   transparent dressings: protection of debrided wounds from microorganisms
   pressure dressings: provides hemostasis
   wound irrigations: removes dead tissue and drainage from wounds
   wound suctioning: removes drainage from wounds to prevent microbial growth
9. circular: anchors bandage at its beginning or end; may be used on small body parts
   spiral: covers body areas of uniform shape
   spiral reverse: covers body areas not of uniform shape
   recurrent: covers distal ends of body parts
   figure-8: covers and supports jointed areas
   spica: covers large body areas similar to a figure-8
10. abdominal or straight: supports abdominal muscles
    breast: supports breasts or chest muscles
    scultetus: supports abdomen or secures dressings; can be sized to shape
    single T: supports perineal dressings; used mostly for women
    double T: supports perineal dressings; used mostly for men

CHAPTER 45 SELF-TEST

1. heat, cold, heat, heat, cold, heat, cold
2. 1) reduced or absent sensitivity to or perception of pain or temperature; 2) edema or abnormal thickening of the skin, such as with scarring; 3) presence of localized infection
3. 1) current or past history of cardiac problems; 2) reduced or absent sensitivity to or perception of pain or temperature; 3) diminished circulation in the body part
4. Mrs. Chung: heat because it relieves pain
   Jack: cold because it will vasoconstrict and reduce edema
   Mr. Arthur: heat because it will relax muscle spasms
   Mrs. Connor: heat because it will enhance healing and relieve pain
5. Apply a thin layer of petroleum jelly on intact skin around the edges of a wound. Remove heat and moist compress after 20–30 minutes.
6. Dry the skin; place the lamp at the correct distance from the wound; assess the client's skin every 5 minutes; make sure the client is not uncomfortable; remove the lamp in 20 minutes.
7. Seal the ice bag tightly; wrap in a cloth case; remove the ice bag promptly.

CHAPTER 46 SELF-TEST

1. Stage I: Skin is pinkish-red, mottled but does return to normal color when pressure relieved.
   Stage II: Skin is red with edema and induration; may be cracked, blistered, or broken.
   Stage III: Skin is broken, exudate is present.

Stage IV: Skin is broken with extensive damage to underlying subcutaneous and muscle tissues.

2. Friction is the rubbing of one surface against another. Shearing force is the pulling of the skin in one direction and the movement of the subcutaneous tissues in the opposite direction.
3. 1) poor nutrition; 2) muscle atrophy or loss of subcutaneous tissue; 3) age; 4) impaired circulation; 5) anemia; 6) skin exposure to continuous moisture; 7) neurologic impairments; 8) steroid therapy; 9) immobility
4. underweight, neurologic impairment, immobility, potential incontinence and prolonged exposure of skin to irritants
5. frequent change of body position, proper padding of bony prominences, use of protective mattress surface, frequent skin inspection, meticulous skin cleanliness, high-protein food intake, increased fluid intake

UNIT X CASE STUDY

1. Impaired skin integrity
2. The client's wounds heal without the complications of hemorrhage, infection, or disfigurement.
3. 1) Turn and reposition at least once every two hours.
   2) Massage skin over the bony prominences when repositioning.
   3) Place a protective mattress cover under the client or use a therapeutic bed to decrease pressure against the skin.
   4) Cushion bony prominences if the client sits in a chair.
   5) Apply foam or sheepskin heel and elbow protectors.
   6) Avoid positioning the client on the involved areas.
   7) Keep skin dry and clean.
4. Absorb drainage from the open wound.
5. 1) Wash hands.
   2) Expose the wound.
   3) Don clean gloves.
   4) Untie the Montgomery straps.
   5) Remove old dressing and discard in plastic container or bag.
   6) Remove and discard gloves.
   7) Open sterile packages of absorbent pads.
   8) Don sterile gloves.
   9) Apply pads to open wound.
   10) Retie Montgomery straps.
   11) Remove and discard gloves.
6. The coccyx is Stage III; the heel is Stage II.
7. Hydrogen peroxide acts as a debriding agent, removing dead tissue. This permits tissue regeneration.
8. Povidone-iodine is a disinfectant used to prevent growth of microorganisms in the wound; when the dressing dries, it acts as a debriding agent.
9. It acts as a barrier to microorganisms but permits passage of air to the wound, thus promoting tissue regeneration. The wound may be easily inspected through the transparent dressing, thus facilitating wound monitoring.
10. The moist heat will increase circulation to the area, help reduce edema and inflammation, and relax the muscles, thus relieving pain.
11. An application of a water-impermeable ointment or jelly will protect the skin from maceration. Frequent monitoring of the heat application is the best guard against thermal injury.

CHAPTER 47 SELF-TEST

1. Preoperative assessment is done to identify factors that will affect the outcome of surgery.
2. 1) vital signs: establish baseline data for later comparison
   2) general appearance: identifies any impairments or problems that may alter outcome of surgery as well as establishes baseline data for later comparison
   3) height and weight: establishes baseline data for later comparison
3. 1) level of consciousness: determines the client's ability to communicate effectively for exchange of information
   2) mental status: determines client's ability to comprehend instructions, make sound judgments, and communicate his thoughts and feelings effectively
   3) mood: suggests client's ability to cope with surgery
   4) anxiety level: identifies client's concerns so that appropriate anxiety-relief measures may be instituted
   5) self-esteem and self-image: suggests client's emotional responses to surgery
4. Informed consent protects the client's right for information regarding his treatment. The physician is responsible for providing the information and obtaining the signed consent. The nurse is responsible for ensuring that information is properly given and the consent form is signed.
5. 1) to achieve or maintain the client's optimal state of health
   2) to prevent intra- or postoperative complications
   3) to prepare for the use of anesthesia
6. a. Mr. Perez. Nursing diagnosis: Knowledge deficit related to postoperative discharge. Nursing measure: Explain to Mr. Perez that he will be remaining in the hospital and why.
   b. Mrs. Stuart. Nursing diagnosis: Anxiety related to impending surgery. Nursing measure: Help client understand that she is anxious and why; then suggest anxiety-relief behaviors.
   c. Mr. Ford. Nursing diagnosis: Potential for injury related to sedation. Nursing measure: Inform client that he should call for help if he wishes to get out of bed; raise the siderails.

CHAPTER 48 SELF-TEST

1. Stage 2: restlessness, muscle twitching, shivering, rigid posturing; increased pulse and blood pressure; rapid, irregular respirations; retching or vomiting
   Stage 1: eye opening, responding to questions, experiences pain, attempts to move or sit up; talks restlessly
2. 1) surgical procedure and results, findings
   2) unusual events that occurred during surgery
   3) type, amount, and duration of anesthesia
   4) vital signs during surgery; most recent vital signs
   5) amount and type of fluids infused; what is presently infusing
   6) amount of blood lost and amount of blood replaced
   7) position of drains placed during surgery
   8) types of body fluids draining
   9) volume of urinary output during procedure (if indwelling catheter in place)
   10) any special observations that must be made
   11) physician's orders that must be implemented immediately
3. cardiovascular: Monitor pulse and blood pressure.
   respiratory: Monitor respirations.

gastrointestinal: Monitor presence of retching or vomiting; listen for client's report of nausea.
integumentary: Inspect incision site (or dressing).
metabolic: Monitor temperature.
renal: Measure urinary output.

4. immune
   Nursing diagnosis: Potential for infection related to disruption of integument. Nursing measures: Maintain careful asepsis.
   respiratory
   Nursing diagnosis: Ineffective airway clearance related to accumulated secretions. Nursing measures: Initiate preventive pulmonary physiotherapy, specifically coughing, deep breathing, incentive spirometry.
   gastrointestinal
   Nursing diagnosis: Fluid volume deficit related to inability to drink and eat because of nausea, fluid loss because of vomiting. Nursing measures: Monitor and maintain intravenous fluid therapy as per the physician's orders; monitor for the return of bowel sounds and gradually introduce oral fluids as the client is able to drink.
   Nursing diagnosis: Alteration in bowel elimination: constipation related to sluggish peristalsis following anesthesia. Nursing measure: Monitor for return of bowel sounds and withhold oral fluids until sounds are auscultated; encourage ambulation to stimulate peristalsis.
   musculoskeletal
   Nursing diagnosis: Impaired physical mobility related to pain or surgical injury. Nursing measures: Encourage client to move all extremities in bed as soon as he is awake and aware; begin progressive ambulation as per the physician's orders.
   integumentary
   Nursing diagnosis: Impaired skin integrity related to surgical incision. Nursing measures: Monitor incision for signs of infection or delayed healing.
   renal
   Nursing diagnosis: Alteration in urinary output: retention-related effects of anesthesia. Nursing measures: Monitor output; ensure adequate fluid intake; catheterize as per physician's order if urinary output is absent or low.

5. atelectasis: inadequate pulmonary function during anesthesia; inadequate lung expansion; immobility; ineffective cough
   hemorrhage: disrupted sutures or dislodged clots in the surgical region
   thrombophlebitis of the leg: venous stasis from anesthesia and immobility; surgical trauma to the vessel wall
   pulmonary embolus: dislodged clots from thrombi caused by immobilization, preexisting coagulation disorders, or stasis of blood during anesthesia
   nausea and vomiting: depression of peristalsis by anesthesia or narcotics; abdominal distention
   urinary retention: depression of bladder tone by anesthesia; local manipulation of tissues
   wound infection: contaminated surgical wound; failure of aseptic technique

UNIT XI CASE STUDY

1. Knowledge deficit related to impending surgery
2. The client understands the preparations for surgery and the expected events following surgery as evidenced by his verbalization of such to the nurse.

3. Key points:
   - Explain purpose of physical preparations (enemas, preoperative medications, insertion of indwelling catheter, intravenous infusion).
   - Teach postoperative leg exercises, pulmonary physiotherapy (coughing, deep breathing and use of incentive spirometer, if use is anticipated).
   - Explain purpose of postop tubes or procedures (nasogastric intubation, progressive ambulation, diet).
4. Enemas until clear remove any residual stool from the rectum to prepare it for surgery.
5. Food and fluids are withheld to clear the gastrointestinal system and prevent possible aspiration of contents if the client should vomit.
6. Intravenous fluids are given to ensure sufficient fluid intake while the client is NPO.
7. The indwelling catheter keeps the bladder deflated; when surgery is performed in the pelvis, this prevents accidental injury to the bladder.
8. S: Reports pain.

   O: Upon return from PAR, sleepy but able to identify self and surroundings. Temp = 98.4°F; P = 68; R = 16; BP = 122/68. IV infusing at 75 ml/hour; infusion site without redness or swelling. Nasogastric tube draining greenish-brown fluid with dark specks. Incision dry and approximated. Urinary catheter draining straw-colored urine.

   A: Potential for injury related to post-operative drowsiness. Potential for infection related to undressed incision, indwelling catheter, and intravenous infusion site. Alteration in comfort: pain related to surgery

   P: Maintain siderails in up position; monitor frequently. Maintain asepsis when monitoring wound, venipuncture site, emptying urine collector.
9. The client recovers from surgery without the complications of hemorrhage, infection, or altered elimination function.

   The client's postoperative pain is controlled so that he maintains comfort as evidenced by his verbal and nonverbal responses.
10. Set the pump to infuse about 152 ml/hour.
11. Another bag must be added at 1900.
12. 1500 Assess vital signs; record.
    Monitor IV infusion and venipuncture site.
    Monitor NG output.
    Inspect incision.
    Remove indwelling urinary catheter.
    Administer pain medication.
    Encourage coughing and deep breathing.
    Assist client to comfortable position.

    1600 Assess vital signs; record.
    Monitor IV, NG.
    Assess pain.

    1700 Assess vital signs; record.
    Monitor IV, NG.
    Assist client to a sitting and then standing position; return him to position of comfort.
    Inspect incision.
    Guide client to use the incentive spirometry; encourage coughing.
    Encourage client to void, if possible.

    1800 Assess vital signs; record.
    Monitor IV, NG.
    Assess pain.
    Encourage client to void if he hasn't yet.

1900 Monitor IV, NG.
Inspect incision.
Assess pain; administer pain medication if necessary.
Have the client use the incentive spirometry; encourage coughing.
Encourage client to void if he hasn't already.
Assist client to turn to comfortable position.
1930 Monitor IV; prepare next bag.
2000 Add second IV infusion bag.
Monitor NG.
Encourage the client to void if he hasn't already.
2100 Monitor IV, NG.
Inspect incision.
Have the client use the incentive spirometry; encourage coughing.
Encourage client to void if he hasn't already.
Assess pain.
Assist client to turn to comfortable position.
2200 Assess vital signs; record.
Assess pain.
Encourage client to void if he hasn't already.
2300 Assess pain; administer pain medication if necessary.
Have the client use the incentive spirometry; encourage coughing.
Assist client to turn to comfortable position.

13. The nurse will monitor the client's urinary output, paying particular attention to the time of the first voiding after the catheter is out.
14. First check the suction to ensure proper function; obtain an irrigation set and gently irrigate the tube to clear any obstructions.
15. Splint around the abdominal incision with a pillow or bath blanket. His most effective cough may follow administration of pain medication by about one hour.
16. Explain firmly how getting out of bed will help his recovery. Postpone the client's getting out of bed until about one hour after he has received a pain medication. Have a second nurse help you; the client may be worried about his safety.

CHAPTER 49 SELF-TEST

1. Mrs. Kersey: bargaining
   Mr. Peterson: depression alternating with acceptance
   Mr. O'Brien: denial
   Mrs. Tranh: anger and depression
2. respiratory: Respirations become difficult for the dying person; they become irregular, noisy, rapid, shallow. May have a death rattle, a coarse, loud bubbling sound.
   circulatory: Circulation slows; pulse becomes faint and irregular; blood pressure drops.
   metabolic: Rate is slowed; body temperature is lower than normal.
   musculoskeletal: Muscles relax; person feels very fatigued.
   gastrointestinal: Anorexia, dehydration, weight loss; loss of gag reflex and ability to swallow; slowed peristalsis results in gastric or bowel distention, constipation, or incontinence.
   renal or urinary: Urine output diminishes; bladder is distended, urinary retention and incontinence result.

neurologic: Longer periods of sleep; gradually lowering levels of consciousness; neurologic reflexes fade; pain sensation fades.
visual: Acuity fades.

3. the cessation of heart beat, respirations, and blood pressure
4. the cessation of brain cell activity as confirmed by an electroencephalogram that measures brain wave activity
5. hospice: holistic health care services that offer comfort rather than curing and permit and encourage person to control his dying process
   home care: provides physical and emotional support from nurses or other health care providers; coordinates support services
   respite care: provides relief to the primary caregiver in the home by supplying a temporary caregiver
6. shock and disbelief: Expresses denial; reports a "numb" sensation, physical symptoms of tight feeling in the chest or throat, dry mouth; has rapid pulse; sighs and cries.
   developing awareness (stage of pain): Feels intense painful longing, loneliness, yearning to be with the loved one again; experiences hopelessness; becomes preoccupied with thoughts of the lost one.
   resolution or restitution: Accepts reality of death; may discard belongings of the loved one; finds new relationships.

CHAPTER 50 SELF-TEST

1. rigor mortis: muscle contraction, joint immobilization
   algor mortis: cooling of body tissues
   livor mortis: pooling of blood in body tissues because of gravity; causes discoloration
   autolysis: lytic actions of tissue enzymes that cause tissue destruction
2. determines the exact nature of the disease or the cause of death
3. The physician is responsible for obtaining permission from the family of the deceased; the physician explains the purpose and value of the autopsy. The nurse emotionally supports the family and supports the need for the autopsy.
4. Postmortem care: Close eyelids and secure shut; position the body in straight alignment; insert dentures, close the mouth, and secure the jaw shut; remove tubing; remove soiled dressings or tape; place absorbent pads between the buttocks; remove jewelry; wash soiled body areas; comb or brush hair; place clean clothing on the body; permit viewing time for the family; attach identification tags to the designated body parts; place the body in a shroud.

UNIT XII CASE STUDY

1. Altered body image related to hair loss
2. anticipatory grieving
3. The Carr family grieves their loss in a healthy and constructive way so that they may continue with their collective and individual lives.
4. Jason accepts the inevitability of his death; he is giving his belongings to those people he loves the most so that they will remember him.
5. Respite care provides the caregiver some time away from an ill person. That time is spent in whatever fashion is necessary for the caregiver.

6. Provide ample opportunity for ventilation of feelings.
   Suggest the family plan activities in which Jason can fully participate and will strengthen their family bonds.
   Suggest each family member spend time with Jason.
   Encourage well family members to spend time away from the family, pursuing their own interests, with their own friends.

CHAPTER 51 SELF-TEST

1. Gross examination is the inspection of volume, color, transparency or opacity, viscosity, shape or form, and other characteristics of appearance.
   Microscopic examination is the inspection under a microscope to identify those characteristics not visible to the naked eye, such as cell structure or presence of microorganisms.
   A chemical examination is the analysis of the composition of substances to determine the quantities of usual components or the presence of unusual components.
2. A smear is a thin layer of a liquid or semi-liquid substance that is placed on a slide for microscopic examination; a culture is the placement of a small amount of a substance on a nutrient media to isolate and grow microorganisms.
3. 1) Know the nature of the test.
   2) Know why the client is having the test.
   3) Ensure appropriate preparations.
   4) Collect specimen at the correct time.
   5) Collect specimen in the correct container without contamination.
   6) Label the container correctly.
   7) Send the specimen to the appropriate laboratory for testing.
4.

Specimen	Type of Test	Purpose	Special Client Preparation?
nose secretions	culture	identify microorganism causing infection; determine treatment	client education; positioned upright with head tilted back
sputum	culture	identify microorganism causing infection; determine treatment	client education; client must cough deeply
gastric secretion	analysis	determines acidity or alkalinity of secretions	client education; client must be NPO for 8 hours
	occult blood analysis	identifies undetected bleeding	NG tube in place
venous blood	biochemical analysis	identifies chemical components	client education; may need to be fasting; antiseptic cleansing of puncture site

(continued)

Specimen	Type of Test	Purpose	Special Client Preparation?
capillary blood	biochemical analysis	identifies microscopic structure of chemical components	client education; may need to be fasting; antiseptic cleansing of puncture site
arterial blood	gaseous analysis	identifies concentration of gases in blood	client education; oxygen administration is discontinued unless physician orders otherwise; antiseptic cleansing of puncture site
wound drainage	culture	identifies microorganisms present; determines treatment	client education
midstream urine	culture	identifies microorganisms present; determines treatment	client education; antiseptic cleansing of perineum and urethra
stools	occult blood analysis	determines if client is bleeding in GI tract	client education

CHAPTER 52 SELF-TEST

1. E, C, F, H, B, I, D, J, A, G
2. a. To Mr. Martinez: "A thoracentesis is the removal of fluid through a long needle that is placed into the chest cavity. You will sit leaning against a table; the physician will sterilize the skin where the needle enters and then administer a small amount of anesthesia in the area to deaden the skin. When the physician inserts the needle, you will feel pressure and perhaps some pain. After the needle is inserted, the physician will drain some (or all) of the fluid from the area and then remove the needle. A dressing will be used to cover the puncture site. During the procedure, you must sit quietly and avoid coughing."
   b. To Ms. Curtis: "You must remove your clothing from the waist down for this exam. You will lay on your back with your hips and knees bent and your feet; you will be covered with a sheet. When the physician is ready for the exam, I will position the sheet so that your external genitalia are visible. The physician will place an instrument called a speculum into your vagina; it may be uncomfortable. The physician will wipe the inside of your vagina with a swab to obtain some tissue; this will be placed on a slide for examination under a microscope. The purpose of the microscope exam is to determine if the tissue cells are normal."
   c. To Mr. Charles: "Six (or twelve) wires, called leads, will be secured to your chest wall. The machine detects the electrical activity of your heart and records it on a length of paper. You will not feel anything and no electrical current is transmitted to your body."

d. To Mr. and Mrs. Karl: "After your baby is positioned with his back curved, the physician will wipe a disinfectant solution over the skin of his spine and inject a small amount of anesthesia to deaden the area. As the nurse holds your baby, the physician will inject a needle into a space between his vertebrae (spinal bones) to remove a small amount of the fluid located there. The test does not hurt the baby although he may be angry because he will be held still through the procedure. The results of the spinal fluid examination by the laboratory will help the physician determine why your child is ill."

e. To Mrs. Chester: "You will lie on your back on a narrow bed; this bed will slowly move through a large machine that takes x-rays every minute or so. The technician may ask you to hold your breath at intervals. The test will take about an hour."

3. a. For a liver biopsy, the client must sign an informed consent document. Vital signs are taken and recorded before the exam. After voiding, he may receive a sedative prior to the biopsy. The client will remove his pajama top. He will be positioned supine with his right hand raised above his head and positioned behind his neck.

b. For an angiogram, the client must sign an informed consent document. She may be NPO. Vital signs are taken and recorded before the exam. All jewelry or prostheses are removed. After the client voids, a sedative is given. The client is transferred via a stretcher for the examination, which is done in radiology.

c. For a bone marrow biopsy, the client must sign an informed consent document. After the client voids, a sedative may be given. The client is placed in supine position if the sternum or anterior iliac crest site is used; the client is placed prone or lateral if the posterior iliac crest site is used. The client is draped to expose the puncture site.

d. For an electroencephalogram, the client shampoos his hair; a sedative may be given.